Pediatric Cancer

Editor

ROSHNI DASGUPTA

SURGICAL ONCOLOGY
CLINICS OF NORTH AMERICA

www.surgonc.theclinics.com

Consulting Editor
TIMOTHY M. PAWLIK

April 2021 • Volume 30 • Number 2

ELSEVIER

1600 John F. Kennedy Boulevard • Suite 1800 • Philadelphia, Pennsylvania, 19103-2899

http://www.theclinics.com

SURGICAL ONCOLOGY CLINICS OF NORTH AMERICA Volume 30, Number 2
April 2021 ISSN 1055-3207, ISBN-13: 978-0-323-76266-3

Editor: John Vassallo (j.vassallo@elsevier.com)
Developmental Editor: Diana Ang

Surgical Oncology Clinics of North America (ISSN 1055-3207) is published quarterly by Elsevier Inc., 360 Park Avenue South, New York, NY 10010-1710. Months of publication are January, April, July, and October. Business and Editorial Offices: 1600 John F. Kennedy Blvd., Ste. 1800, Philadelphia, PA 19103-2899. Customer Service Office: 3251 Riverport Lane, Maryland Heights, MO 63043. Periodicals postage paid at New York, NY and additional mailing offices. Subscription prices are $315.00 per year (US individuals), $750.00 (US institutions) $100.00 (US student/resident), $352.00 (Canadian individuals), $784.00 (Canadian institutions), $100.00 (Canadian student/resident), $456.00 (foreign individuals), $784.00 (foreign institutions), and $205.00 (foreign student/resident). Foreign air speed delivery is included in all *Clinics* subscription prices. All prices are subject to change without notice. **POSTMASTER**: Send address changes to *Surgical Oncology Clinics of North America*, Elsevier Health Science Division, Subscription Customer Service, 3251 Riverport Lane, Maryland Heights, MO 63043. **Customer Service: 1-800-654-2452 (US and Canada). 314-447-8871 (outside US and Canada). Fax: 314-447-8029. E-mail: journalscustomerservice-usa@elsevier.com (for print support); journalsonline support-usa@elsevier.com (for online support)**.

Reprints. For copies of 100 or more, of articles in this publication, please contact the Commercial Reprints Department, Elsevier Inc., 360 Park Avenue South, New York, New York 10010-1710. Tel. 212-633-3874; Fax: 212-633-3820; E-mail: reprints@elsevier.com.

Surgical Oncology Clinics of North America is covered in *MEDLINE/PubMed (Index Medicus)* and *EMBASE/ Excerpta Medica, Current Contents/Clinical Medicine, and ISI/BIOMED.*

Contributors

CONSULTING EDITOR
_____

TIMOTHY M. PAWLIK, MD, MPH, MTS, PhD, FACS, FRACS (Hon.)
Professor and Chair, Department of Surgery, The Urban Meyer III and Shelley Meyer Chair
for Cancer Research, Professor of Surgery, Oncology, Health Services Management and
Policy, Surgeon in Chief, The Ohio State University Wexner Medical Center, Columbus,
Ohio, USA

EDITOR
_____

ROSHNI DASGUPTA, MD, MPH
Professor of Surgery, Division of Pediatric General and Thoracic Surgery, Cincinnati
Children's Hospital Medical Center, University of Cincinnati, Cincinnati, Ohio, USA

AUTHORS
_____

JENNIFER H. ALDRINK, MD
Division of Pediatric Surgery, Department of Surgery, Nationwide Children's Hospital, The
Ohio State University College of Medicine, Columbus, Ohio, USA

MARY AUSTIN, MD
Department of Surgical Oncology, Division of Surgery, The University of Texas MD
Anderson Cancer Center, Houston, Texas, USA

RETO M. BAERTSCHIGER, MD, PhD
Assistant Professor, Division of General and Thoracic Surgery, The Hospital for Sick
Children, University of Toronto, Toronto, Ontario, Canada

DEBORAH F. BILLMIRE, MD
Department of Pediatric Surgery, Riley Hospital for Children at Indiana University Health,
Indianapolis, Indiana, USA

KAREN BURNS, MD
Associate Professor of Pediatrics, University of Cincinnati College of Medicine, Pediatric
Oncologist, Cincinnati Children's Hospital Medical Center, Cincinnati, Ohio, USA

EMILY CHRISTISON-LAGAY, MD
Associate Professor, Division of Pediatric Surgery, Department of Surgery, Yale School of
Medicine, New Haven, Connecticut, USA

NIKKE CROTEAU, MD
Department of Surgery, Pediatric Service, Memorial Sloan Kettering Cancer Center, New
York, New York, USA

PIOTR CZAUDERNA, MD
Professor, Department of Surgery and Urology for Children and Adolescents, Medical
University of Gdansk, Gdansk, Poland

ROSHNI DASGUPTA, MD, MPH
Professor of Surgery, Division of Pediatric General and Thoracic Surgery, Cincinnati Children's Hospital Medical Center, University of Cincinnati, Cincinnati, Ohio, USA

ANDREW M. DAVIDOFF, MD
Full Member and Chairman, Department of Surgery, St. Jude Children's Research Hospital, Memphis, Tennessee, USA

SIMONE DE CAMPOS VIEIRA ABIB, MD, PhD
Professor of Pediatric Surgery, Federal University of São Paulo (UNIFESP) – Paulista School of Medicine, Head of Pediatric Surgical Oncology, Pediatric Oncology Institute – GRAACC/UNIFESP

PETER F. EHRLICH, MD, MSc
Professor of Surgery, University of Michigan, C.S. Mott Children's Hospital Section of Pediatric Surgery, Ann Arbor, Michigan, USA

JOERG FUCHS, MD
Department of Pediatric Surgery and Pediatric Urology, University Children's Hospital Tuebingen, Tuebingen, Germany

HANNA GARNIER, MD, PhD
Department of Surgery and Urology for Children and Adolescents, Medical University of Gdansk, Gdańsk, Poland

EISO HIYAMA, MD, PhD
Professor, Department of Pediatric Surgery, Hiroshima University Hospital, Hiroshima, Japan

JONATHAN KARPELOWKSY, MBBCh, PhD
Associate Professor, Pediatric Oncology and Thoracic Surgery, The Children's Hospital at Westmead, Children's Cancer Research Unit, Kids Research Institute, Faculty of Medicine and Health, The University of Sydney, Sydney, Australia

MICHAEL P. LaQUAGLIA, MD, FACS
Department of Surgery, Pediatric Service, Memorial Sloan Kettering Cancer Center, New York, New York, USA

TIMOTHY B. LAUTZ, MD
Assistant Professor of Surgery, Northwestern Feinberg School of Medicine, Pediatric Surgeon, Ann & Robert H. Lurie Children's Hospital of Chicago, Chicago, Illinois, USA

CAITLYN LOO, BS
Division of Pediatric Surgery, Michael E. DeBakey Department of Surgery, Texas Children's Surgical Oncology Program, Texas Children's Liver Tumor Program, Dan L. Duncan Cancer Center, Baylor College of Medicine, Houston, Texas, USA; School of Medicine, Royal College of Surgeons in Ireland, Dublin, Ireland

NATALIE M. LOPYAN, MD
Pediatric Critical Care Fellow, C.S. Mott Children's Hospital Section of Pediatric Surgery, Ann Arbor, Michigan, USA

REBECKA MEYERS, MD
Professor, Division of Pediatric Surgery, University of Utah, Primary Children's Hospital, Salt Lake City, Utah, USA

JED NUCHTERN, MD, FACS
Department of Surgery, Baylor College of Medicine, Houston, Texas, USA

STEPHANIE F. POLITES, MD
Division of Pediatric Surgery, Department of Surgery, Mayo Clinic, Rochester, Minnesota, USA

DAVID A. RODEBERG, MD
Department of Surgery, Brody School of Medicine, East Carolina University, Greenville, North Carolina, USA

TIMOTHY N. ROGERS, MBBCh, FCS(SA), FCS(paed), FRCS(paed)
Department of Pediatric Surgery, University Hospitals Bristol NHS Foundation Trust, Bristol, United Kingdom

ERIN E. ROWELL, MD
Associate Professor of Surgery, Northwestern Feinberg School of Medicine, Pediatric Surgeon, Ann & Robert H. Lurie Children's Hospital of Chicago, Chicago, Illinois, USA

ANDREAS SCHMIDT, MD
Department of Pediatric Surgery and Pediatric Urology, University Children's Hospital Tuebingen, Tuebingen, Germany

GUIDO SEITZ, MD
Department of Pediatric Surgery, University Hospital Marburg, Baldingerstraße, Marburg, Germany

GREG M. TIAO, MD
Professor and Chief, Division of Pediatric Surgery, Cincinnati Children's Hospital and Medical Center, Cincinnati, Ohio, USA

SANJEEV A. VASUDEVAN, MD
Division of Pediatric Surgery, Michael E. DeBakey Department of Surgery, Texas Children's Surgical Oncology Program, Texas Children's Liver Tumor Program, Dan L. Duncan Cancer Center, Baylor College of Medicine, Houston, Texas, USA

STEVEN W. WARMANN, MD
Department of Pediatric Surgery and Pediatric Urology, University Children's Hospital Tuebingen, Tuebingen, Germany

BRENT R. WEIL, MD, MPH
Department of Pediatric Surgery, Boston Children's Hospital, Boston, Massachusetts, USA

CHRISTOPHER B. WELDON, MD, PhD
Associate Professor of Surgery, Harvard Medical School, Senior Surgeons' Chair, Associate in Surgery and Anesthesiology, Boston Children's Hospital, Boston, Massachusetts, USA

MARC W.H. WIJNEN, MD
Professor, Department of Surgery, Princess Maxima Center, Utrecht, the Netherlands

Contents

Gastrointestinal stromal tumors and neuroendocrine tumors in adult and pediatric populations differ immensely. Despite these established differences, the extreme rarity of gastrointestinal stromal tumors and neuroendocrine tumors in the pediatric population has resulted in the lack of consensus management guidelines, making optimal surgical approaches unclear. Comprehensive management principles to guide surgical approaches in adult literature are extensive. However, these are still lacking for pediatric patients. International cooperation to develop standardized pediatric-specific guidelines is urgently warranted in the future. This article highlights the vast differences between adult and pediatric parameters and provides recommendations on optimal and novel surgical approaches in children.

Differentiated thyroid carcinomas are rare in young children but represent almost 10% of all malignancies diagnosed in older adolescents. Differentiated thyroid carcinoma in children is more likely to demonstrate nodal involvement and is associated with higher recurrence rates than seen in adults. Decisions regarding extent of surgical resection are based on clinical and radiologic features, cytology, and risk assessment. Total thyroidectomy and compartment-based resection of involved lymph node basins form the cornerstone of treatment. The use of molecular genetics to inform treatment strategies and the use of targeted therapies to unresectable progressive disease is evolving.

The most recent advance in the care of children diagnosed with hepatoblastoma and hepatocellular carcinoma is the Pediatric Hepatic International Tumor Trial, which opened to international enrollment in 2018. It is being conducted as a collaborative effort by the pediatric multicenter trial groups in North America, Europe, and the Far East. This international effort was catalyzed by a new unified global risk stratification system for

surgical staging and resection, and developing novel methods to monitor for disease relapse.

Rhabdomyosarcoma is the commonest soft tissue sarcoma in children. Clinicians need vigilance to recognize the different signs and symptoms this tumor can present with because of variable sites of origin. Diagnosis requires a safe biopsy that obtains sufficient tissue for pathologic, genetic, and biological characterization of the tumor. Treatment depends on accurate staging with imaging and surgical sampling of draining lymph nodes. A multidisciplinary team assigns patients to risk-based therapy. Patients require chemotherapy and usually a combination of complex, site-specific surgery and/or radiotherapy. Outcomes for localized rhabdomyosarcoma continue to improve but new treatments are required for metastatic and relapsed disease.

Pediatric nonrhabdomyosarcoma soft tissue sarcomas (NRSTSs) encompass a heterogeneous group of mesenchymal tumors with more than 50 histologic variants. The incidence of NRSTS is greater than rhabdomyosarcoma; however, each histologic type is rare. The treatment schema for all NRSTSs is largely surgical. The treatment is a risk-adapted approach based on tumor size, localization, tumor grade, and presence of metastases. Low-grade tumors are mainly managed by surgery alone, whereas for high-grade tumors a multimodal treatment concept is necessary. The multimodal treatment consists of tumor biopsy, chemotherapy, local treatment (surgery ± radiotherapy), and immunotherapy in selected conditions.

Melanoma is the most common skin cancer in children, often presenting in an atypical fashion. The incidence of melanoma in children has been declining. The mainstay of therapy is surgical resection. Sentinel lymph node biopsy often is indicated to guide therapy and determine prognosis. Completion lymph node dissection is recommended in selective cases after positive sentinel lymph node biopsy. Those with advanced disease receive adjuvant systemic treatment. Because children are excluded from melanoma clinical trials, management is based on pediatric retrospective data and adult clinical trials. This review focuses on epidemiology, presentation, surgical management, adjuvant therapy, and outcomes of pediatric melanoma.

Decisions regarding the role of surgery in pulmonary metastasis need to take into account histology and biology of the cancer. Response to chemotherapy and radiotherapy, balanced with toxicities, factors into decisions about metastasectomy. The less sensitive the tumor is to adjuvant therapy, the more likely that metastasectomy may be beneficial. Broad principles include the following: the aims of resection are localized resections with clear margins, with the aim of preserving adequate lung volume; unnecessary toxic therapy sometimes is avoided with accurate diagnosis; tumor type is of utmost importance; and number of metastases and the disease-free interval are not contraindications to metastasectomy.

Survivors of pediatric cancer are at increased risk for infertility and premature hormonal failure. Surgeons caring for children with cancer have an important role to play in understanding this risk, as well as advocating for and performing appropriate fertility preservation procedures. Fertility preservation options in males and females vary by pubertal status and include nonexperimental (oocyte harvest, ovarian tissue cryopreservation, sperm cryopreservation) and experimental (testicular tissue cryopreservation) options. This review summarizes the basics of risk assessment and fertility preservation options and explores unique considerations in pediatric fertility preservation.

Minimally invasive approaches to pediatric cancer surgery are increasingly used, not only for the benefits of smaller incisions, but also for better field visualization and precise dissection. Advances in technology and surgeon experience have facilitated this trend. However, the appropriate indications for its use remain to be determined, and oncologic principles should not be compromised. We discuss the current and potential future uses, and new technologies that are being developed and introduced to assist with and enhance the role of minimally invasive surgery in the management of children with cancer.

SURGICAL ONCOLOGY CLINICS OF NORTH AMERICA

SERIES OF RELATED INTEREST

Surgical Clinics of North America
http://www.surgical.theclinics.com
Thoracic Surgery Clinics
http://www.thoracic.theclinics.com
Advances in Surgery
http://www.advancessurgery.com

THE CLINICS ARE AVAILABLE ONLINE!
Access your subscription at:
www.theclinics.com

Foreword

Pediatric Cancer

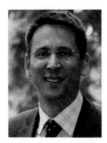

Timothy M. Pawlik, MD, MPH, MTS, PhD, FACS, FRACS (Hon.)
Consulting Editor

This issue of the *Surgical Oncology Clinics of North America* focuses on the management of Pediatric Cancer. Despite advances over the last several decades, pediatric cancer remains among the top causes of death in children. While the profession of pediatrics has a tradition of treating a broad range of diseases, a specific focus on pediatric oncology was established in the mid-twentieth century. Specifically, Dr Odile Schweisguth is generally recognized as the first pediatric oncologist, after she was appointed to the Consultant post in 1948 at the Institute Gustave Roussy to establish a new pediatric section at this renowned cancer center in France.[1] Dr Schweisguth established an independent pediatric oncology ward that focused exclusively on the care of children with cancer. In turn, pediatric surgical oncology itself evolved as a clear subspecialty field within pediatric surgery. The treatment of pediatric cancers has evolved over time with marked improvements in survival for various malignant diagnoses. The advances in pediatric oncology have been derived from a broad systematic integrated multidisciplinary approach to the care of patients with childhood cancer. As clinical modalities and regimens have evolved, so has our understanding of the basic molecular biology of tumors. Amidst all of this, the surgeon has remained a critical and central member of the treatment team. Importantly, surgical treatment continues to change and evolve, with the role of surgery constantly being redefined.[2] In light of this, I am grateful to have Dr Roshni Dasgupta as the guest editor of this important issue of *Surgical Oncology Clinics of North America*. Dr Dasgupta is a professor with the University of Cincinnati College of Medicine. Dr Dasgupta obtained her medical degree at the University of Toronto and subsequently completed her residency at Massachusetts General Hospital. She completed a Rhodes Scholarship at the University of Oxford in Oxford, England, followed by a Pediatric Surgery Fellowship at the Hospital for Sick Children in Toronto, Canada. Dr Dasgupta is the current chair of the American Pediatric Surgical Association Cancer Committee, as well as the Pediatric Surgical Oncology Research Collaborative. As such, Dr Dasgupta is imminently

Surg Oncol Clin N Am 30 (2021) xiii–xiv
https://doi.org/10.1016/j.soc.2021.02.001
1055-3207/21/© 2021 Published by Elsevier Inc.

qualified to be the guest editor of this important issue of *Surgical Oncology Clinics of North America*.

The issue covers many important topics, including the treatment and surgical management of patients with a wide range of pediatric tumors. In particular, an impressive team of experts details the state-of-the-art management of various abdominal tumors, including neuroendocrine cancer, GIST (gastrointestinal stromal tumor), liver, and, among others, renal tumors. In addition, other important cancers that are prevalent in pediatric populations, such as melanoma and thyroid cancer, are covered. Furthermore, the role of minimally invasive and newer surgical techniques in the pediatric cancer population is addressed. Fertility considerations, which can be particularly germane to pediatric patients with cancer, are also discussed in detail.

I owe Dr Dasgupta a great debt of gratitude for her work to identify such a wonderful group of pediatric oncology leaders to contribute to this issue of *Surgical Oncology Clinics of North America*. This team of authors has done a skillful job in highlighting the important and relevant aspects of caring for children with cancer. I am convinced that this issue of *Surgical Oncology Clinics of North America* will serve faculty and trainees well in understanding the latest state-of-the-art practices related to the care of pediatric cancer. I would like to thank Dr Dasgupta and all the contributing authors again for an outstanding issue of the *Surgical Oncology Clinics of North America*.

Timothy M. Pawlik, MD, MPH, MTS, PhD, FACS, FRACS (Hon.)
Department of Surgery
The Urban Meyer III and Shelley Meyer Chair for Cancer Research
Departments of Surgery, Oncology, and Health Services Management and Policy
The Ohio State University Wexner Medical Center
395 West 12th Avenue, Suite 670
Columbus, OH 43210, USA

E-mail address:
tim.pawlik@osumc.edu

REFERENCES

1. Carachi R, Grosfeld JL. A brief history of pediatric oncology. In: The surgery of childhood tumors. Springer; 2016. p. 1–5.
2. Von Allmen D. Pediatric surgical oncology: a brief overview of where we have been and the challenges we face. Semin Pediatr Surg 28(6):150864.

Preface

An Introduction to Pediatric Surgical Oncology

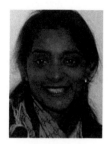

Roshni Dasgupta, MD, MPH
Editor

Cancer is the leading disease-related cause of death in children and adolescents. Pediatric surgical oncology has emerged as a newer subspecialty within the field of pediatric surgery. The explosion in precision medicine paralleled in adult oncology has revolutionized the management of patients with pediatric cancer. This paradigm shift in the genetic classification of tumors has advanced the ability to predict prognosis and tailor treatment regimens accordingly. Multimodal therapy is the norm for most pediatric tumors; however, with accurate risk stratification, certain tumors may be observed, or treated with surgery only, to mitigate the late effects of treatment. As the management of pediatric oncology patients becomes more complex, it is essential to develop specific surgical expertise in the nuances of pediatric solid tumor management. The contributors to this issue are international experts in their fields. Their participation underscores the need for collaboration within the field of pediatric surgical oncology. Due to the rarity of pediatric tumors and their diverse biological characteristics, it is integral to pool data and develop standardized regimens to allow for trials that are powered to improve outcomes.

This issue summarizes the most common solid tumors in pediatric oncology, including Wilms tumor, neuroblastoma, rhabdomyosarcoma, non–rhabdomyosarcoma sarcomas, hepatoblastoma, and germ cell tumors. While primarily focusing on the pediatric patient, there are treatment suggestions for the adult patient who may develop pediatric malignancies. Also included are articles that will be familiar to adult surgical oncologists, such as the treatises on melanoma, thyroid, adrenal, neuroendocrine tumors, and management of metastatic disease, all of which have overlap with adult regimens; however, an effort was made focus on the aspects of tumor biology and treatment, which differ in the pediatric patient. An article on fertility options emphasizes the unique concerns of the prepubertal patient and late effects of cytotoxic chemotherapy. Finally, included is a discourse on use of minimally invasive techniques and implementation of new

Surg Oncol Clin N Am 30 (2021) xv–xvi
https://doi.org/10.1016/j.soc.2021.01.001
1055-3207/21/© 2021 Published by Elsevier Inc.

technologies. These include the use of targeted fluorescent molecules and operative planning with advanced imaging. Due to the unique characteristics of pediatric cancers and physiology of the patients, specialized expertise is required to ensure excellent surgical outcomes while reducing long-term adverse effects.

Roshni Dasgupta, MD, MPH
Division of Pediatric General and Thoracic Surgery
Cincinnati Children's Hospital Medical Center
University of Cincinnati
3333 Burnet Avenue
Cincinnati, OH 45229, USA

E-mail address:
roshni.dasgupta@cchmc.org

Pediatric Gastrointestinal Stromal Tumors and Neuroendocrine Tumors
Advances in Surgical Management

Hanna Garnier, MD, PhD[a], Caitlyn Loo, BS[b,c],
Piotr Czauderna, MD, PhD[a], Sanjeev A. Vasudevan, MD[b,*]

KEYWORDS

- NET • Neuroendocrine tumors • GIST • Gastrointestinal stromal tumors
- Pediatric oncology • Pediatric surgery

KEY POINTS

- Gastrointestinal stromal tumors (GIST) and neuroendocrine tumors (NET) in adult and pediatric populations differ immensely.
- Despite these established differences, the extreme rarity of GIST and NET in the pediatric population has resulted in the lack of consensus management guidelines, making optimal surgical approaches unclear.
- Surgery is adopted as the mainstay treatment for both pediatric GIST and NET with optimal approaches depending on tumor site.
- Pediatric GIST involves chronic management of disease burden to preserve quality of life as disease progression is often indolent with low mortality rates.
- Pediatric NET requires multi-disciplinary management with extensive long term follow-up and frequent screening.

INTRODUCTION

Gastrointestinal stromal tumors (GIST) and neuroendocrine tumors (NET) are extremely rare within the pediatric population. Although it is possible for GIST and

[a] Department of Surgery and Urology for Children and Adolescents, Medical University of Gdansk, Marii Skłodowskiej-Curie 3a, Gdańsk 80-210, Poland; [b] Division of Pediatric Surgery, Michael E. DeBakey Department of Surgery, Texas Children's Surgical Oncology Program, Texas Children's Liver Tumor Program, Dan L. Duncan Cancer Center, Baylor College of Medicine, 7200 Cambridge Street, 7th Floor, Houston, TX 77030, USA; [c] School of Medicine, Royal College of Surgeons in Ireland, 123 St Stephens Green, Saint Peter's, Dublin D02 YN77, Ireland
* Corresponding author. Texas Children's Hospital - Main Campus, 6701 Fannin, Suite 1210 Houston, TX 77030, USA
E-mail address: sanjeevv@bcm.edu

Surg Oncol Clin N Am 30 (2021) 219–233
https://doi.org/10.1016/j.soc.2020.11.001
1055-3207/21/© 2020 Elsevier Inc. All rights reserved.

NET to occur simultaneously, this is exceedingly rare with only one published case in the literature.[1] Accordingly, these malignancies usually occur in isolation. Comprehensive management principles to guide surgical approaches in adult literature are extensive. However, these are still lacking for pediatric patients. As such, this review individually highlights the unique differences between adult and pediatric subtypes in GIST and NET, which sheds light on the pressing need for standardized management principles specific to these young patients. At the same time, we offer insights into surgical approaches that may be adopted when encountering pediatric patients with these uncommon malignancies.

GASTROINTESTINAL STROMAL TUMORS IN CHILDREN

GIST are neoplasms of mesenchymal origin that are believed to arise from interstitial cells of Cajal or their precursors.[2] In the current literature, three subtypes exist: (1) adult GIST; (2) pediatric or wild-type GIST (P/WT-GIST); and (3) most recently described, young adult GIST.[3] Unlike their counterparts, P/WT-GIST are distinct in almost all facets, expressing differences in clinical behavior, molecular profile, prognosis, and therapeutic sensitivities.[4–7] Despite this, current management approach is adapted from adult guidelines because of the lack of principles specific to P/WT-GIST.[8–10] This is partly explained by the extreme rarity of P/WT-GIST, which is approximated by Surveillance, Epidemiology, and End Results and other reports to be 0.02 to 0.11 cases per million annually.[11,12] Because the exact incidence is unknown, this poses an extreme challenge for consolidation and preparation of a centralized management strategy. Consequently, because of the lack of understanding and universal guidelines, P/WT-GIST often go undiagnosed or misdiagnosed because of their vague indolent symptoms.[7] Moreover, because many patients have potentially long lifespans and often live for decades with this background malignancy, the focus for surgical management shifts from an absolute cure to chronic management of disease burden and the associated symptoms for prolonged event-free survival (EFS).[13]

Classification

The classification of P/WT-GIST arose because 85% of patients lacked the hallmark *KIT/PDGRA* mutations compared with only 10% to 15% in adult GIST.[14,15] Since then, genetic evaluation has continued to reveal further unique molecular signatures, particularly in succinate dehydrogenase (SDH).[16] This has linked P/WT-GIST to the GIST-related cancer syndromes Carney triad and Carney-Stratakis syndrome, and has even led to the proposal of a new molecular classification based on SDH status, which encompass SDH-competent, SDH-mutant, and SDH-epimutant.[17–20]

Clinical Features

In less than 15% of P/WT-GIST that are SDH-competent, tumor and patient demographic features overlap with *KIT/PDGRA*-positive adult GIST tumors and should be treated according to adult guidelines.[13,20–22]

However, pediatric reports of GIST encompassing SDH-mutant and epimutants show unique clinical presentations compared with adults. Patients were overwhelmingly female, with a median age of 13 years old.[20,23] Because their lesions were 90% gastric in origin showing epithelioid or mixed histology, common presentations included anemia, epigastric pain, or gastric-specific symptoms.[24,25] Most significantly, patients presented with multifocal tumors and metastasis, especially to the lymph nodes in 45% of cases.[13] Additionally, multiple recurrences were common with 27%, 76%, and 84% of patients experiencing recurrence over 1, 5, and 10 years after diagnosis, respectively.[26] Despite this, because of the indolent nature of neoplastic progression, patients with P/WT-GIST have a prolonged survival with few patients succumbing to their disease and a 16-year survival after diagnosis.[22,27]

Imaging, Diagnosis, and Staging

In adults, computed tomography (CT) is the gold standard for initial investigation and monitoring of treatment response.[9,10,28] However, because of the young age of patients with P/WT-GIST and their need for lifelong screening (discussed later), it is important to minimize radiation exposure. As a result, alterative imaging, such as MRI and contrast-enhancing ultrasound, are preferred.[29] In fact, these same imaging principles are adopted for the staging work-up, with the inclusion of thorough investigations for lymph node, liver, and peritoneum seeding because of frequent metastasis at presentation (**Fig. 1**).[29]

However, diagnosis is still established through histologic analysis and immunohistochemical staining of tumor specimens.[9,10] Endoscopic ultrasound–guided fine-needle aspirate for masses larger than 1 cm is highly recommended because it yields a diagnostic rate of 62% to 93%.[30,31] On the contrary, traditional endoscopic forceps are discouraged because of the poor diagnostic rates and associated bleeding complications.[32–34] Percutaneous image-guided biopsy should also be avoided and only adopted on a case-by-case basis because of the risk of tumor spillage.[10] This must be approached with extreme caution because spillage is significantly associated with recurrence in P/WT-GIST.[35,36] For this reason, if endoscopic ultrasound–guided fine-needle aspirate is not feasible, it may be prudent to conduct a primary surgical resection for pathologic diagnosis.[9,10]

Surgical Management

Currently, guidelines for the management and treatment of P/WT-GIST are based on case reports and limited series because data supporting consensus guidelines for P/

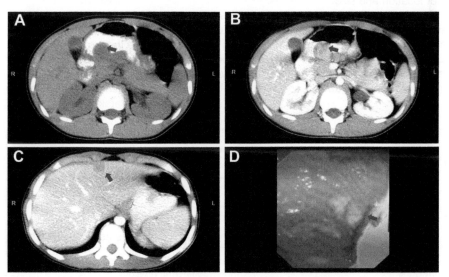

Fig. 1. A 12-year-old girl with abdominal pain diagnosed with multiple gastric tumors with lymph node metastases and a single liver metastasis. (*A*) Tumor and lymph nodes metastases (*red arrow*). (*B*) Tumor and lymph nodes metastases (*red arrow*). (*C*) Liver metastases (*red arrow*). (*D*) Tumor mass visualized during gastroscopy (*red arrow*).

W-GIST are lacking. However, surgical resection remains the mainstay treatment of all GIST including P/WT-GIST.[7,9,10,26]

Generally, a laparoscopic approach is adopted in lesions with favorable anatomic locations between 2 and 5 cm in size.[37] However, if these principles are adopted, tumor pseudocapsule must be preserved and resection specimens must be removed using a plastic bag to prevent spillage and port site seeding.[8] Additionally, if tumors run the risk of intraoperative rupture, especially in larger lesions greater than 5 cm, laparoscopic approach is strongly discouraged and open surgery should be considered instead.[10]

In adult GIST, complete R0 en bloc surgical resection for localized nonmetastatic tumors is the gold standard treatment and is achieved in 85% of patients.[38] Because GIST has the potential to occur anywhere along the gastrointestinal tract, surgical interventions are often site-dependent and are outlined in the latest guidelines (**Table 1**).[10] These are selectively applied to P/WT-GIST with the addition of sampling and possible dissection of lymph node draining basins and enlarged nodes because of frequent metastasis. In addition, surgical principles for P/WT-GIST are aimed at organ-sparing resection of primary tumor.[39] In P/WT-GIST, tumors are predominantly found in the stomach and usually occur in the antrum or lesser curvature.[38] As such, current literature focuses on gastric interventions.

Laparoscopic wedge resection has been adopted globally as the principle procedure for gastric GIST. However, a major difficulty with this approach lies in determining the appropriate resection margin often resulting in excessive gastric resection.[40] Additionally, certain tumor locations and morphology make laparoscopic wedge resection challenging especially when located close to the gastroesophageal junction (GOJ) or pyloric ring. This potentially results in partial gastrectomy being adopted instead because of risk of strictures and stenosis.[41] Despite this, no defined strategy exists to guide surgeons on selection of the appropriate resection technique. However, case reports and studies have independently outline various techniques based on tumor location and size.

Laparoscopic endoscopic cooperative surgery allows for a standardized gastric submucosal tumor resection independent of tumor location and site.[42] In this technique, endoscopic submucosal resection is performed around the tumor, which is followed by laparoscopic seromuscular dissection and tumor removal. Because tumor lesions are removed intra-abdominally, this procedure is limited to submucosal tumors without ulceration and bleeding. Unfortunately, laparoscopic endoscopic

Table 1
Surgical guidelines for localized GIST in adults

Site of GIST	Surgical Intervention
Esophageal	Resection Enucleation
Gastric	Wedge resection Segmental resection Partial/total gastrectomy (rarely indicated)
Duodenal	Wedge resection
Intestinal	Segmental resection
Colorectal	Segmental resection Local transanal excision (for small lesions)[a]

[a] Conduct sphincter-sparing approach wherever possible.

cooperative surgery has a higher risk of tumor rupture and peritoneal seeding because of tumor manipulation during surgery. As a result, other techniques, such as nonexposed endoscopic wall inversion surgery (NEWS), are ideal for intraluminal lesions because resection is conducted without exposure to the peritoneal cavity.[43] NEWS is an laparoscopic endoscopic cooperative surgery–related procedure and involves intraluminal submucosal incision on the laparoscopic side. Then, a spacer is used to push the tumor into the gastric lumen, allowing it to be excised endoscopically into the stomach and removed transorally. However, NEWS is not suitable for tumors of more than 3 cm, or those close to the GOJ or pyloric ring. These limitations are similar to endoluminal endoscopic full-thickness resection (EFTR) microsurgery, which has also been outlined in adult patients with GIST originating from the muscularis propria.[44] EFTR involves endoscopically precutting the surrounding mucosa and submucosa to expose the tumor. Then, dissection of the muscularis propria around the tumor is performed, followed by dissection of the serous membrane. If patients are eligible, this technique could be highly successful because a study has demonstrated promising results, achieving a complete resection rate of 100% with 0% recurrence after 1 year.

To overcome the limitations of NEWS and EFTR, laparoscopic wedge resection with the serosal and muscular layers incision technique is adopted.[45] In this novel technique, incisions are made into the serosal and muscular layers around the tumor laparoscopically. After the circumference of the tumor is excised, the tumor appearance shifts from intraluminal to extraluminal where a wedge resection is performed for its removal. This technique is optimal for challenging lesions located close to the GOJ or pyloric ring. Most advantageously, serosal and muscular layers incision technique does not require endoscopic submucosal dissection expertise and devices. Because it also does not require full-thickness gastric perforation as the mucosal and submucosal layers are left intact, the risk of tumor seeding is also prevented.

Postsurgical Outcomes

It is generally accepted that complete resection without tumor rupture is successful in halting disease progression. However, Weldon and colleagues[26] have demonstrated that EFS in P/WT-GIST is significantly more closely related to tumor biology compared with surgical factors, such as resection margins. Although reoperation is generally a common consideration with metastasis and recurrence, this might not be indicated for P/WT-GIST because subsequent resections were significantly associated with decreased postoperative EFS. National Comprehensive Cancer Network guidelines also outline that reresection is generally not indicated for microscopically positive margins, even in adult GIST.[8]

Although this might be concerning especially because disease progression and recurrence are common in P/WT-GIST, patients are afforded low mortality rates of less than 10%.[46] For this reason, P/WT-GIST must be considered in the paradigm of chronic disease with long-term management focusing on disease control, symptom management, and preserving quality of life. Therefore, indications for aggressive or repeat resections and their associated long-term sequelae must be critically evaluated against the potential benefit.

Novel Therapies and Follow-Up

Contrary to the immensely successful conventional tyrosine kinase inhibitor therapy adopted in adult GIST, P/WT-GIST continue to show nonresponse, inability to improve recurrence-free survival, and is associated with dedifferentiation.[39,47] Thankfully, various therapeutic agents are being trialed and may have a promising application in P/WT-GIST.[48–50]

Considering the limitations of medical therapy and nature of the disease, cure is not likely. Thus it is imperative that patients with P/WT-GIST be monitored and surveilled frequently and consistently with lifelong follow-up to ensure the long-term survival of these young patients.[29]

NEUROENDOCRINE TUMORS IN CHILDREN

NET originate from neuroendocrine cells present in almost every organ in the human body. Their characteristic features and immunoprofiles allow them to be classified into one group regardless of their anatomic location. Similar to P/WT-GIST, most available data are not specific to the pediatric population because of its extreme rarity. The incidence rate of NET between 0 and 29 years of age is estimated at approximately 2.8 cases per million.[51] NET incidence in children varies between 0.1 (ovary, thyroid gland, cervix, foregut) and 0.6 (lungs) per million population. Moreover, only 5% to 10% of pediatric pancreatic tumors with incidence of only 0.018/100,000 in the United States are found to be NET.[52] Ninety percent of pediatric NET are benign and mainly solitary. They originate from pancreatic islet cells with insulinomas and gastrinomas being most common; somatostatinomas and VIPomas are exceedingly rare in children.[53]

Pediatric NET show gender and genetic predispositions. NET are observed more frequently in females, with appendix NET and pediatric bronchial carcinoid tumors showing female preponderance.[54–56] Multiple endocrine neoplasia type 1 (MEN1) and von Hippel-Lindau disease are the most frequent hereditary predispositions.[57] Other syndromes include: neurofibromatosis type 1, tuberous sclerosis, Lynch syndrome, and familial adenomatous polyposis.[58] In particular, pancreatic NET, especially gastrinomas, seem to be associated with genetic syndromes, such as MEN1. Therefore, genetic predisposition should be suspected when multiple primary tumors are present or specific clinical features are noticed.[59]

Classification

NET are widely distributed throughout the body. Hence, most of the clinical features are unique to the site of the origin and/or hormone overexcretion. The World Health Organization proposed a new diagnostic system based on results from various studies. This has significantly changed the diagnostic processes and treatment approaches in NET (**Table 2**).[60,61]

Clinical Features

Although most NET are initially asymptomatic, patient symptoms strongly correlate with tumor localization, its size, and hormonal secretion.[62] In adults, the most common sites are small intestine, rectum, and lungs.[63] This is in contrast to children and young adults, with the most common sites being the lungs and appendix.[64]

Bronchial carcinoids usually have an endobronchial location causing persistent cough, wheezing, shortness of breath, hemoptysis, or chest pain. As such, they are frequently misdiagnosed as benign conditions. Unlike adults, children are almost always symptomatic, with the most common presentation being obstructive pneumonia and recurrent pulmonary infections.[65]

In pediatric patients, NET of the appendix is usually found incidentally but can often present with symptoms of acute appendicitis in 63% to 75% of cases.[66,67] Despite this, appendiceal NET is only responsible for about 0.16% to 2.3% of appendectomies.[68]

Table 2
NEN 2018 WHO classification of selected NEN by site, category, family, and tumor type[14]

Site	Category	Family	Type	Grade	Current Terminology
Lung	NEN	NET	Pulmonary NET	G1	Carcinoid
				G2	Atypical carcinoid
		NEC	Small cell lung carcinoma (pulmonary NEC, small cell type)		Small cell lung carcinoma
			Pulmonary NEC, large cell type		Large cell NE carcinoma
Uterus (corpus and cervix)	NEN	NET	Uterine NET	G1	Carcinoid
				G2	Atypical carcinoid
				G3	Atypical carcinoid
		NEC	Uterine NEC, small cell type		Small cell carcinoma
			Uterine NEC, large cell type		Large cell NE carcinoma
Pancreas	NEN	NET	Pancreatic NET	G1	PanNET G1
				G2	PanNET G2
				G3	PanNET G3
		NEC	Pancreatic NEC, small cell type		Small cell NE carcinoma
			Pancreatic NET, large cell type		Large cell NE carcinoma

Abbreviations: NEC, neuroendocrine carcinoma; NEN, neuroendocrine neoplasm; WHO, World Health Organization.
Data from Hirota S, Isozaki K, Moriyama Y, et al. Gain-of-Function Mutations of c-kit in Human Gastrointestinal Stromal Tumors. Science. 1997;279.

Pancreatic NET are usually associated with abdominal mass, pain, and vomiting. Various hormonal symptoms are associated with pancreatic NET, such as hypoglycemia ± seizures in insulinoma, peptic ulcers in gastrinoma, or diarrhea in VIPoma.[58] Carcinoid syndrome is an extremely rare presentation of NET in children, in contrast to 0.7% of adults at presentation.[56] In around 60% of patients, NET secreting vasoactive substances involve the heart and cause carcinoid heart disease, resulting in right heart failure.[69]

Imaging, Diagnosis, and Staging

CT, MRI, PET, somatostatin receptor imaging, and hybrid PET/CT or PET/MRI are used to localize, grade, stage, and classify NET (**Fig. 2**). Contrast-enhanced CT is highly accurate for neoplasms larger than 2 cm, with a broad sensitivity range of 63% to 82%.[70] Because of better soft tissue contrast, MRI better visualizes some NET tumors with sensitivity and specificity of 93% and 88% in pediatric NET, respectively.[71] In MRI, pancreatic insulinomas and gastrinomas reveal T1 and T2 prolongation.[72] Somatostatin receptor imaging with radiolabeled somatostatin analogue octreotide (OctreoScan) is especially useful for visualization of gastrinomas, glucagonomas, and VIPomas with sensitivity between 75% and 100%.[73]

Recently, a new somatostatin analogue 68Ga-DOTA-tyrosine3-octreotide (DOTA-TOC) PET/CT has shown a higher detection rate and is an excellent tracer for and planning of NET patient management.[74] Its low toxicity, low radiation exposure, fast administration, and clearance time make it the most reliable diagnostic modality for

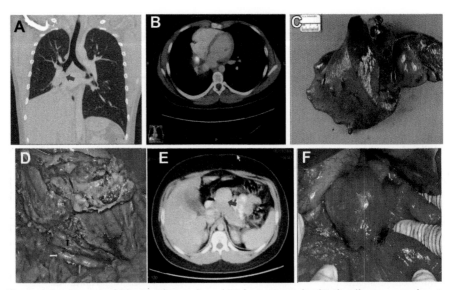

Fig. 2. (*A*) A 16-year-old boy with cough and Right Lower Lobe (RLL) collapse secondary to Right Medial Lobe (RML)/RLL endobronchial mass (*red arrow*). (*B*) Octreotide scan shows positive uptake within the mass. (*C*) Patient underwent thoracotomy with RML/RLL lobectomy with endobronchial carcinoid seen extruding from opened bronchus (*red arrow*). (*D*) An 8-year-old boy with hypoglycemia episodes found to have an insulin-secreting tumor in the body/tail of the pancreas distal to the inferior mesenteric vein (IMV) junction with the splenic vein (SV); laparoscopic splenic-sparing distal pancreatectomy performed with mass (*red arrow*) elevated off of the SV (*blue arrow*) and splenic artery (*black arrow*) and dissection taken to the IMV/SV junction (*white arrow*). (*E*) A 10-year-old boy with chronic constipation, diagnosed with pancreatic NET of head of pancreas; tumor mass (*red arrow*). (*F*) No metastases presented, and patient underwent central pancreatectomy.

the pediatric population. Thus, 68Ga-DOTATATE PET/CT should be adopted as the first-line diagnostic tool.

Although pathologic diagnosis is crucial for the treatment selection and prediction of the prognosis and the risk of progression, noninvasive laboratory tests can also be used in NET detection and follow-up. Serum chromogranin A is the most effective marker, with high levels strongly correlating with NET presence, especially in low-grade NET.[75] Additionally, higher serum levels of pancreastatin are also associated with poor prognosis, and is able to distinguish patients at high risk of recurrence.[76] Another useful marker in diagnosis and therapy monitoring is 5-hydroxyindoleacetic acid, showing specificity of up to 100%.[77] Other NET tumor markers described in the literature include: serotonin, neurokinin A, N-terminal pro–B-type natriuretic peptide, and neurone-specific enolase.[78]

Surgical Management and Postsurgical Outcomes

Because of the good long-term results, surgical management of pediatric NET is considered the first-line therapy for local-stage disease and is site-dependent.[79]

For appendiceal NET, various surgical interventions are described. Of the 0.3% of appendectomies confirmed at NET, 38% of patients underwent an ileocolic resection or right hemicolectomy.[80] The indications for more aggressive treatment included larger tumor size, extended invasiveness, and presence of tumor at resection margin.

Because some consider appendicectomy alone to be the most adequate treatment in children irrespective of NET size, lymph nodes involvement, tumor limited to the appendix, or mesenteric involvement, the need for a secondary colectomy is in question.[81] Others also suggest that simple appendectomy is only sufficient for tumors less than 1 cm or 1.6 cm, and right hemicolectomy should be recommended otherwise.[82] The North American Neuroendocrine Society reports that the 5-year mortality from appendiceal NET reached 29.5% for tumors 2 cm or greater. Thus, right hemicolectomy is recommended in those cases.[83] Additionally, although the "2-cm rule" is not applicable to adult duodenal, small bowel, and rectal tumors, which are often metastatic at smaller sizes, this is debatable in children.[84]

Pancreatic NET are extremely rare in children, hence data related to surgical management in this group are limited. Although surgery remains the crucial treatment, controversy still exists. Tumors less than 2 cm of size and those that are nonfunctioning are often considered to be left under observation because only 6% of them are confirmed to be malignant.[85] Because pediatric NET can localize in any part of the pancreas, surgical approach depends once again on tumor location.[86] The gold standard for surgical treatment of pancreatic head NET in adults and children is pancreaticoduodenectomy (Whipple procedure), with pylorus preservation (Traverso-Longmire modification).[52,87] In more distally located tumors, open or laparoscopic resection using distal pancreatomy, central pancreatectomy, or even tumor excision is applied.[58] Intraoperative ultrasound is helpful because some tumors tend to be multifocal. Complications, such as pancreatic leak, pancreatic deficiencies, and delayed gastric emptying, must also be avoided in pancreatic resections because they are associated with significant morbidity.[52]

Surgical treatment of pediatric bronchial carcinoid tumors is less controversial. Conservative procedures are the treatment of choice, because they are performed successfully by experienced thoracic surgeons. If possible, lung-sparing resections, such as sleeve resections or bronchoplasties, should be performed because the oncologic result is similar to pneumonectomy and offers a better quality of life.[88] In the pediatric population typical carcinoid tumors have a favorable prognosis following definitive surgical resection.[56]

Novel Therapies and Follow-Up

Unfortunately, surgical intervention in metastatic NET is not sufficient. Therefore, the main nonsurgical treatment options include somatostatin analogues, molecularly targeted therapies, cytotoxic therapies, and peptide receptor radionuclide therapy (PRRT). Increased expression of somatostatin receptors in NET tumors leads to targeted therapy with somatostatin analogues, such as octreotide and lanreotide.[89] They have shown an antitumor effect with regards to tumor progression and overall survival, especially in patients with metastatic midgut carcinoid tumors.[90]

Standard cytotoxic chemotherapy is believed to have limited benefits in metastatic NET. However, these may still be selectively effective. Temozolomide is an effective agent in the pediatric population with recurrent medulloblastoma/primitive neuroectodermal tumor.[91] Additionally, the combination of capecitabine and temozolomide was also shown to be effective in patients with grade 3 NET.[92] PRRT is another form of molecular targeted therapy approved as the standard of care treatment in progressive midgut NET. Good response of PRRT with 90Y and 177LU DOTA conjugated somatostatin analogues was reported.[93]

Although pediatric NET are rare, they do occur and may be associated with significant morbidity. Most patients are successfully treated with surgical tumor excision and no further management other than follow-up is required. Long-term follow-up is strongly recommended, especially in bronchial NET because of their frequent recurrences.[94] Despite this, the definition of adequate follow-up for NET is still not clear. However, most papers suggest a complex frequent follow-up in the first 3 to 5 years after resection.[95] For carcinoids that are less than 2 cm and localized to the appendix, no further follow-up is required after appendectomy.[55] Because of proven genetic predisposition of NET more frequent screening is indicated in cases of genetic syndromes MEN-1, von Hippel-Lindau disease, tuberous sclerosis, or familial adenomatous polyposis. Even still, the 5-year overall survival in NET remains in the range of 78%, with NET localized in the colon/rectum, appendix, and thyroid tumor locations having an even better 5-year overall survival of greater than 95%.[96]

SUMMARY AND FUTURE WORK

P/WT-GIST and pediatric NET are extremely rare malignancies that show uniquely distinct clinical features from their adult counterparts. Although surgery is adopted in both malignancies as the mainstay treatment, the wide range of site-dependent presentations and lack of pediatric-specific consensus treatment protocols makes it challenging to identify the most efficient surgical approach. As a result, international cooperation to develop standardized pediatric-specific guidelines is urgently warranted in the future. This will optimize the outcome and quality of life for these young patients.

CLINICS CARE POINTS

- Surgical management of pediatric GIST is the mainstay as medical treatments continue to show non-response and are associated with increased complications.
- Repeat resections for pediatric GIST recurrence is often not indicated as they are significantly associated with decreased postoperative EFS.
- Pediatric NET are associated with gender and genetic predispositions such as multiple endocrine neoplasia type 1 and von Hippel-Lindau disease.
- Surgical manegement of pediatric NET is considered first-line therapy and is largely site-dependent.

DISCLOSURE

The authors declare no commercial or financial conflict of interest.

REFERENCES

1. Kitajima R, Morita Y, Furuhashi S, et al. Simultaneous occurrence of an ampullary neuroendocrine tumor and multiple duodenal/jejunal gastrointestinal stromal tumors in a patient with neurofibromatosis type 1. Nihon Shokakibyo Gakkai Zasshi 2019;116(7):583–91.
2. Kindbolm L, Remotti HE, Aldenborg F, et al. Gastrointestinal pacemaker cell tumor (GIPACT). Am J Pathol 1998;152(5):1259–69.
3. NS IJ, Drabbe C, den Hollander D, et al. Gastrointestinal stromal tumours (GIST) in young adult (18-40 years) patients: a report from the Dutch GIST registry. Cancers (Basel) 2020;12(3):730.
4. Janeway KA, Weldon CB. Pediatric gastrointestinal stromal tumor. Semin Pediatr Surg 2012;21(1):31–43.
5. Mullassery D, Weldon CB. Pediatric/"wildtype" gastrointestinal stromal tumors. Semin Pediatr Surg 2016;25(5):305–10.

6. Pappo AS, Janeway KA. Pediatric gastrointestinal stromal tumors. Hematol Oncol Clin North Am 2009;23(1):15–34, vii.

7. Quiroz HJ, Willobee BA, Sussman MS, et al. Pediatric gastrointestinal stromal tumors: a review of diagnostic modalities. Transl Gastroenterol Hepatol 2018;3:54.

8. National Comprehensive Cancer Network. (2020). Soft Tissue Sarcoma (Version 1.2021). Available at: https://www.nccn.org/professionals/physician_gls/pdf/sarcoma.pdf

9. Casali PG, Abecassis N, Aro HT, et al. Gastrointestinal stromal tumours: ESMO-EURACAN clinical practice guidelines for diagnosis, treatment and follow-up. Ann Oncol 2018;29(Suppl 4):iv68–78.

10. Landi B, Blay JY, Bonvalot S, et al. Gastrointestinal stromal tumours (GISTs): French Intergroup Clinical Practice Guidelines for diagnosis, treatments and follow-up (SNFGE, FFCD, GERCOR, UNICANCER, SFCD, SFED, SFRO). Dig Liver Dis 2019;51(9):1223–31.

11. Pappo AS, Janeway K, Laquaglia M, et al. Special considerations in pediatric gastrointestinal tumors. J Surg Oncol 2011;104(8):928–32.

12. Benesch M, Wardelmann E, Ferrari A, et al. Gastrointestinal stromal tumors (GIST) in children and adolescents: a comprehensive review of the current literature. Pediatr Blood Cancer 2009;53(7):1171–9.

13. Parab TM, DeRogatis MJ, Boaz AM, et al. Gastrointestinal stromal tumors: a comprehensive review. J Gastrointest Oncol 2019;10(1):144–54.

14. Hirota S, Isozaki K, Moriyama Y, et al. Gain-of-function mutations of c-kit in human gastrointestinal stromal tumors. Science 1997;279:577–80.

15. Heinrich MC, Corless CL, Duensing A, et al. PDGFRA activating mutations in gastrointestinal stromal tumors. Science 2003;299:708–10.

16. Belinsky MG, Rink L, von Mehren M. Succinate dehydrogenase deficiency in pediatric and adult gastrointestinal stromal tumors. Front Oncol 2013;3:117.

17. McWhinney SR, Pasini B, Stratakis C. Familial gastrointestinal stromal tumors and germ-line mutations. N Engl J Med 2007;357:1054–6.

18. Settas N, Faucz FR, Stratakis CA. Succinate dehydrogenase (SDH) deficiency, Carney triad and the epigenome. Mol Cell Endocrinol 2018;469:107–11.

19. Pasini B, McWhinney SR, Bei T, et al. Clinical and molecular genetics of patients with the Carney-Stratakis syndrome and germline mutations of the genes coding for the succinate dehydrogenase subunits SDHB, SDHC, and SDHD. Eur J Hum Genet 2008;16(1):79–88.

20. Boikos SA, Pappo AS, Killian JK, et al. Molecular subtypes of KIT/PDGFRA wild-type gastrointestinal stromal tumors: a report from the National Institutes of Health gastrointestinal stromal tumor clinic. JAMA Oncol 2016;2(7):922–8.

21. Miettinen M, Sarlomo-Rikala M, Sobin LH, et al. Esophageal stromal tumors. Am J Surg Pathol 2000;24:211–22.

22. Miettinen M, Lasota J, Sobin LH. Gastrointestinal stromal tumors of the stomach in children and young adults. Am J Surg Pathol 2005;29:1373–81.

23. Wada R, Arai H, Kure S, et al. Wild type" GIST: clinicopathological features and clinical practice. Pathol Int 2016;66(8):431–7.

24. Wang YM, Gu ML, Ji F. Succinate dehydrogenase-deficient gastrointestinal stromal tumors. World J Gastroenterol 2015;21(8):2303–14.

25. Miettinen M, Wang ZF, Sarlomo-Rikala M, et al. Succinate dehydrogenase-deficient GISTs: a clinicopathologic, immunohistochemical, and molecular genetic study of 66 gastric GISTs with predilection to young age. Am J Surg Pathol 2011;35:1712–21.

26. Weldon CB, Madenci AL, Boikos SA, et al. Surgical management of wild-type gastrointestinal stromal tumors: a report from the National Institutes of Health pediatric and wildtype GIST clinic. J Clin Oncol 2017;35(5):523–8.

27. Agaram NP, Laquaglia MP, Ustun B, et al. Molecular characterization of pediatric gastrointestinal stromal tumors. Clin Cancer Res 2008;14(10):3204–15.

28. Meyer M, Hohenberger P, Apfaltrer P, et al. CT-based response assessment of advanced gastrointestinal stromal tumor: dual energy CT provides a more predictive imaging biomarker of clinical benefit than RECIST or Choi criteria. Eur J Radiol 2013;82(6):923–8.

29. Herzberg M, Beer M, Anupindi S, et al. Imaging pediatric gastrointestinal stromal tumor (GIST). J Pediatr Surg 2018;53(9):1862–70.

30. Mekky MA, Yamao K, Sawaki A, et al. Diagnostic utility of EUS-guided FNA in patients with gastric submucosal tumors. Gastrointest Endosc 2010;71(6):913–9.

31. Akahoshi K, Oya M, Koga T, et al. Clinical usefulness of endoscopic ultrasound-guided fine needle aspiration for gastric subepithelial lesions smaller than 2 cm. J Gastrointestin Liver Dis 2014;23(4):405–12.

32. Cantor MJ, Davila RE, Faigel DO. Yield of tissue sampling for subepithelial lesions evaluated by EUS: a comparison between forceps biopsies and endoscopic submucosal resection. Gastrointest Endosc 2006;64(1):29–34.

33. Hunt GC, Smith PP, Faigel DO. Yield of tissue sampling for submucosal lesions evaluated by EUS. Gastrointest Endosc 2003;57(1):68–72.

34. Buscaglia JM, Nagula S, Jayaraman V, et al. Diagnostic yield and safety of jumbo biopsy forceps in patients with subepithelial lesions of the upper and lower GI tract. Gastrointest Endosc 2012;75(6):1147–52.

35. Holmebakk T, Hompland I, Bjerkehagen B, et al. Recurrence-free survival after resection of gastric gastrointestinal stromal tumors classified according to a strict definition of tumor rupture: a population-based study. Ann Surg Oncol 2018; 25(5):1133–9.

36. Holmebakk T, Nishida T, Rutkowski P, et al. Defining rupture in gastrointestinal stromal tumor: semantics and prognostic value. Ann Surg Oncol 2019;26(7): 2304–5.

37. De Vogelaere K, Van Loo I, Peters O, et al. Laparoscopic resection of gastric gastrointestinal stromal tumors (GIST) is safe and effective, irrespective of tumor size. Surg Endosc 2012;26(8):2339–45.

38. Mei L, Du W, Idowu M, et al. Advances and challenges on management of gastrointestinal stromal tumors. Front Oncol 2018;8:135.

39. Neppala P, Banerjee S, Fanta PT, et al. Current management of succinate dehydrogenase-deficient gastrointestinal stromal tumors. Cancer Metastasis Rev 2019;38(3):525–35.

40. Choi SM, Kim MC, Jung GJ, et al. Laparoscopic wedge resection for gastric GIST: long-term follow-up results. Eur J Surg Oncol 2007;33(4):444–7.

41. Hwang SH, Park DJ, Kim YH, et al. Laparoscopic surgery for submucosal tumors located at the esophagogastric junction and the prepylorus. Surg Endosc 2009; 23(9):1980–7.

42. Hiki N, Yamamoto Y, Fukunaga T, et al. Laparoscopic and endoscopic cooperative surgery for gastrointestinal stromal tumor dissection. Surg Endosc 2008; 22(7):1729–35.

43. Matsumoto S, Hosoya Y, Lefor AK, et al. Non-exposed endoscopic wall-inversion surgery for pediatric gastrointestinal stromal tumor: a case report. Asian J Endosc Surg 2019;12(3):322–5.

44. Huang J, Xian XS, Huang LY, et al. Endoscopic full-thickness resection for gastric gastrointestinal stromal tumor originating from the muscularis propria. Rev Assoc Med Bras (1992) 2018;64(11):1002–6.

45. Fujishima H, Etoh T, Hiratsuka T, et al. Serosal and muscular layers incision technique in laparoscopic surgery for gastric gastrointestinal stromal tumors. Asian J Endosc Surg 2017;10(1):92–5.

46. Lima M, Gargano T, Ruggeri G, et al. Laparoscopic resection of a rare gastrointestinal stromal tumor in children. Springerplus 2015;4:73.

47. Malik F, Santiago T, Bahrami A, et al. Dedifferentiation in SDH-deficient gastrointestinal stromal tumor: a report with histologic, immunophenotypic, and molecular characterization. Pediatr Dev Pathol 2019;22(5):492–8.

48. Hadoux J, Favier J, Scoazec JY, et al. SDHB mutations are associated with response to temozolomide in patients with metastatic pheochromocytoma or paraganglioma. Int J Cancer 2014;135(11):2711–20.

49. Courtney KD, Infante JR, Lam ET, et al. Phase I dose-escalation trial of PT2385, a first-in-class hypoxia-inducible factor-2a antagonist in patients with previously treated advanced clear cell renal cell carcinoma. J Clin Oncol 2018;36:867–74.

50. MacKenzie ED, Selak MA, Tennant DA, et al. Cell-permeating alpha-ketoglutarate derivatives alleviate pseudohypoxia in succinate dehydrogenase-deficient cells. Mol Cell Biol 2007;27(9):3282–9.

51. Navalkele P, O'Dorisio MS, O'Dorisio TM, et al. Incidence, survival, and prevalence of neuroendocrine tumors versus neuroblastoma in children and young adults: nine standard SEER registries, 1975-2006. Pediatr Blood Cancer 2011; 56(1):50–7.

52. Vasudevan SA, Ha TN, Zhu H, et al. Pancreaticoduodenectomy for the treatment of pancreatic neoplasms in children: a pediatric surgical oncology research collaborative study. Pediatr Blood Cancer 2020;67:e28425.

53. Nasher O, Hall NJ, Sebire NJ, et al. Pancreatic tumours in children: diagnosis, treatment and outcome. Pediatr Surg Int 2015;31(9):831–5.

54. Diets IJ, Nagtegaal ID, Loeffen J, et al. Childhood neuroendocrine tumours: a descriptive study revealing clues for genetic predisposition. Br J Cancer 2017; 116(2):163–8.

55. Sommer C, Gumy Pause F, Diezi M, et al. A national long-term study of neuroendocrine tumors of the appendix in children: are we too aggressive? Eur J Pediatr Surg 2019;29(5):449–57.

56. Potter SL, HaDuong J, Okcu F, et al. Pediatric bronchial carcinoid tumors: a case series and review of the literature. J Pediatr Hematol Oncol 2019;41(1):67–70.

57. Goudet P, Bonithon-Kopp C, Murat A, et al. Gender-related differences in MEN1 lesion occurrence and diagnosis: a cohort study of 734 cases from the Groupe d'etude des Tumeurs Endocrines. Eur J Endocrinol 2011;165(1):97–105.

58. van den Akker M, Angelini P, Taylor G, et al. Malignant pancreatic tumors in children: a single-institution series. J Pediatr Surg 2012;47(4):681–7.

59. Moppett J, Oakhill A, Duncan AW. Second malignancies in children: the usual suspects? Eur J Radiol 2001;38(3):235–48.

60. Tang LH, Basturk O, Sue JJ, et al. A practical approach to the classification of WHO grade 3 (G3) well-differentiated neuroendocrine tumor (WD-NET) and poorly differentiated neuroendocrine carcinoma (PD-NEC) of the pancreas. Am J Surg Pathol 2016;40(9):1192–202.

61. Rindi G, Klimstra DS, Abedi-Ardekani B, et al. A common classification framework for neuroendocrine neoplasms: an International Agency for Research on Cancer

(IARC) and World Health Organization (WHO) expert consensus proposal. Mod Pathol 2018;31(12):1770–86.

62. Farooqui ZA, Chauhan A. Neuroendocrine tumors in pediatrics. Glob Pediatr Health 2019;6. 2333794x19862712.

63. Sackstein PE, O'Neil DS, Neugut AI, et al. Epidemiologic trends in neuroendocrine tumors: an examination of incidence rates and survival of specific patient subgroups over the past 20 years. Semin Oncol 2018;45(4):249–58.

64. Sarvida ME, O'Dorisio MS. Neuroendocrine tumors in children and young adults: rare or not so rare. Endocrinol Metab Clin North Am 2011;40(1):65–80, vii.

65. Dishop MK, Kuruvilla S. Primary and metastatic lung tumors in the pediatric population: a review and 25-year experience at a large children's hospital. Arch Pathol Lab Med 2008;132(7):1079–103.

66. Hatzipantelis E, Panagopoulou P, Sidi-Fragandrea V, et al. Carcinoid tumors of the appendix in children: experience from a tertiary center in northern Greece. J Pediatr Gastroenterol Nutr 2010;51(5):622–5.

67. Prommegger R, Obrist P, Ensinger C, et al. Retrospective evaluation of carcinoid tumors of the appendix in children. World J Surg 2002;26(12):1489–92.

68. Moris D, Tsilimigras DI, Vagios S, et al. Neuroendocrine neoplasms of the appendix: a review of the literature. Anticancer Res 2018;38(2):601–11.

69. Ram P, Penalver JL, Lo KBU, et al. Carcinoid heart disease: review of current knowledge. Tex Heart Inst J 2019;46(1):21–7.

70. Lee DW, Kim MK, Kim HG. Diagnosis of pancreatic neuroendocrine tumors. Clin Endosc 2017;50(6):537–45.

71. Sundin A. Radiological and nuclear medicine imaging of gastroenteropancreatic neuroendocrine tumours. Best Pract Res Clin Gastroenterol 2012;26(6):803–18.

72. Chung EM, Travis MD, Conran RM. Pancreatic tumors in children: radiologic-pathologic correlation. Radiographics 2006;26(4):1211–38.

73. de Herder WW, Kwekkeboom DJ, Valkema R, et al. Neuroendocrine tumors and somatostatin: imaging techniques. J Endocrinol Invest 2005;28(11 Suppl International):132–6.

74. Hennrich U, Benešová M. [(68)Ga]Ga-DOTA-TOC: the first FDA-approved (68) Ga-radiopharmaceutical for PET imaging. Pharmaceuticals (Basel) 2020; 13(3):38.

75. Al-Risi ES, Al-Essry FS. Mula-Abed WS. Chromogranin a as a biochemical marker for neuroendocrine tumors: a single center experience at royal hospital, Oman. Oman Med J 2017;32(5):365–70.

76. Sherman SK, Maxwell JE, O'Dorisio MS, et al. Pancreastatin predicts survival in neuroendocrine tumors. Ann Surg Oncol 2014;21(9):2971–80.

77. Ewang-Emukowhate M, Nair D, Caplin M. The role of 5-hydroxyindoleacetic acid in neuroendocrine tumors: the journey so far. Int J Endocr Oncol 2019;6(2): p.IJE17.

78. Vinik AI, Chaya C. Clinical presentation and diagnosis of neuroendocrine tumors. Hematol Oncol Clin North Am 2016;30(1):21–48.

79. de Lambert G, Lardy H, Martelli H, et al. Surgical management of neuroendocrine tumors of the appendix in children and adolescents: a retrospective French multicenter study of 114 cases. Pediatr Blood Cancer 2016;63(4):598–603.

80. Ranaweera C, Brar A, Somers GR, et al. Management of pediatric appendiceal carcinoid: a single institution experience from 5000 appendectomies. Pediatr Surg Int 2019;35(12):1427–30.

81. Njere I, Smith LL, Thurairasa D, et al. Systematic review and meta-analysis of appendiceal carcinoid tumors in children. Pediatr Blood Cancer 2018;65(8):e27069.

82. Lobeck IN, Jeste N, Geller J, et al. Surgical management and surveillance of pediatric appendiceal carcinoid tumor. J Pediatr Surg 2017;52(6):925–7.
83. Boudreaux JP, Klimstra DS, Hassan MM, et al. The NANETS consensus guideline for the diagnosis and management of neuroendocrine tumors: well-differentiated neuroendocrine tumors of the jejunum, ileum, appendix, and cecum. Pancreas 2010;39(6):753–66.
84. Huang LC, Poultsides GA, Norton JA. Surgical management of neuroendocrine tumors of the gastrointestinal tract. Oncology (Williston Park) 2011;25(9): 794–803.
85. Wong KP, Tsang JS, Lang BH. Role of surgery in pancreatic neuroendocrine tumor. Gland Surg 2018;7(1):36–41.
86. Waters AM, Russell RT, Maizlin II, et al. Comparison of pediatric and adult solid pseudopapillary neoplasms of the pancreas. J Surg Res 2019;242:312–7.
87. Lambert A, Schwarz L, Borbath I, et al. An update on treatment options for pancreatic adenocarcinoma. Ther Adv Med Oncol 2019;11. 1758835919875568.
88. Rizzardi G, Marulli G, Bortolotti L, et al. Sleeve resections and bronchoplastic procedures in typical central carcinoid tumours. Thorac Cardiovasc Surg 2008; 56(1):42–5.
89. Yau H, Kinaan M, Quinn SL, et al. Octreotide long-acting repeatable in the treatment of neuroendocrine tumors: patient selection and perspectives. Biologics 2017;11:115–22.
90. Barrows S, Cai B, Copley-Merriman C, et al. Systematic literature review of the antitumor effect of octreotide in neuroendocrine tumors. World J Metaanal 2018;6.
91. Cefalo G, Massimino M, Ruggiero A, et al. Temozolomide is an active agent in children with recurrent medulloblastoma/primitive neuroectodermal tumor: an Italian multi-institutional phase II trial. Neuro Oncol 2014;16(5):748–53.
92. Rogowski W, Wachuła E, Gorzelak A, et al. Capecitabine and temozolomide combination for treatment of high-grade, well-differentiated neuroendocrine tumour and poorly-differentiated neuroendocrine carcinoma: retrospective analysis. Endokrynol Pol 2019;70(4):313–7.
93. Kolasińska-Ćwikła A, Łowczak A, Maciejkiewicz KM, et al. Peptide receptor radionuclide therapy for advanced gastroenteropancreatic neuroendocrine tumors: from oncology perspective. Nucl Med Rev Cent East Eur 2018;21(2). https://doi.org/10.5603/NMR.2018.0019.
94. Rizzardi G, Marulli G, Calabrese F, et al. Bronchial carcinoid tumours in children: surgical treatment and outcome in a single institution. Eur J Pediatr Surg 2009; 19(4):228–31.
95. Lamarca A, Clouston H, Barriuso J, et al. Follow-up recommendations after curative resection of well-differentiated neuroendocrine tumours: review of current evidence and clinical practice. J Clin Med 2019;8(10):1630.
96. Singh S, Moody L, Chan DL, et al. Follow-up recommendations for completely resected gastroenteropancreatic neuroendocrine tumors. JAMA Oncol 2018;4(11): 1597–604.

Management of Differentiated Thyroid Carcinoma in Pediatric Patients

Emily Christison-Lagay, MD[a],*, Reto M. Baertschiger, MD, PhD[b]

KEYWORDS

- Thyroid cancer • Thyroid carcinoma • Papillary thyroid cancer
- Follicular thyroid cancer • Pediatric • Molecular genetics • Lymphadenectomy
- Cervical lymph node dissection

KEY POINTS

- Differentiated thyroid carcinomas (DTC) are rare in young children but represent almost 10% of all malignancies diagnosed in older adolescents.
- DTC in children is more likely to demonstrate nodal involvement and is associated with higher recurrence rates than seen in adults.
- Total thyroidectomy and compartment-based resection of involved lymph node basins form the cornerstone of treatment.

INTRODUCTION

Although fewer than 2% of thyroid cancers develop in children, thyroid cancer accounts for 6% of all childhood cancers and is the leading cause of pediatric endocrine malignancy.[1] Reported rates of pediatric thyroid cancer have more than doubled over the last 40 years, although this rise seems to be plateauing.[2] Papillary thyroid cancer (PTC), the most common subtype of thyroid cancer, accounts for the greatest increase in number of detected cases. Smaller increases have also been observed in follicular thyroid cancer (FTC).[1]

Historic recommendations for the treatment of pediatric thyroid neoplasms were derived from adult practice; however, important clinical and molecular features distinguish differentiated thyroid cancer (DTC) in children from adults.[3,4] Clinically, pediatric PTC is more likely to present with regional lymph node involvement, extrathyroidal extension, and pulmonary metastases than adult-onset PTC.[5–8] Despite this, children are less likely to die from disease, with disease-specific mortality less than 2%.[8] These

[a] Division of Pediatric Surgery, Department of Surgery, Yale University School of Medicine, 330 Cedar Street, PO Box 208062, New Haven, CT, USA; [b] Division of General and Thoracic Surgery, The Hospital for Sick Children, Room 1524, 555 University Ave, Toronto, ON M5G 1X8, Canada
* Corresponding author.
E-mail address: Emily.christison-lagay@yale.edu

Surg Oncol Clin N Am 30 (2021) 235–251
https://doi.org/10.1016/j.soc.2020.11.013   surgonc.theclinics.com

differences were first formally recognized in 2015, when the American Thyroid Association (ATA) published guidelines outlining the evaluation and treatment of thyroid nodules (TN) and DTC in children.[4] However, because national pediatric or oncologic databases lack sufficient granularity to provide nuanced insight into pediatric thyroid cancer, coupled with the absence of a pediatric thyroid-specific database, many recommendations within those guidelines were formulated by expert consensus. This summary article reviews the current recommendations of the ATA and more recent progress into the epidemiology and molecular genetics of DTC that may inform future guidelines.

BACKGROUND AND INCIDENCE

Pediatric DTC arises from the thyroid follicular cell and its histologic classification mirrors that in adults. PTC and PTC variants (follicular variant, diffuse sclerosing variant, cribriform-morula variant, solid variant, and tall cell variant), and FTC comprise the category of DTC. PTC and its variants comprise most (>80%) pediatric thyroid cancers in a recent Surveillance, Epidemiology, and End Results database analysis, followed by FTC (10%) and medullary thyroid cancer (8%).[1] As patients transition into adolescence, the incidence and relative rates of PTC increase, whereas those of medullary thyroid cancer decline. Age-standardized DTC incidence rates (per million) are 0.04 for ages 0 to 4 years, 0.43 for ages 5 to 9 years, 3.50 for ages 10 to 14 years, and 15.6 for children 15 to 19 years.[9] After the first decade of life, the female/male preponderance increases to 4.4:1 per 100,000. DTC is the second most common cancer of adolescent girls.[10]

THYROID CANCER IN THE PEDIATRIC PATIENT WITH A THYROID NODULE

Pediatric TN demonstrate a higher risk of malignancy (20%–25%) than TN found in adults (5%–15%), although recent epidemiologic studies have identified TN in up to 5% of children suggesting that the rates of thyroid cancer in small, asymptomatic nodules may be lower than historically reported.[11,12] Most children diagnosed with thyroid disease have no identifiable risk factors, despite that several populations are at increased risk. Exposure to 10 to 30 Gy of ionizing radiation is associated with an approximately 2% annual chance of DTC, beginning 5 years after exposure and peaking at 15 to 30 years.[13] A family history of benign thyroid disease doubles the risk for pediatric DTC, whereas a family history of DTC quadruples the risk. Up to a third of patients with Hashimoto thyroiditis develop TN and these patients may have a 100-fold greater risk of thyroid malignancy than the general population.[14] A variety of genetic disorders may predispose to TN and DTC including: familial adenomatoid polyposis, Carney complex, Werner syndrome, *DICER1* syndrome, *PTEN* hamartoma tumor syndrome, McCune-Albright syndrome, and Peutz-Jeghers syndromes.[4]

EVALUATION OF A THYROID NODULE

TN most commonly present as asymptomatic masses noted by the child, parents, or a pediatrician during a well-child visit. Less commonly nodules cause symptomatic dysphagia, dyspnea, or cervical lymphadenopathy. A thorough thyroid examination includes careful palpation of the central and lateral neck. Large, firm, or fixed nodules, or those associated with lymphadenopathy are concerning for malignancy, but most malignant nodules do not exhibit these features. Following detection or suspicion of TN, a dedicated thyroid and neck ultrasound (US) should be performed.[4] Features of malignancy on US include hypoechogenicity, invasive margins, increased intranodular blood flow, and microcalcifications.[15,16] In contrast to malignant nodules, benign TN are more often isoechoic, partially cystic, with sharp or noninfiltrative margins, absent calcifications, and lack of blood flow.[17,18] Cystic composition of greater than 50% of a nodule is the most reliable feature identifying low risk of malignancy.[19]

Several scoring systems facilitate selection of TN that should undergo fine-needle aspiration (FNA) in adults and have demonstrated good performance in the pediatric population.[20,21] The most popular of these scoring systems, the Thyroid Imaging Reporting and Data System (TI-RADS), comments on 10 US patterns to assign risk of malignancy (**Fig. 1**).[22,23] Most adult criteria contributing to risk assignation are applicable to children with several notable exceptions. In adults, FNA is recommended for TI-RADS 3, 4, and 5 categories if the nodule is greater than or equal to 2.5 cm, 1.5 cm, or 1 cm, respectively; no size criteria has been studied in children.[24] Diffuse sclerosing variant PTC is more common in the pediatric population and presents as nonnodular, diffuse infiltration of the thyroid associated with widespread microcalcifications giving a "snow-storm" appearance on US. Lateral lymph node involvement is common.[25] Current ATA Pediatric Guidelines preceded development of the TI-RADS scoring system and recommend FNA for vascular, calcified, solid, and/or pericapsular nodules based on clinical context rather than size alone.[4]

Fine-Needle Aspiration

FNA is the preferred method to diagnose DTC; however, before FNA all patients should have a serum thyroid-stimulating hormone (TSH) sent to evaluate for the presence of hyperthyroidism.[26] Hyperfunctioning "hot" nodules have a low risk of malignancy; therefore, if TSH is suppressed, a thyroid uptake scan rather than biopsy is indicated to confirm the diagnosis.[27] For the remainder of "cold" nodules, FNA is sensitive, specific, and accurate, although there is a risk for false-negative FNA in nodules greater than 4 cm.[11,28]

FNA results are categorized according to the Bethesda System for Reporting Thyroid Cytopathology: (I) nondiagnostic or unsatisfactory, (II) benign, (III) atypia of undetermined significance or follicular lesion of undetermined significance (AUS/FLUS), (IV) follicular/Hürthle neoplasm or suspicious for follicular/Hürthle neoplasm (FN/SFN), (V) suspicious for malignancy, and (VI) malignant (**Table 1**).[29] The risk of malignancy in each Bethesda category seems to be higher for children than for adults, although the risk varies by reporting institution, suggesting FNA results must be interpreted in the context of individual institutional indices for accuracy.[30–32]

Lymph Node Evaluation

In addition to evaluation of the nodule itself, examination of the cervical lymph nodes is essential in risk stratifying DTC and determining operative management. In children, nodal architecture and shape are better predictors of lymph node involvement than size.[18] Concerning features on US include round shape, irregular margins, calcifications, cystic change, peripheral vascularity, loss of fatty hilum, and heterogeneous echotexture. Interpretation of US images varies with expertise; therefore, sonographic lymph node evaluation should be performed by a radiologist with experience in pediatric head and neck imaging because less experienced sonographers can miss nodal involvement.[33] FNA should be performed on any suspicious lymph nodes in the lateral neck as confirmation of metastatic involvement before lateral neck dissection.[4]

Other Imaging

Additional imaging may be considered in patients with evidence of lymph node metastasis. Chest radiograph or computed tomography are used to rule out macronodular

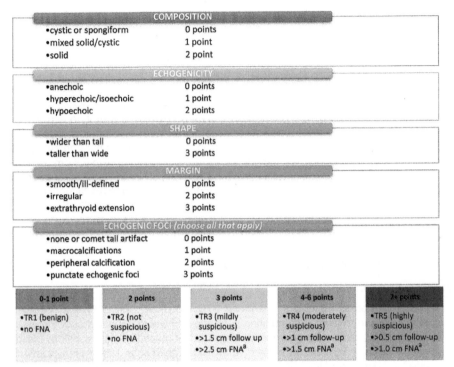

COMPOSITION	
•cystic or spongiform	0 points
•mixed solid/cystic	1 point
•solid	2 point

ECHOGENICITY	
•anechoic	0 points
•hyperechoic/isoechoic	1 point
•hypoechoic	2 points

SHAPE	
•wider than tall	0 points
•taller than wide	3 points

MARGIN	
•smooth/ill-defined	0 points
•irregular	2 points
•extrathryoid extension	3 points

ECHOGENIC FOCI (choose all that apply)	
•none or comet tail artifact	0 points
•macrocalcifications	1 point
•peripheral calcification	2 points
•punctate echogenic foci	3 points

0-1 point	2 points	3 points	4-6 points	7+ points
•TR1 (benign) •no FNA	•TR2 (not suspicious) •no FNA	•TR3 (mildly suspicious) •>1.5 cm follow up •>2.5 cm FNA[a]	•TR4 (moderately suspicious) •>1 cm follow-up •>1.5 cm FNA[a]	•TR5 (highly suspicious) •>0.5 cm follow-up •>1.0 cm FNA[a]

Fig. 1. TI-RADS Classification and recommendations. [a] No size criteria exist in children. (*Courtesy of* Kate Christison-Lagay, PhD, New Haven, CT.)

lung disease and computed tomography of the neck can aid in the assessment of anatomic relationships between important neurovascular structures of the neck and deposits of bulky disease.[34,35] Neither nuclear scintigraphy nor [18]fluorodeoxyglucose PET play a role during initial evaluation.

OPERATIVE RECOMMENDATIONS FOR NONDIAGNOSTIC, BENIGN, AND INDETERMINATE NODULES

Operative recommendations in patients with nondiagnostic, indeterminate, or benign nodules is based on individual DTC risk, the likelihood of a false-negative FNA, the risks of operative intervention, symptomatology, and patient/family tolerance for diagnostic ambiguity.[4] Patients with nondiagnostic cytology (Bethesda I) may choose repeat FNA. To avoid atypical cellular artifact because of the previous biopsy, conventional practice has been to allow at least 3 months to pass between each biopsy attempt, although several recent studies in adults have challenged the necessity of this interval.[36] Other options include continued US surveillance or lobectomy. Bedside cytologic examination of the aspirate at the time of the procedure can reduce the likelihood of an insufficient biopsy.

Children with benign cytopathology (Bethesda II) and nodules less than 4 cm should be followed by serial US tracking TN growth. Operative intervention is warranted in the presence of rapid TN growth or compressive symptoms.[4] Lesions greater than 4 cm have a higher false-negative rate and lobectomy should be offered even if cytology is

Table 1
Bethesda system for reporting thyroid cytopathology

Bethesda Category	Cytopathologic Category	Malignancy Rate, %	Suggested Treatment
I	Nondiagnostic/inadequate	1–5	Repeat FNA (other options: continued US surveillance, lobectomy)
II	Benign	0–10	Serial US if small, lobectomy if >4 cm
III	Atypia/follicular lesion of undetermined significance	20–30	Molecular genetics, lobectomy if no concerning mutation, thyroidectomy if BRAF or fusion mutation
IV	Follicular neoplasm	30–60	Molecular genetics, lobectomy if no concerning mutation, thyroidectomy if BRAF or fusion mutation
V	Suspicious for malignancy	70–86	Total thyroidectomy ± central neck dissection
VI	Malignant	97–100	Total thyroidectomy ± central neck dissection

benign. Many large nodules cause dysphagia or dyspnea or are aesthetically unappealing and patients opt for resection independent of cytology.

Because of the increased risk for DTC in children with AUS/FLUS, lobectomy is often recommended over repeat biopsy. Recently, a report from Cherella and colleagues found that almost a third of AUS/FLUS nodules were benign on repeat FNA, suggesting that repeat biopsy may be a reasonable approach.[33,37] If lobectomy is selected and DTC is confirmed intraoperatively or on final histology, a completion thyroidectomy is performed. Intraoperative frozen section may be of help in diagnosing classic PTC but has no benefit in follicular variant PTC or FTC, because the latter requires evaluation of the entire lesion to detect vascular invasion (VI) and/or capsular invasion (CI).[38,39]

The risk of DTC seems to be greater than 50% in children with FN/SFN cytology (Bethesda IV).[40–43] Lobectomy has historically been the standard of care, but the role of oncogene panels in assisting with operative planning is an area of active investigation. In high-volume centers in which oncogene panels are routinely performed on fine-needle aspirate, a positive result may augment the positive predictive value of malignancy in pediatric PTC. For example, if a BRAF mutation or gene fusion (RET/PTC or NTRK3/ETV6) is detected in the AUS/FLUS or FN/SFN category, total thyroidectomy (TT) is warranted based on the high risk of PTC.[44,45] However, malignancy may be less likely in a solitary, isoechoic, smooth-margined TN harboring a RAS mutation or PAX8-PPARG rearrangement. In these instances a lobectomy may be preferable.[45] For FNA suspicious for malignancy or revealing malignant cytology (Bethesda V or VI), the risk for DTC is near 100% and TT with or without central neck dissection (CND) is recommended.[46]

OPERATIVE RECOMMENDATIONS FOR MALIGNANT NODULES AND LYMPH NODE METASTASES

TT is the cornerstone of the management of DTC. The ability to achieve long-term recurrence-free survival is directly related to the adequacy of the initial operative resection.[4] Unlike the adult population in which thyroid lobectomy may be adequate for small (<4 cm) low-risk tumors, TT is currently recommended by the ATA for all children with PTC based on the high incidence of bilateral (30%) or multifocal (65%) disease.[4,47,48] Patients with preoperatively detected or clinically apparent central lymph node metastases should undergo therapeutic CND of level VI nodes (**Fig. 2**).[4,5,47] Thyroid lobectomy is associated with 10-fold greater recurrence rates and inadequate lymph node dissections in patients with clinically positive nodes increases the need for subsequent intervention three-fold.[4,5,7,47] Studies in adults have shown that compartment-focused lymph node dissections reduce recurrence compared with "berry picking"; these studies have generally been applied to children.[49] Several high-volume centers have reported the need to reoperate for persistent and relapsed disease treated less aggressively at a lower-volume institution.[50,51] Although a compartment-oriented central neck lymphadenectomy theoretically increases the risks of hypoparathyroidism and recurrent laryngeal nerve injury, these complications are minimized when performed by a high-volume surgeon.[48,50–53] It is imperative that the correct operation be performed initially because anatomic planes are absent or distorted in reoperative fields thus increasing the risk of complications.[54]

Modified radical neck dissection is reserved for biopsy-proven metastatic DTC in the lateral compartment (levels II, III, IV, and V) and improves disease-free survival.[47,51,55]

COMPLICATIONS

A convincing series of data have demonstrated a volume-outcome relationship between surgeon experience at thyroidectomy and patient complications and length of stay in children.[53,56] As a result, the ATA recommends thyroidectomy should be performed by an experienced thyroid surgeon (>30 cases/year) or as a multidisciplinary approach between a pediatric surgeon and an adult endocrine/head and neck surgeon.[56,57] In a cross-sectional analysis of the Healthcare Cost and Utilization Project, pediatric patients undergoing TT had a general complication rate of 17.6% and an endocrine-specific (including hypocalcemia, voice disturbance, and recurrent

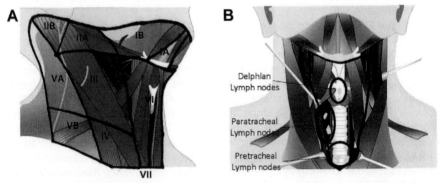

Fig. 2. (A) Cervical lymph node levels I-VII. (B) Depiction of central lymph nodes with thyroid removed. (*Courtesy of* Kate Christison-Lagay, PhD, New Haven, CT.)

laryngeal nerve injury) complication rate of 16.3%. These numbers were reduced by more than half if the operation was performed by a high-volume surgeon.[56]

A recent analysis of 1654 patients undergoing TT in the KID database identified a recurrent laryngeal nerve injury rate of 1.8%.[58] Young children seem particularly at risk for nerve injury with a reported incidence of vocal cord paralysis of 14.3% in children less than 1 year.[59,60] Several recent retrospective studies from high-volume institutions report inadvertent nerve injury rates of 0.4% to 2.8% based on loss of signal during intraoperative nerve monitoring or postoperative laryngoscopy.[48,50,51]

Rates of transient hypocalcemia ranging from 7% to 59% are widely discordant across studies, caused in part by a lack of consensus in defining metrics and study-specific variations in patient extent of disease and extent of routine surgical dissection.[56,61–63] A diagnosis of permanent hypoparathyroidism should not be made before the sixth postoperative month, based on a need for continued calcium ± calcitriol supplementation.[61] The reported incidence of permanent hypoparathyroidism also varies: running higher in population-based or multicenter pediatric studies (5.5%–25%)[58,64] and lower in single-institution studies (0.6%–8.0%).[65,66] Some centers find it useful to obtain either an intraoperative or postoperative intact parathyroid hormone level to help prognosticate need for and likely duration of calcium supplementation.[67,68]

Injuries to other regional nerves during lateral neck dissection (including the sympathetic chain, vagus, spinal accessory nerve, and hypoglossal nerve) are rare events.[50,69,70]

RISK OF RECURRENCE

The risk of recurrence in children with PTC is hard to pinpoint given the lack of standardization of treatment, the potentially long latency period to recurrence, and that adolescents comprise a particularly mobile segment of the population who may have temporally and geographically dis-synchronous care. Most studies report recurrence rates of 20% to 40% at 10 years unadjusted for initial stage of disease.[5,59,60,71] Children with palpable cervical nodal metastases are more likely than those without clinical node involvement to present with distant metastasis and experience persistent and/or recurrent disease over time.[7,72] In general, younger age, larger tumor size, solid architecture pattern, extensive tumor fibrosis, VI, disseminated psammoma bodies, extrathyroidal extension, node-positive disease with a high metastatic ratio index (>0.45), metastatic disease within the central compartment (level VI), macroscopic nodal disease, and extranodal extension are associated with a greater risk for ipsilateral or bilateral N1b disease.[51,60,72,73]

SURVIVAL

Overall survival is excellent, with 5-year survival rates of 99.8% in children with DTC confined to the thyroid and 97.1% of those with regional metastatic disease.[5,74,75] Studies with long-term follow-up indicate that children with DTC have increased mortality from second malignancies, possibly related to radioactive iodine use.[5,76,77]

RADIOACTIVE IODINE TREATMENT FOLLOWING INITIAL SURGERY

The historic practice of treating all children with DTC with ^{131}I following initial operative resection has been replaced with a stratified approach aimed at minimizing ^{131}I exposure in patients deemed low risk for persistent postsurgical disease.[4] [131]I therapy is indicated for patients with pulmonary metastases or small-volume nonresectable residual cervical disease.[8,78] Most experts also advocate ^{131}I therapy for children with extensive regional nodal involvement (extensive N1a or N1b disease).[79] Up to a third of children with distant metastasis have persistent but stable disease following radioactive iodine therapy resulting in a more favorable progression-free survival in children compared with adults with persistent DTC.[8,9,80]

THYROID-STIMULATING HORMONE SUPPRESSION AND THYROGLOBULIN SURVEILLANCE

Postoperative TSH suppression is indicated for children with any type of DTC, although there is a paucity of data guiding degree of suppression. If thyroglobulin (Tg) rises while the patient is on levothyroxine, disease relapse is likely to become clinically apparent.[81,82] The decision to pursue further therapy is based on the degree of Tg elevation, the trend in Tg over time, and the results of imaging studies. When imaging fails to confirm disease, the clinical importance of biochemical recurrence in children is not yet clear.[81,82]

TREATMENT OF PERSISTENT OR RECURRENT PAPILLARY THYROID CANCER

Treatment of persistent or recurrent disease should be individualized and careful consideration given to the potential risks and benefits of therapy. Patients with small cervical foci or patients with cervical disease that cannot be visualized with cross-sectional imaging may be considered for (repeat) therapeutic ^{131}I but may also often be safely observed while maintaining TSH suppression. Macroscopic cervical disease should be removed surgically if this can be safely accomplished.

Children with pulmonary metastases may continue to experience post-therapy targeted ^{131}I effects for years and an undetectable Tg level should not be the focus of treatment efforts. A third of patients exhibit persistent, stable disease following radioactive iodine therapy; therapy should be directed at those with evidence of progression.[4]

CONTROVERSIES IN SURGICAL MANAGEMENT

There is no consensus on the optimal extent of resection of PTC sonographically confined to the thyroid. Large database studies have measured success of various operative approaches using an end point of death from disease, but outcomes in PTC are best measured by disease recurrence (a parameter not collected in national databases) over a span of decades. Furthermore, pediatric literature lacks the granularity of adult studies that distinguish structural from biochemical recurrence.[83] Proponents of lobectomy cite equivalent survival in patients, and an increased rate of permanent hypocalcemia and recurrent laryngeal nerve injury in patients undergoing TT.[3,8] Countering this argument is evidence for a lower recurrence rate after TT, and the observation that at least 40% of pediatric PTC is multifocal.[84] Few institutional series have had sufficient patient volume to report recurrence rates based on extent of disease or modified by operative approach. In addition to TT, some experts believe a prophylactic CND should be considered for all children with PTC to reduce the risk of persistent or recurrent disease. These recommendations are based on the observation of nodal involvement in more than half of resected PTC specimens in centers that routinely perform CND, and on several small studies suggesting that the addition of prophylactic CND decreases recurrence rates to 5% at 10 years.[5,47,51,85,86] CND in theory increases the risk of transient and permanent hypoparathyroidism (because the inferior parathyroids typically lie in the middle of a regional lymph node "packet" and must be either sacrificed or reimplanted) and these sequelae are the most frequently cited counterarguments to prophylactic central neck lymphadenectomy.[61,64,66,87] In patients with unifocal lateralized disease, several studies in adults suggest that ipsilateral, prophylactic CND may provide the same benefit as bilateral CND while decreasing the rate of hypoparathyroidism, but this has not been studied in children.[88] When considering operative strategy, the potential morbidity of bilateral CND must be weighed against the indolent nature of PTC. Prophylactic CND should be performed only by surgeons with extensive experience operating in the central neck. Multiple adult groups have reported on the use of near-infrared autofluorescence to help identify (and thus preserve) parathyroid tissue (either in eutopic position or as an aide in autotransplantation), a potentially promising, although largely untested, practice in children.[89,90]

FOLLICULAR THYROID CARCINOMA

Fewer than 10% of pediatric DTC are follicular carcinomas. The diagnosis of FTC is based on the identification of CI and/or VI on permanent histologic sectioning. The 2015 ATA Guidelines divide FTC into those with CI alone, minimal (<4 vessels) VI, and extensive VI ($\geq$4 vessels).[30] As opposed to PTC, which are frequently multifocal, FTC are typically unifocal tumors without extrathyroidal extension. Any patient with multifocal FTC should be evaluated for *PTEN* hamartoma tumor syndrome or a *DICER1* mutation.[91,92] Unlike PTC, FTC spreads hematogenously to lung and bone and rarely metastasizes to regional lymph nodes. The presence of lymph node involvement in a patient diagnosed as FTC should raise the possibility that the lesion is a follicular variant PTC.[93]

FTC has a different sonographic appearance than PTC. It is frequently larger, isoechoic, and often demonstrates a hypoechoic rim.[94,95] Because of the need for permanent histology to evaluate for CI or VI, FNA cytology is largely unhelpful in diagnosing FTC.

The recommended treatment of angioinvasive FTC ($\geq$4 vessels VI) or FTC greater than or equal to 4 cm is TT and radioactive iodine.[96,97] Treatment of minimally invasive FTC is controversial because it seems to mimic a benign lesion.[98,99] Studies of minimally invasive FTC in children have also demonstrated indolent behavior and have suggested that lobectomy followed by close follow-up and TSH suppression may be sufficient.[93] However, a separate study that included children with minimally invasive FTC with VI observed recurrence in three of nine children. Thirty-year disease-specific survival is 100%.[100]

FUTURE DIRECTIONS: MOLECULAR GENETICS AND TARGETED THERAPEUTICS

Molecular genetic testing provides techniques to better characterize TN; however, data in children are limited. Large-volume pediatric centers often use "positive" results of gene panels to inform a conversation about the likelihood of malignancy and to help tailor the surgical approach for individual children.[45] Compared with adult PTC, childhood PTC has a higher prevalence of gene rearrangements (50% in children vs 15% in adults) and a lower frequency of point mutations (30% of children vs 70% of adults).[45] Gene fusions in DTC occur most commonly between *RE*arranged during *T*ransfection (*RET*) and a variety of other genes, resulting in some 20 *RET/PTC* rearrangements.[45,101,102] *RET/PTC1* and *RET/PTC3* are the most common rearrangements in sporadic and radiation-induced pediatric PTC. The *BRAF* gene is the most common location for a point mutation in pediatric PTC.[45,103] In adults, *BRAF* mutations may be associated with more aggressive phenotype characterized by an increased likelihood for lymph node metastasis, extrathyroidal extension, risk for recurrence, and resistance to iodine.[104] In contrast, *BRAF* mutations in children have not been associated with a greater risk for recurrence but they more frequently have metastatic lymph nodes, an observation that may have implications for the extent of initial surgical resection.[105–108] As genetic testing becomes routinely incorporated into the early diagnostic testing, staging, operative decision making, and adjuvant therapy plans may be based on individual precision medicine, incorporating these tumor characteristics into clinical care.

An increasing number of multikinase inhibitors (tyrosine kinase inhibitors) that target protein tyrosine kinase–dependent pathways are being developed for adult patients with iodine-refractory disease. Sorafenib and lenvatinib have been used in adult trials with some favorable results and have been approved for compassionate use in a small number of children with DTC.[109–112]

SUMMARY

DTC are rare in young children but represent almost 10% of all malignancies diagnosed in older adolescents, with PTC comprising most cases. Compared with PTC in adults, PTC in children is more frequently bilateral and associated with nodal metastasis and higher rates of recurrence. Operative resection remains integral to treatment, and local recurrence is directly affected by operative approach to regional metastatic disease. TT with central lymph node dissection is the treatment of choice for PTC with clinically evident lymph node involvement in the central neck. The role of prophylactic CND for patients with microscopic disease in the central neck requires further investigation. Lateral lymph node involvement should be addressed with modified radical neck dissection. The role of novel targeted therapies in high-risk patients with disseminated disease, and the use of molecular profiling of indeterminate lesions are areas of ongoing inquiry.

CLINICS CARE POINTS

- Preoperative workup of a thyroid nodule should begin with a dedicated thyroid ultrasound. Concerning features on ultrasound should prompt and extended ultrasound of the lymph nodes of the lateral neck.

- Biopsy via Fine Needle Aspiration should be performed on any concerning nodules. A minimum of thyroid lobectomy should be offered to Bethesda III/IV nodules and total thyroidectomy should be offered to Bethesda V/VI nodules.

- A compartment based lymph node dissection should be performed if positive lymph nodes are identified preoperatively.

- Radioactive Iodine should be offered to patients at risk for persistent disease.

DISCLOSURE

The authors have no relevant commercial or financial conflicts of interest. The work related to this review was unfunded.

REFERENCES

1. Dermody S, Walls A, Harley EH. Pediatric thyroid cancer: An update from the SEER database 2007-2012. Int J Pediatr Otorhinolaryngol 2016;89:121–6.

2. Henley SJ, Ward EM, Scott S, et al. Annual report to the nation on the status of cancer, part I: National cancer statistics. Cancer 2020;126(10):2225–49.
3. Hogan AR, Zhuge Y, Perez EA, et al. Pediatric thyroid carcinoma: incidence and outcomes in 1753 patients. J Surg Res 2009;156(1):167–72.
4. Francis GL, Waguespack SG, Bauer AJ, et al. Management guidelines for children with thyroid nodules and differentiated thyroid cancer. Thyroid 2015;25(7):716–59.
5. Hay ID, Gonzalez-Losada T, Reinalda MS, et al. Long-term outcome in 215 children and adolescents with papillary thyroid cancer treated during 1940 through 2008. World J Surg 2010;34(6):1192–202.
6. Sugino K, Nagahama M, Kitagawa W, et al. Papillary thyroid carcinoma in children and adolescents: long-term follow-up and clinical characteristics. World J Surg 2015;39(9):2259–65.
7. Machens A, Lorenz K, Nguyen Thanh P, et al. Papillary thyroid cancer in children and adolescents does not differ in growth pattern and metastatic behavior. J Pediatr 2010;157(4):648–52.
8. La Quaglia MP, Black T, Holcomb GW 3rd, et al. Differentiated thyroid cancer: clinical characteristics, treatment, and outcome in patients under 21 years of age who present with distant metastases. A report from the Surgical Discipline Committee of the Children's Cancer Group. J Pediatr Surg 2000;35(6):955–9 [discussion: 960].
9. Pawelczak M, David R, Franklin B, et al. Outcomes of children and adolescents with well-differentiated thyroid carcinoma and pulmonary metastases following (1)(3)(1)I treatment: a systematic review. Thyroid 2010;20(10):1095–101.
10. Vergamini LB, Frazier AL, Abrantes FL, et al. Increase in the incidence of differentiated thyroid carcinoma in children, adolescents, and young adults: a population-based study. J Pediatr 2014;164(6):1481–5.
11. Wu XC, Chen VW, Steele B, et al. Cancer incidence in adolescents and young adults in the United States, 1992-1997. J Adolesc Health 2003;32(6):405–15.
12. Mussa A, De Andrea M, Motta M, et al. Predictors of Malignancy in Children with Thyroid Nodules. J Pediatr 2015;167(4):886–892 e1.
13. Hayashida N, Imaizumi M, Shimura H, et al. Thyroid ultrasound findings in children from three Japanese prefectures: Aomori, Yamanashi and Nagasaki. PLoS One 2013;8(12):e83220.
14. Chow EJ, Friedman DL, Stovall M, et al. Risk of thyroid dysfunction and subsequent thyroid cancer among survivors of acute lymphoblastic leukemia: a report from the Childhood Cancer Survivor Study. Pediatr Blood Cancer 2009;53(3):432–7.
15. Won JH, Lee JY, Hong HS, et al. Thyroid nodules and cancer in children and adolescents affected by Hashimoto's thyroiditis. Br J Radiol 2018;9:20180014.
16. Leboulleux S, Girard E, Rose M, et al. Ultrasound criteria of malignancy for cervical lymph nodes in patients followed up for differentiated thyroid cancer. J Clin Endocrinol Metab 2007;92(9):3590–4.
17. Lyshchik A, Drozd V, Demidchik Y, et al. Diagnosis of thyroid cancer in children: value of gray-scale and power doppler US. Radiology 2005;235(2):604–13.
18. Gannon AW, Langer JE, Bellah R, et al. Diagnostic Accuracy of Ultrasound with Color Flow Doppler in Children with Thyroid Nodules. J Clin Endocrinol Metab 2018. https://doi.org/10.1210/jc.2017-02464.
19. Essenmacher AC, Joyce PH Jr, Kao SC, et al. Sonographic evaluation of pediatric thyroid nodules. Radiographics 2017;37(6):1731–52.

20. Bauer AJ. Thyroid nodules in children and adolescents. Curr Opin Endocrinol Diabetes Obes 2019;26(5):266–74.
21. Martinez-Rios C, Daneman A, Bajno L, et al. Utility of adult-based ultrasound malignancy risk stratifications in pediatric thyroid nodules. Pediatr Radiol 2018;48(1):74–84.
22. Lim-Dunham JE, Toslak IE, Reiter MP, et al. Assessment of the American College of Radiology Thyroid Imaging Reporting and Data System for thyroid nodule malignancy risk stratification in a pediatric population. AJR Am J Roentgenol 2018;7:1–7.
23. Horvath E, Silva CF, Majlis S, et al. Prospective validation of the ultrasound based TIRADS (Thyroid Imaging Reporting And Data System) classification: results in surgically resected thyroid nodules. Eur Radiol 2017;27(6):2619–28.
24. Tessler FN, Middleton WD, Grant EG, et al. ACR thyroid imaging, reporting and data system (TI-RADS): White Paper of the ACR TI-RADS Committee. J Am Coll Radiol 2017;14(5):587–95.
25. Vargas-Uricoechea H, Meza-Cabrera I, Herrera-Chaparro J. Concordance between the TIRADS ultrasound criteria and the BETHESDA cytology criteria on the nontoxic thyroid nodule. Thyroid Res 2017;10:1.
26. Chereau N, Giudicelli X, Pattou F, et al. Diffuse sclerosing variant of papillary thyroid carcinoma is associated with aggressive histopathological features and a poor outcome: results of a large multicentric study. J Clin Endocrinol Metab 2016;101(12):4603–10.
27. Baxter KJ, Short HL, Thakore MA, et al. Cost comparison of initial lobectomy versus fine-needle aspiration for diagnostic workup of thyroid nodules in children. J Pediatr Surg 2017;52(9):1471–4.
28. Niedziela M, Breborowicz D, Trejster E, et al. Hot nodules in children and adolescents in western Poland from 1996 to 2000: clinical analysis of 31 patients. J Pediatr Endocrinol Metab 2002;15(6):823–30.
29. McCoy KL, Jabbour N, Ogilvie JB, et al. The incidence of cancer and rate of false-negative cytology in thyroid nodules greater than or equal to 4 cm in size. Surgery 2007;142(6):837–44 [discussion: 844.e1-3].
30. Cibas ES, Ali SZ. The 2017 Bethesda system for reporting thyroid cytopathology. Thyroid 2017;27(11):1341–6.
31. Haugen BR, Alexander EK, Bible KC, et al. 2015 American Thyroid Association Management Guidelines for Adult Patients with Thyroid Nodules and Differentiated Thyroid Cancer: The American Thyroid Association Guidelines Task Force on Thyroid Nodules and Differentiated Thyroid Cancer. Thyroid 2016;26(1):1–133.
32. Amirazodi E, Propst EJ, Chung CT, et al. Pediatric thyroid FNA biopsy: Outcomes and impact on management over 24 years at a tertiary care center. Cancer Cytopathol 2016;124(11):801–10.
33. Cherella CE, Angell TE, Richman DM, et al. Differences in thyroid nodule cytology and malignancy risk between children and adults. Thyroid 2019;29(8):1097–104.
34. Monteiro R, Han A, Etiwy M, et al. Importance of surgeon-performed ultrasound in the preoperative nodal assessment of patients with potential thyroid malignancy. Surgery 2018;163(1):112–7.
35. Kouvaraki MA, Shapiro SE, Fornage BD, et al. Role of preoperative ultrasonography in the surgical management of patients with thyroid cancer. Surgery 2003;134(6):946–54 [discussion: 954–5].

36. Waguespack SG, Francis G. Initial management and follow-up of differentiated thyroid cancer in children. J Natl Compr Canc Netw 2010;8(11):1289–300.
37. Baloch ZW, LiVolsi VA. Post fine-needle aspiration histologic alterations of thyroid revisited. Am J Clin Pathol 1999;112(3):311–6.
38. Baloch Z, LiVolsi VA, Jain P, et al. Role of repeat fine-needle aspiration biopsy (FNAB) in the management of thyroid nodules. Diagn Cytopathol 2003;29(4):203–6.
39. Antic T, Taxy JB. Thyroid frozen section: supplementary or unnecessary? Am J Surg Pathol 2013;37(2):282–6.
40. Kesmodel SB, Terhune KP, Canter RJ, et al. The diagnostic dilemma of follicular variant of papillary thyroid carcinoma. Surgery 2003;134(6):1005–12 [discussion: 1012].
41. Norlen O, Charlton A, Sarkis LM, et al. Risk of malignancy for each Bethesda class in pediatric thyroid nodules. J Pediatr Surg 2015;50(7):1147–9.
42. Buryk MA, Simons JP, Picarsic J, et al. Can malignant thyroid nodules be distinguished from benign thyroid nodules in children and adolescents by clinical characteristics? A review of 89 pediatric patients with thyroid nodules. Thyroid 2015;25(4):392–400.
43. Monaco SE, Pantanowitz L, Khalbuss WE, et al. Cytomorphological and molecular genetic findings in pediatric thyroid fine-needle aspiration. Cancer Cytopathol 2012;120(5):342–50.
44. Smith M, Pantanowitz L, Khalbuss WE, et al. Indeterminate pediatric thyroid fine needle aspirations: a study of 68 cases. Acta Cytol 2013;57(4):341–8.
45. Prasad ML, Vyas M, Horne MJ, et al. NTRK fusion oncogenes in pediatric papillary thyroid carcinoma in northeast United States. Cancer 2016;122(7):1097–107.
46. Bauer AJ. Molecular genetics of thyroid cancer in children and adolescents. Endocrinol Metab Clin North Am 2017;46(2):389–403.
47. Welch Dinauer CA, Tuttle RM, Robie DK, et al. Extensive surgery improves recurrence-free survival for children and young patients with class I papillary thyroid carcinoma. J Pediatr Surg 1999;34(12):1799–804.
48. Handkiewicz-Junak D, Wloch J, Roskosz J, et al. Total thyroidectomy and adjuvant radioiodine treatment independently decrease locoregional recurrence risk in childhood and adolescent differentiated thyroid cancer. J Nucl Med 2007;48(6):879–88.
49. Baumgarten H, Jenks CM, Isaza A, et al. Bilateral papillary thyroid cancer in children: Risk factors and frequency of postoperative diagnosis. J Pediatr Surg 2020. https://doi.org/10.1016/j.jpedsurg.2020.02.040.
50. Musacchio MJ, Kim AW, Vijungco JD, et al. Greater local recurrence occurs with "berry picking" than neck dissection in thyroid cancer. Am Surg 2003;69(3):191–6 [discussion: 196–7].
51. Baumgarten HD, Bauer AJ, Isaza A, et al. Surgical management of pediatric thyroid disease: Complication rates after thyroidectomy at the Children's Hospital of Philadelphia high-volume Pediatric Thyroid Center. J Pediatr Surg 2019;54(10):1969–75.
52. Rubinstein JC, Herrick-Reynolds K, Dinauer C, et al. Recurrence and complications in pediatric and adolescent papillary thyroid cancer in a high-volume practice. J Surg Res 2020;249:58–66.
53. Thompson GB, Hay ID. Current strategies for surgical management and adjuvant treatment of childhood papillary thyroid carcinoma. World J Surg 2004;28(12):1187–98.

54. Sosa JA, Tuggle CT, Wang TS, et al. Clinical and economic outcomes of thyroid and parathyroid surgery in children. J Clin Endocrinol Metab 2008;93(8): 3058–65.

55. Mazzaferri EL, Kloos RT. Clinical review 128: Current approaches to primary therapy for papillary and follicular thyroid cancer. J Clin Endocrinol Metab 2001;86(4):1447–63.

56. Jarzab B, Handkiewicz Junak D, Wloch J, et al. Multivariate analysis of prognostic factors for differentiated thyroid carcinoma in children. Eur J Nucl Med 2000;27(7):833–41.

57. Sosa JA, Bowman HM, Tielsch JM, et al. The importance of surgeon experience for clinical and economic outcomes from thyroidectomy. Ann Surg 1998;228(3): 320–30.

58. Tuggle CT, Roman SA, Wang TS, et al. Pediatric endocrine surgery: who is operating on our children? Surgery 2008;144(6):869–77 [discussion: 877].

59. Fridman M, Krasko O, Branovan DI. Factors affecting the approaches and complications of surgery in childhood papillary thyroid carcinoma. Eur J Surg Oncol 2019;45(11):2078–85.

60. Hanba C, Svider PF, Siegel B, et al. Pediatric thyroidectomy. Otolaryngol Head Neck Surg 2017;156(2):360–7.

61. Spinelli C, Strambi S, Rossi L, et al. Surgical management of papillary thyroid carcinoma in childhood and adolescence: an Italian multicenter study on 250 patients. J Endocrinol Invest 2016;39(9):1055–9.

62. Enomoto Y, Enomoto K, Uchino S, et al. Clinical features, treatment, and long-term outcome of papillary thyroid cancer in children and adolescents without radiation exposure. World J Surg 2012;36(6):1241–6.

63. Chen Y, Masiakos PT, Gaz RD, et al. Pediatric thyroidectomy in a high volume thyroid surgery center: Risk factors for postoperative hypocalcemia. J Pediatr Surg 2015;50(8):1316–9.

64. Freire AV, Ropelato MG, Ballerini MG, et al. Predicting hypocalcemia after thyroidectomy in children. Surgery 2014;156(1):130–6.

65. Jumaily JS, Noordzij JP, Dukas AG, et al. Prediction of hypocalcemia after using 1- to 6-hour postoperative parathyroid hormone and calcium levels: an analysis of pooled individual patient data from 3 observational studies. Head Neck 2010; 32(4):427–34.

66. Nordenstrom E, Bergenfelz A, Almquist M. Permanent Hypoparathyroidism After Total Thyroidectomy in Children: Results from a National Registry. World J Surg 2018. https://doi.org/10.1007/s00268-018-4552-7.

67. Scholz S, Smith JR, Chaignaud B, et al. Thyroid surgery at Children's Hospital Boston: a 35-year single-institution experience. J Pediatr Surg 2011;46(3): 437–42.

68. Morris LF, Waguespack SG, Warneke CL, et al. Long-term follow-up data may help manage patient and parent expectations for pediatric patients undergoing thyroidectomy. Surgery 2012;152(6):1165–71.

69. McLeod IK, Arciero C, Noordzij JP, et al. The use of rapid parathyroid hormone assay in predicting postoperative hypocalcemia after total or completion thyroidectomy. Thyroid 2006;16(3):259–65.

70. Tsai SD, Mostoufi-Moab S, Bauer S, et al. Clinical utility of intraoperative parathyroid hormone measurement in children and adolescents undergoing total thyroidectomy. Front Endocrinol (Lausanne) 2019;10:760.

71. McMullen C, Rocke D, Freeman J. Complications of bilateral neck dissection in thyroid cancer from a single high-volume center. JAMA Otolaryngol Head Neck Surg 2017;143(4):376–81.

72. Shaha AR. Complications of neck dissection for thyroid cancer. Ann Surg Oncol 2008;15(2):397–9.

73. Rubinstein JC, Dinauer C, Herrick-Reynolds K, et al. Lymph node ratio predicts recurrence in pediatric papillary thyroid cancer. J Pediatr Surg 2018. https://doi.org/10.1016/j.jpedsurg.2018.10.010.

74. Borson-Chazot F, Causeret S, Lifante JC, et al. Predictive factors for recurrence from a series of 74 children and adolescents with differentiated thyroid cancer. World J Surg 2004;28(11):1088–92.

75. Chéreau N, Buffet C, Trésallet C, et al. Recurrence of papillary thyroid carcinoma with lateral cervical node metastases: Predictive factors and operative management. Surgery 2016;159(3):755–62.

76. SEER Cancer Statistics Review, 1975-2007. Available at: http://seer.cancer.gov/statfacts/html/thyro.html#survival. Accessed April 11, 2016.

77. Durante C, Haddy N, Baudin E, et al. Long-term outcome of 444 patients with distant metastases from papillary and follicular thyroid carcinoma: benefits and limits of radioiodine therapy. J Clin Endocrinol Metab 2006;91(8):2892–9.

78. Brown AP, Chen J, Hitchcock YJ, et al. The risk of second primary malignancies up to three decades after the treatment of differentiated thyroid cancer. J Clin Endocrinol Metab 2008;93(2):504–15.

79. Marti JL, Jain KS, Morris LG. Increased risk of second primary malignancy in pediatric and young adult patients treated with radioactive iodine for differentiated thyroid cancer. Thyroid 2015;25(6):681–7.

80. Brink JS, van Heerden JA, McIver B, et al. Papillary thyroid cancer with pulmonary metastases in children: long-term prognosis. Surgery 2000;128(6):881–6 [discussion: 886–7].

81. Jarzab B, Handkiewicz-Junak D, Wloch J. Juvenile differentiated thyroid carcinoma and the role of radioiodine in its treatment: a qualitative review. Endocr Relat Cancer 2005;12(4):773–803.

82. Biko J, Reiners C, Kreissl MC, et al. Favourable course of disease after incomplete remission on (131)I therapy in children with pulmonary metastases of papillary thyroid carcinoma: 10 years follow-up. Eur J Nucl Med Mol Imaging 2011;38(4):651–5.

83. Kloos RT, Mazzaferri EL. A single recombinant human thyrotropin-stimulated serum thyroglobulin measurement predicts differentiated thyroid carcinoma metastases three to five years later. J Clin Endocrinol Metab 2005;90(9):5047–57.

84. Mazzaferri EL, Robbins RJ, Spencer CA, et al. A consensus report of the role of serum thyroglobulin as a monitoring method for low-risk patients with papillary thyroid carcinoma. J Clin Endocrinol Metab 2003;88(4):1433–41.

85. Lang BH, Wong KP, Wan KY. Postablation stimulated thyroglobulin level is an important predictor of biochemical complete remission after reoperative cervical neck dissection in persistent/recurrent papillary thyroid carcinoma. Ann Surg Oncol 2013;20(2):653–9.

86. Rachmiel M, Charron M, Gupta A, et al. Evidence-based review of treatment and follow up of pediatric patients with differentiated thyroid carcinoma. J Pediatr Endocrinol Metab 2006;19(12):1377–93.

87. Jarzab B, Handkiewicz-Junak D. Differentiated thyroid cancer in children and adults: same or distinct disease? Hormones (Athens) 2007;6(3):200–9.

88. Savio R, Gosnell J, Palazzo FF, et al. The role of a more extensive surgical approach in the initial multimodality management of papillary thyroid cancer in children. J Pediatr Surg 2005;40(11):1696–700.
89. Yu YR, Fallon SC, Carpenter JL, et al. Perioperative determinants of transient hypocalcemia after pediatric total thyroidectomy. J Pediatr Surg 2017;52(5):684–8.
90. Moo TA, Umunna B, Kato M, et al. Ipsilateral versus bilateral central neck lymph node dissection in papillary thyroid carcinoma. Ann Surg 2009;250(3):403–8.
91. McWade MA, Thomas G, Nguyen JQ, et al. Enhancing parathyroid gland visualization using a near infrared fluorescence-based overlay imaging system. J Am Coll Surg 2019;228(5):730–43.
92. Kahramangil B, Dip F, Benmiloud F, et al. Detection of parathyroid autofluorescence using near-infrared imaging: a multicenter analysis of concordance between different surgeons. Ann Surg Oncol 2018;25(4):957–62.
93. Rutter MM, Jha P, Schultz KA, et al. DICER1 mutations and differentiated thyroid carcinoma: evidence of a direct association. J Clin Endocrinol Metab 2016;101(1):1–5.
94. Schultz KAP, Rednam SP, Kamihara J, et al. PTEN, DICER1, FH, and their associated tumor susceptibility syndromes: clinical features, genetics, and surveillance recommendations in childhood. Clin Cancer Res 2017;23(12):e76–82.
95. Daniels GH. Follicular thyroid carcinoma: a perspective. Thyroid 2018;28(10):1229–42.
96. Jeh SK, Jung SL, Kim BS, et al. Evaluating the degree of conformity of papillary carcinoma and follicular carcinoma to the reported ultrasonographic findings of malignant thyroid tumor. Korean J Radiol 2007;8(3):192–7.
97. Hoang JK, Lee WK, Lee M, et al. US Features of thyroid malignancy: pearls and pitfalls. Radiographics 2007;27(3):847–60 [discussion: 861–5].
98. Grubbs EG, Rich TA, Li G, et al. Recent advances in thyroid cancer. Curr Probl Surg 2008;45(3):156–250.
99. Asari R, Koperek O, Scheuba C, et al. Follicular thyroid carcinoma in an iodine-replete endemic goiter region: a prospectively collected, retrospectively analyzed clinical trial. Ann Surg 2009;249(6):1023–31.
100. Zou CC, Zhao ZY, Liang L. Childhood minimally invasive follicular carcinoma: clinical features and immunohistochemistry analysis. J Paediatr Child Health 2010;46(4):166–70.
101. Robinson A, Schneider D, Sippel R, et al. Minimally invasive follicular thyroid cancer: treat as a benign or malignant lesion? J Surg Res 2017;207:235–40.
102. Enomoto K, Enomoto Y, Uchino S, et al. Follicular thyroid cancer in children and adolescents: clinicopathologic features, long-term survival, and risk factors for recurrence. Endocr J 2013;60(5):629–35.
103. Agrawal N, Akbani R, Aksoy BA, et al. Integrated genomic characterization of papillary thyroid carcinoma. Cell 2014;159(3):676–90.
104. Fenton CL, Lukes Y, Nicholson D, et al. The ret/PTC mutations are common in sporadic papillary thyroid carcinoma of children and young adults. J Clin Endocrinol Metab 2000;85(3):1170–5.
105. Penko K, Livezey J, Fenton C, et al. BRAF mutations are uncommon in papillary thyroid cancer of young patients. Thyroid 2005;15(4):320–5.
106. Caronia LM, Phay JE, Shah MH. Role of BRAF in thyroid oncogenesis. Clin Cancer Res 2011;17(24):7511–7.
107. Alzahrani AS, Murugan AK, Qasem E, et al. Single point mutations in pediatric differentiated thyroid cancer. Thyroid 2017;27(2):189–96.

108. Hardee S, Prasad ML, Hui P, et al. Pathologic characteristics, natural history, and prognostic implications of BRAF(V600E) mutation in pediatric papillary thyroid carcinoma. Pediatr Dev Pathol 2017;20(3):206–12.
109. Brose MS, Nutting CM, Jarzab B, et al. Sorafenib in radioactive iodine-refractory, locally advanced or metastatic differentiated thyroid cancer: a randomised, double-blind, phase 3 trial. Lancet 2014;384(9940):319–28.
110. Schlumberger M, Tahara M, Wirth LJ, et al. Lenvatinib versus placebo in radioiodine-refractory thyroid cancer. N Engl J Med 2015;372(7):621–30.
111. Waguespack SG, Sherman SI, Williams MD, et al. The successful use of sorafenib to treat pediatric papillary thyroid carcinoma. Thyroid 2009;19(4):407–12.
112. Mahajan P, Dawrant J, Kheradpour A, et al. Response to lenvatinib in children with papillary thyroid carcinoma. Thyroid 2018;28(11):1450–4.

Liver Tumors in Pediatric Patients

Rebecka Meyers, MD[a],*, Eiso Hiyama, MD, PhD[b], Piotr Czauderna, MD[c], Greg M. Tiao, MD[d]

KEYWORDS

- Hepatoblastoma • Hepatocellular carcinoma • PRETEXT
- Undifferentiated embryonal sarcoma of the liver • Biliary rhabdomyosarcoma
- Malignant rhabdoid tumor of the liver • Mesenchymal hamartoma
- Focal nodular hyperplasia • Infantile hemangioma

KEY POINTS

- The most common liver tumors by age are benign congenital and infantile hemangiomas in newborns/infants, malignant hepatoblastoma in an infants/toddlers, and malignant hepatocellular carcinoma in teenagers.
- Hepatoblastoma is usually chemosensitive and with surgical resection has a favorable prognosis.
- Hepatocellular carcinoma occurs most commonly as a de novo tumor in an otherwise healthy liver.
- Hepatocellular carcinoma is relatively chemoresistant; therefore, complete surgical resection is central to achieving favorable outcomes.
- The Pediatric Hepatic International Tumor Trial is a collaborative multicenter trial prospectively investigating all stages of pediatric hepatoblastoma and pediatric hepatocellular carcinoma.

INTRODUCTION

In contrast with adults, about two-thirds of hepatic tumors in children are malignant. The 2014 international consensus classification of pediatric liver tumors is shown in **Box 1** (International Consensus Classification Pediatric Liver Tumors). The differential diagnosis includes epithelial tumors, mixed epithelial and mesenchymal tumors, and

[a] Division Pediatric Surgery, University of Utah, Primary Children's Hospital, 100 North Mario Capecchi Drive, Suite 3800, Salt Lake City, UT 84113, USA; [b] Department of Pediatric Surgery, Hiroshima University Hospital, 1-2-3, Kasumi, Minami-Ku, Hiroshima 734-8551, Japan; [c] Department of Surgery and Urology for Children and Adolescents, Medical University of Gdansk, Marii Skłodowskiej-Curie 3a, 80-210 Gdańsk, Poland; [d] Division Pediatric Surgery, Cincinnati Children's Hospital and Medical Center, 3333 Burnet Ave, Cincinnati, Ohio 45229, USA
* Corresponding author.
E-mail address: rebecka.meyers@hsc.utah.edu

Surg Oncol Clin N Am 30 (2021) 253–274
https://doi.org/10.1016/j.soc.2020.11.006
surgonc.theclinics.com

Box 1
Pediatric tumors of the liver, international consensus classification

EPITHELIAL TUMORS
  Hepatocellular
    Benign and tumor like conditions
      Hepatocellular adenoma (adenomatosis)
      Focal nodular hyperplasia (FNH)
      Macroregenerative nodule
    Premalignant lesions
      Dysplastic nodules
    Malignant
      Hepatoblastoma, HB (epithelial variants)
        Pure Fetal with low mitotic activity
        Fetal, mitotically active
        Pleomorphic, poroly differentiated
        Embryonal
        Small cell component, IN1-negative/ INI1-positive
        Epithellal mixed (any/all above)
        Cholangioblastic
        Epithelial macrotrabecular pattern
        Mixed Epithelial and Mesenchymal
        With teratoid features
        Without teratoid features
      Hepatocellular Carcinoma, HCC
        Classic HCC
        Fibrolamellar HCC
      Hepatocellular Neoplasm, not otherwise specified (HcN-NOS), HB with HCC features
  Biliary
    Benign
      Bile duct adenoma, hamartoma, other
    Malignant
      Cholangiocarcinoma
      Combined (hepatocellular cholangiocarcinoma)

MESENCHYMAL TUMORS
  Benign
    Vascular tumors (Infantile hepatic hemangioma, Rapidly involuting congenital hemangioma)
    Mesenchymal hamartoma
    Pecoma
  Malignant
    Embryonal Sarcoma
    Rhabdomyosarcoma
    Vascular (Epithelioid hemagnioendothelioma, Angiosarcoma)

OTHER MALIGNANCIES
  Tumors of uncertain origin
    Malignant rhabdoid tumor of the liver (INI-1 negative)
    Nested epithelial stromal tumor
    Other
      Germ cell tumors
      Desmoplastic small round cell tumor (DSRCT)
      Peripheral primitive neuroectodermal tumor (pPNET)
  Metastatic (and Secondary)
    Metastatic solid tumors (Neuroblastoma, Wilms, other)
    Hepatic Involvement Hematologic Malignancy (Acute Myeloid Leukemia, Megakaryoblastic Leukemia (M7), Hemophagocystic Lymphohistiocytosis (HLH), Langerhahn's Cell Histiocytosis (LCH))

Data from Lopez-Terrada D, Alaggio R, DeDavila MT et al. Towards an international pediatric liver tumor consensus classification: Proceedings of the Los Angeles COG International Pathology Pediatric Liver Tumors Symposium. Modern Pathology, 2014; 26; 19-28 PMID: 24008558.

mesenchymal tumors, including some rare sarcomas, germ cell tumors, and metastatic or secondary tumors.[1] The 2 most common malignant primary hepatic tumors are hepatoblastoma (HB) and hepatocellular carcinoma (HCC), with HB accounting for 90% of malignant tumors in children younger than 5 years of age.[2] Curiously, although the incidence of HB has doubled from about 0.1 in 100,000 in the 1980s to about 0.2 in 100,000 in 2008, the incidence of HCC in children in the United States has remained constant at 0.5 in 100,000.[3] Occasional epithelial liver tumors are seen in intermediate age children with histologic heterogeneity and features of both HB and HCC.

Malignant mesenchymal tumors of the liver are more rare than epithelial liver tumors with malignant rhabdoid tumor of the liver seen in infants, whereas biliary rhabdomyosarcoma and undifferentiated embryonal sarcoma of the liver (UESL) are seen in school age children.[4] Angiosarcomas are exceedingly rare.

Over the last 4 decades, effective chemotherapeutic regimens have been introduced and, in combination with modern surgical techniques, have resulted in significant improvement in the prognosis. HB risk stratification and treatment in the legacy trials of the pediatric trial groups were based on different risk classifications for stage, metastasis, and histology.[5] In the past decade, the 4 major trial groups formed a cooperative consortium, the Children's Hepatic tumors International Collaboration (CHIC), which had a primary objective of developing a common global approach to risk stratification. In 2018, based on these consensus definitions and staging, the Pediatric Hepatic International Tumor Trial (PHITT) opened to international enrollment.

PATIENT EVALUATION OVERVIEW
Diagnosis

The most common signs of a pediatric liver tumor are abdominal distension and a palpable mass. In the rare case of prediagnosis tumor rupture there will be peritoneal irritation and anemia. Serum alpha-fetoprotein (AFP) is the most important clinical marker for HB, and is monitored both as a response to treatment and for relapse.[6–8] Malignant rhabdoid tumors do not express AFP and have a worse prognosis.[9,10] Elevated AFP may be associated with germ cell tumors and benign liver tumors, such as mesenchymal hamartoma and infantile hemangioma, but in these situations the AFP elevation is less pronounced.[11]

Radiographic Imaging

Imaging is either by contrast-enhanced abdominal computed tomography (CT) scan or by MRI. MRI enhanced by hepatocyte specific contrast agents (eg, Eovist) may improve differential diagnosis and are especially helpful in the detection of small multifocal nodules not reliably seen with a CT scan[12] (**Fig. 1**); MR with Eovist showing multifocal nodules). Metastases when present are usually to the lungs and diagnosed by a chest CT scan. In 1990, the European based International Childhood Liver Tumors Strategy Group (SIOPEL) introduced radiology based staging called PRE-Treatment EXTent of disease (PRETEXT). The PRETEXT groups (I, II, III, and IV) have remained constant; however, the PRETEXT Annotation Factors (V, P, E, F, R, C, N, and M) have evolved over time[12,13] (**Fig. 2**). Definitions of a positive annotation factor for the PHITT study are detailed in Towbin and colleagues[12] (2018) as follows: Positive V = tumor involvement of all 3 hepatic veins or retrohepatic vena cava and/or tumor thrombus in any 1 or more of the main hepatic veins; positive P = tumor involvement of the portal bifurcation, both right and left portal veins, and/or tumor thrombus in either the left or right portal; positive E = contiguous organ involvement such as the diaphragm, abdominal wall, colon, and stomach; positive F = multifocal tumor

A   B

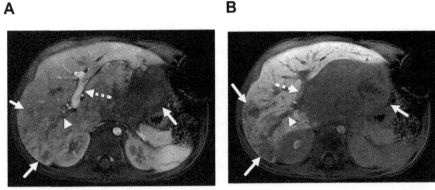

Fig. 1. HB, PRETEXT II, positive P and F. (*A*) Hepatocyte specific contrast enhanced MRI, axial T1-weighted image obtained in the portal venous phase of enhancement after administration of a hepatocyte specific contrast agent shows enhancement of the left portal vein (*dashed arrow*), thrombosis of the right portal vein (*arrowhead*), and multifocal tumor (*arrows*). (*B*) The multifocal tumor is seen better on the hepatocyte phase of imaging (annotations point to the same landmarks).

nodules; positive R = tumor rupture before diagnosis; positive N = enlarged lymph nodes; positive C = tumor involvement of the caudate lobe; and positive M = distant metastatic, usually lung nodules.

Biopsy

For tumors that are not clearly benign or resectable at diagnosis, the recommended approach is image-guided, coaxial core needle biopsy with embolization of the biopsy tract.[14,15]

HEPATOBLASTOMA
Risk Stratification

The PRETEXT/POST-TEXT groups (I, II, III, and IV) and metastatic disease (M) have been shown to be highly predictive of outcome.[16–19] Building on this foundation, the CHIC unified global risk stratification was developed, which adds other risk factors including AFP level, patient age at diagnosis, and the PRETEXT annotation factors VPEFR[5,10,20] (**Fig. 3**). A recent single institution series validated the discriminatory power of the CHIC stratification.[21] Accurate PRETEXT grouping (I, II, III, or IV) and PRETEXT annotation factor (VPEFR/M) assessment is vital for patient assignment to the appropriate risk group.[12]

Chemotherapy

Contemporary chemotherapy regimens have all been variations on a backbone of cisplatin and sometimes doxorubicin. The evolution of these chemotherapeutic approaches has shown a decrease in toxicity for localized disease and an increased intensity for high-risk tumors.[4,11,22] Details and outcomes of the most recently published studies are presented elsewhere in this article, under the discussion of outcomes.

Surgical Guidelines and Interventional Treatment Options

Although new, uniform, PRETEXT-based, international surgical guidelines are now in place, historically the recommended timing of surgical resection of HB has varied

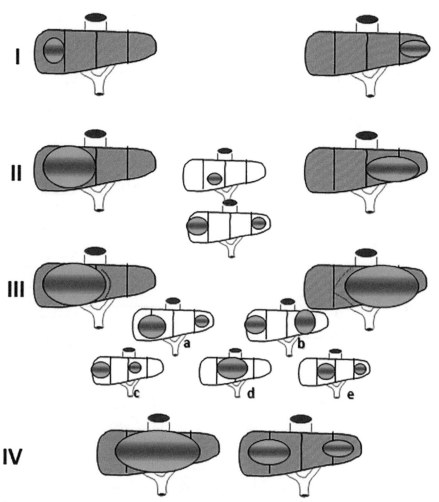

Fig. 2. PRETEXT group, pretreatment extent of disease. Extent of parenchyma involvement at diagnosis. POST-TEXT Group, Posttreatment Extent of Disease, Extent of parenchyma involvement after chemotherapy. I, 3 contiguous sections tumor free; II, 2 contiguous sections tumor free; III, 1 contiguous sections tumor free; IV, no contiguous sections tumor free. In addition, any group may have 1 or more. Annotation factors: V, involvement vena cava, all 3 hepatic veins; P, involvement portal bifurcation, both R and L; E, contiguous extrahepatic tumor; F, multifocal tumor; R, tumor rupture before diagnosis; C, caudate lobe; N, lymph node involvement; M, metastasis, distant extrahepatic tumor.

among the major trial groups.[4,23,24] In North America, consideration for surgical resection of tumors at diagnosis resulted in a surgical-based staging system: stage 1 successfully resected at diagnosis, stage 2 resected at diagnosis with microscopic residual, stage 3 unresectable at diagnosis, or gross residual/rupture/biopsy only, and stage 4, metastatic disease. In Europe since 1990 all children received preoperative chemotherapy and staging has been based on PRETEXT.

Resection rates have increased over time through intensification of chemotherapy for high-risk tumors and an increased use of vascular reconstruction and liver

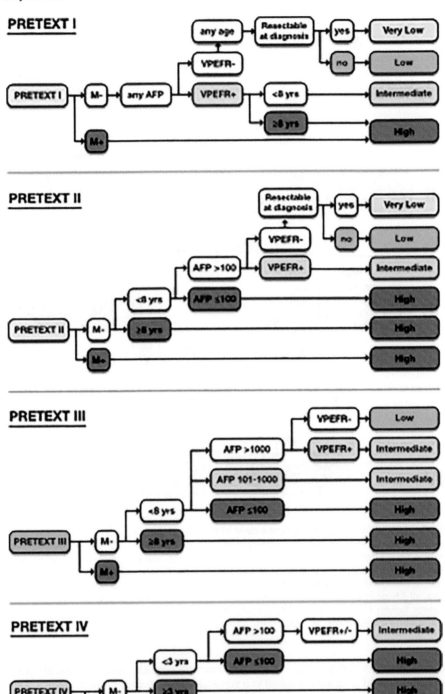

Fig. 3. Children's Hepatic tumor International Collaboration (CHIC) hepatoblastoma risk stratification. Color highlights of groups within each tree indicate which prognostic factor determined patient assignment to the ultimate group assignment: very low, low, intermediate, or high-risk group.

transplantation for unresectable tumors[25–27] (**Table 1**). One important observation has been that the majority of the chemotherapy response occurs in the first few cycles and continuing chemotherapy beyond this point induces drug resistance genes and increased toxicity.[28,29]

The PHITT trial introduced common, international, PRETEXT-based, surgical resection guidelines.[4,29] Resection is recommended at diagnosis for PRETEXT I and II tumors, with negative VPEFR/M annotation factors, if preoperative radiographic imaging shows 1 cm or more of uninvolved parenchyma between the tumor and the middle hepatic vein, inferior vena cava, and remaining portal vein. Resection at diagnosis should not require extension across Cantlie's line. Trial guidelines recommend that PRETEXT II, III, and IV tumors with less than 1 cm of a radiographic margin from the middle hepatic vein, and/or a positive VPEFR/M annotation factor, be biopsied and receive preoperative chemotherapy. Early communication with a transplant-capable liver center is encouraged for tumors with anticipated POST-TEXT unresectable vascular involvement and POST-TEXT IV multifocal tumors.

Extreme resections required in large central tumors with major vascular involvement of all 3 hepatic veins, the retrohepatic vena cava, and/or both portal veins are done by experienced liver surgeons as a potential alternative to orthotopic liver transplantation. This point is especially important for patients with extensive tumors and chemoresistant metastatic disease in which orthotopic liver transplantation cannot be offered.[30,31] When the surgical resection is performed after a confirmed effective chemotherapy response, SIOPEL experience suggests that a positive microscopic resection margin may not portend a worse prognosis.[32] Most investigators agree that POST-TEXT IV multifocal tumors require transplantation to prevent local relapse from occult nodules. It is important for all treating teams to realize that children who present with unresectable tumors may become resectable with neoadjuvant chemotherapy and careful POST-TEXT oncologic reevaluation is needed before deciding on the resection strategy.[22,29,31]

Surgical Complications

Intraoperative complications may include hemorrhage, air embolism and subsequent cardiac arrest. The most common postoperative complications are bleeding, impairment of blood flow in or out of the liver remnant, bile blockage or bile leak, liver failure, infection and ileus.[4] The potential causes of postoperative liver failure include a small

Table 1
HB increased surgical resection rates over time

	Years	Patient Group	Resection Rate (%)	Liver Transplantation, n (%)
INT-0098	1988–1992	Children's Oncology Group stage III/IV	57	0 (0)
SIOPEL 1	1989–1994	High risk[a]	53	6 (5)
SIOPEL 2	1994–1998	High risk[a]	67	7 (12)
SIOPEL 3HR	1998–2006	High risk[a]	74	34 (21)
SIOPEL 4	2005–2009	High risk[a]	97	16 (27)
AHEP-0731	2009–2012	Intermediate risk[b]	96	33 (32)

[a] PRETEXT IV or any PRETEXT with +VPEM or SCU histology.
[b] PRETEXT III with +V + P or any PRETEXT IV.
Data from Refs.[4,23,106]

liver remnant, liver devascularization, interruption of hepatic venous drainage, excessive liver warm ischemia owing to prolonged vascular occlusion or massive bleeding, major bile duct obstruction, halogenated anesthetic agents, viral infections, and drug reactions. Bile leak occurs in 10% to 12% of cases and its frequency has not decreased over the years. The prevention of bile leak requires a detailed anatomic knowledge of the potential variations in biliary anatomy, avoiding extensive dissection at the hepatic hilum and a low threshold for performing an intraoperative cholangiogram.

Surgical Management of Lung Metastasis

Children's Oncology Group (COG) studies have shown pulmonary metastectomy to be an effective strategy to achieve complete remission for lesions that fail to resolve on chemotherapy.[33,34] The Japanese trial experience suggests that metastatectomy for residual pulmonary nodules after chemotherapy is effective provided the primary liver tumor can be resected completely.[35] The role of metastatectomy for relapse is less definitive but the bulk of evidence supports surgical resection as a safe and, in the context of multimodal therapy, efficacious approach to manage pulmonary relapse.[8,36] Recently, preoperative intravenous indocyanine green (ICG) has been used to localize occult nodules at the time of metastatectomy and may enhance our ability to clear the lungs of metastatic disease.[37,38]

Transarterial Chemoembolization and Radioembolization

Transarterial chemoembolization or transarterial radioembolization are occasionally used to increase resectability in children who are not liver transplant candidates owing to uncontrolled metastatic disease.[39,40] It has also been used to maintain disease control for those patients who have completed protocol systemic chemotherapy but for whom a donor organ is not yet available.

Hepatoblastoma Outcomes and Combination Therapies

The most recent published trial results for each of the major multicenter trial groups involved in the study of HB are shown in **Table 2**. The most contemporary results for SIOPEL are SIOPEL 4 and 6. SIOPEL 6 was able to decrease ototoxicity and maintain good outcomes in standard risk tumors using 6 cycles cisplatin monotherapy randomized with or without the otoprotectant sodium thiosulfate.[41] SIOPEL 4 study used a neoadjuvant induction of weekly, dose-compressed cisplatin and 3-weekly doxorubicin in high risk (either PRETEXT IV or metastatic) with event-free survival and overall survival of 76% and 83%, respectively, the best results to date for patients presenting with metastatic disease.[42] Results for COG AHEP-0731, which enrolled 225 eligible patients from 2009 to 2018, by treatment strata were as follows: (a) very low risk and low risk, PRETEXT I and II tumors resectable at diagnosis, maintained excellent outcomes with reductions in chemotherapy, (b) intermediate risk showed improved survival and surgical resection rates, compared with historic controls, by adding doxorubicin to their historic regimen and encouraging early involvement of liver specialty surgical centers[43]; and (c) high risk, patients with metastatic disease were randomized to upfront experimental window chemotherapy of either vincristine–irinotecan[44] or vincristine–irinotecan–temsirolimus. There was response to the upfront experimental therapy, but this response was not superior to the C5VD backbone. The Japanese JPLT 2 study, which enrolled 361 patients from 1999 to 2012, showed inferior outcome in the ruptured at diagnosis subset of the low-risk group when ruptured tumors were resected before chemotherapy. This Japanese study achieved outstanding results for cisplatin + pirarubicin responders and did not support intensified chemotherapy or stem cell transplantation for cisplatin + pirarubicin nonresponders.[45] Cross-study

Table 2
Most recently published HB multi-center cooperative trials

Study	Chemotherapy	Patients and PRETEXT	Outcomes

AHEP-0731 2009–2012[25,43,44]	Very low risk: none
	Low risk:C5V postop
	Intermediate risk
	  (SCU or stage III)
	  C5VD
	Mets: VIwindow;
	  VIT Window[a]
		n = 225
		Very low risk/PRETEXT I/II = 8
		Low risk PRETEXT I/II = 47;
		  III = 2;
		Intermediate risk PRETEXT:
		  I/II = 34; III = 54; IV = 14;
		MetsVI: 30
		Mets/VIT[a]: 36 (to be
		  published)
			5-Year EFS/OS
			Very low risk:
			  100%/100%
			Low risk:
			  91%/97%
			Intermediate risk:
			  87%/95%
			MetsVI:
			  49%/62%

HB 99 (GPOH) 1999–2004[24]	SR: IPA; HR: CARBO/VP16	n = 100 SR: 58 HR: 42	3-Year EFS/OS SR: 90%/88% HR: 52%/55%

SIOPEL 4 2005–2009[42]	HR: Block A:
	  Weekly CIS
	  + 3 weekly
	  DOXO;
	  Block B
	  CARBO/DOX
		n = 62
		PRETEXT: I = 2; II = 17;
		  III = 27; IV = 16; Mets: 39
			3-Year EFS/OS
			HR all:76%/83%
			  PRETEXTIV
			  = 75%/88%
			Mets: 77%/79%

SIOPEL 6 2007–2014[41]	SR: CIS vs CIS + STS	n = 109; CIS PRETEXT:
		  I/II = 31; III = 21 CIS
		  + STS PRETEXT: I/II = 41;
		  III = 16
			3-Year EFS/OS
			CIS: 79%/92%
			CIS + STS:
			  82%/98%

JPLT 2 1999–2012[45]	1: low-dose CITA postop only 2: low-dose CITA 3: CITA full dose 4: high dose ± SCT	n = 361; Course 1 PRETEXT I/II rxn@ dx; Course 2 PRETEXT I/II preoperative chemotherapy; Course 3 PRETEXT III/IV; Course 4 metastatic or CITA nonresponder	5-Year EFS/OS 1: 74%/90% 2: 85%/91% 3: 77%/87% 4: 37%/53%

Abbreviations: AFP, alpha fetoprotein; C5V, cisplatin + 5-flurouracil (5FU) + vincristine; C5VD, cisplatin + 5-flurouracil (5FU) + vincristine + doxorubicin; CARBO, carboplatin; CIS, cisplatin; CITA, cisplatin + pirarubicin; DOXO, doxorubicin; EFS, event-free survival; HR, High Risk; IPA, Ifosfamide + cis + adriamycin; OS, overall survival; PFH, pure fetal histology; SCT, Stem Cell Transplant; SCU, Small Cell Undifferentiated; SR, standard risk; STS, sodium thiosulfate otoprotectant; VIT, vincristine–irinotecan–temsirolimus; VP16, etoposide.
[a] VIT window enrolled 2013 to 2016, not yet published.

group comparisons are complicated by the fact that PRETEXT IV nonmetastatic patients were considered intermediate risk by COG and JPLT and high risk by SIOPEL.

Hepatoblastoma with Features of Hepatocellular Carcinoma and Hepatocellular Neoplasm Not Otherwise Specified

Occasionally with expert pathologic review, a consensus diagnosis for histologic subtype cannot be reached because of a variable heterogenous mix of HB, HCC, and undifferentiated histologies. The international consensus conference called these tumors hepatocellular neoplasm, not otherwise specified,[1] although since then they are more often referred to as HB with HCC features. Prokurat and associates[46] and Zhou and coworkers[47] have also reported such tumors, which they respectively called "transitional liver cell tumors" and hepatocellular malignancies not otherwise specified. The median age is about 7 years (range, 4–15 years), AFP is elevated, and response to chemotherapy is common. Historically, there has been no consensus on whether to treat these tumors according to either HB or HCC protocols; the PHITT study protocol recommends that they be treated as HB.

New Developments

Biology

As our understanding of the tumor biology has increased, poor molecular prognostic factors such as NFR2 mutation and a 12-gene signature have been identified.[48,49] Genetic and epigenetic analysis has included Wnt pathway and gene expression analysis, DNA methylation profiling, and *TERT* promoter mutations. Nuclear and cytoplasmic accumulations of β-catenin, whose oncogenic mutations lead to chromosomal instability and aberrant Wnt/β-catenin signaling, are seen in almost all patients with HB and may contribute to tumorigenesis.[48–50]

Indocyanine green navigation surgery

The technique relies on the intravenous administration of ICG before surgery and the intraoperative illumination of the surface of the organ by an infrared camera that simultaneously induces and collects the fluorescence[37,38] (**Fig. 4**). With ICG navigation, tumor nodules otherwise not visible may be seen by green fluorescence at the time of surgery. Usually, ICG (0.5 mg/kg) is injected 24 hours before pulmonary metastatectomy. For the detection of nodules in the liver a higher dose is given several days before surgery because ICG is secreted in the bile and requires time to clear the normal liver. The sensitivity for viable tumor cells is 95%, but the specificity is only about 80% owing to the false-positive fluorescence of inflammatory cells. A limitation of ICG navigation is the inability to detect nodules deep in the parenchyma (deeper than 10–15 mm).

HEPATOCELLULAR CARCINOMA

Most pediatric HCC are de novo tumors and develop in normal livers without underlying chronic liver disease. These de novo HCC include conventional HCC, fibrolamellar HCC, and foci of HCC histology occurring in HB. Comparing pediatric with adult HCC, it has been debated whether pediatric de novo HCC is the same disease as

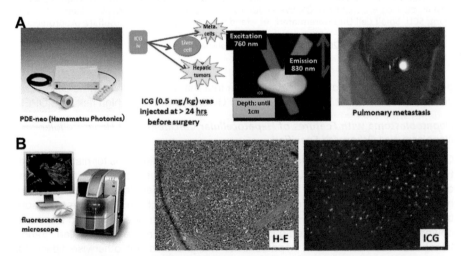

Fig. 4. (*A*) Indocyanine green (ICG) navigation surgery. (*B*) ICG for pulmonary metastasectomy.

HCC in adult cirrhotic livers.[51–53] From a cytogenetic and molecular viewpoint, it seems most likely that the type of HCC and its molecular changes are more important than the age group at which HCC is diagnosed.[53] In a minority of cases of pediatric HCC, the tumor occurs in the background of cirrhosis. Cirrhosis in children is caused by variety of disorders and those with cancer predisposition include tyrosinemia, progressive familial intrahepatic cholestasis syndromes, primary sclerosing cholangitis, congenital portosystemic shunts, glycogen storage disease types I to IV, Fanconi syndrome, and ataxia telangiectasia.[54] As in adults, children with chronic liver disease–induced cirrhosis require surveillance for tumor.

Localized Hepatocellular Carcinoma

In the case of localized, nonmetastatic disease, surgical resection at diagnosis, even by extreme resection or orthotopic liver transplantation, should be considered.[55,56] Contrary to HB, where lymph node metastases are rare, the lymph nodes must be sampled in HCC. In adult HCC, liver transplantation may be restricted to the Milan criteria (single tumor <5 cm; $\leq$3 tumors <3 cm). Milan criteria were originally derived in the context of HCC in adult cirrhotic livers and organ shortage, thus aimed to select patients for optimal success. However, in children it is more common to have large de novo tumors in healthy livers, which, although outside of Milan criteria, have been shown to have a good prognosis with orthotopic liver transplantation.[52] Recent reports show good survival rates of in the range of 75% to 80% at 5 years in selected patients.[56–58] Data from 2 separate Surveillance, Epidemiology, and End Results registry database studies reported that, in children presenting with nonmetastatic HCC, regardless of tumor size, the 5-year survival rate was better after liver transplantation than after resection.[55,57] Although the Surveillance, Epidemiology, and End Results registry data do not include important staging information, the favorable survival suggests that liberalized transplant criteria in children is warranted.

Neoadjuvant Chemotherapy

Various chemotherapy regimens have been used, although the role of chemotherapy in this relatively chemoresistant tumor remains unclear. Results of the SIOPEL-1 study, using neoadjuvant cisplatin and doxorubicin (PLADO), could not be improved in the SIOPEL-2 and -3 studies using neoadjuvant intensified platinum and doxorubicin (SUPER-PLADO), with both studies showing dismal survival rates of 28% and 22% at 5 years.[51,52] Patients who underwent primary surgery or those with complete resection at delayed surgery showed overall survival rates of 40%.[52] The German trial group used ifosfamide, cisplatin, and doxorubicin in the HB-89 trial and carboplatin and ifosfamide in HB-94.[59] The overall survival rates were 33% and 32%, respectively. The more recent HB99 trial showed better (overall survival and event-free survival) 3-year survival rates of 89% and 72%, respectively, in patients with resectable tumors followed by 2 cycles of carboplatin and etoposide. However, in those with metastatic disease or nonresectable tumors, the survival rates were disappointing at 20% and 12%, respectively.[59] These results are in line with a small COG study showing that upfront resections had good survival (5-year event-free survival 88%) with postoperative chemotherapy and the outcome was uniformly poor for advanced stage disease (5-year event-free survival of 10%–23%).[60] Tumor-free margins been have shown to be a strong predictor of favorable outcome,[52] whereas lymphovascular invasion, extrahepatic tumor, and metastatic disease precluding complete resection are poor prognostic factors (5-year event-free survival of 10%).[51] Common pathways for target are vascular endothelial growth factor receptor (sorafenib, bevacizumab, brivanib, sunitib), epidermal growth factor (erlotinib), mammalian target of rapamycin (everolimus, tyrosine kinase receptor for hepatocyte growth factor, cMET [tivantinib]), combined vascular endothelial growth factor and cMET (carbozantinib) and programmed cell death receptor (nivolumab).[53,54] Sorafenib has been used by the German pediatric group in combination with PLADO, which showed tumor regression in a small number of patients with unresectable tumors.[59]

Metastatic Hepatocellular Carcinoma

In children with metastatic HCC, the prognosis is grim. Although there is increasing experience with first- and second-line chemotherapy in adult patients, none of these regimen have translated into prolonged survival. They include treatment with gemcitabine plus oxaliplatin, 5-fluoracil (5-FU) plus cisplatin, cape-citabine plus cisplatin, 5-FU plus mitomycin, 5-FU plus oxaliplatin, gemcitabine plus cisplatin, 5-FU plus interferon, and monotherapy with sorafenib.[54] In the SIOPEL experience the partial tumor response rate to cisplatin and doxorubicin was 33-49%, however many of these patients never became resectable.[52] Only scarce data on the use of gemcitabine plus oxaliplatin in pediatric patients with HCC is available. Some investigators have hypothesized that pediatric HCC is more responsive to chemotherapy than adult HCC, but whether this finding is true for all de novo HCC types in children, or specifically for the hepatocellular neoplasm, not otherwise specified type (HB with HCC features), remains open.[52] Ablative therapies like radiofrequency ablation, percutaneous ethanol ablation, or transarterial chemoembolization, hepatic arterial infusion chemotherapy, and transarterial radioembolization have been widely used in adults, mostly for downstaging to comply with Milan criteria and for bridging to transplantation; however, the experience in children is limited.[61,62] The role of a palliative resection of the primary tumor with the goal to preserve quality of life or even prolong survival is unclear.[62]

Fibrolamellar Hepatocellular Carcinoma

Fibrolamellar HCC is most common in adolescents and young adults and has a slight female preponderance. AFP is usually normal, although the level of transcobalamin I may be elevated.[54] At diagnosis, 35% of patients have vascular invasion and 60% have extrahepatic disease.[63] Although fibrolamellar HCC seems to have a more favorable prognosis in adults, this does not seem to be the case in children.[63–65] A review of SIOPEL fibrolamellar HCC cases showed 31% partial response to super-PLADO, 42% complete resection, and 3-year event-free survival and overall survival rates of 22% and 42%, respectively, which were comparable with conventional pediatric HCC.[65] A recent finding of an RNA transcript and protein incorporating DNAJB1 and PRKACA may provide the basis for a diagnostic marker and could be a future target for therapeutic interventions.[66]

OTHER MALIGNANT LIVER TUMORS IN CHILDREN
Pediatric Hepatic Sarcomas

- *Undifferentiated Embryonal Sarcoma of the Liver (UESL)*. UESL is the third most common malignant pediatric liver tumor usually presenting around 6 to 10 years, it can occur in both younger and older children.[67–69] It has been reported to arise within mesenchymal hamartomas sharing genetic features.[70] UESL has cystic and solid components and the myxoid cystic components may hemorrhage or rupture at diagnosis or with biopsy attempts[68] (**Fig. 5**A). A biopsy should be undertaken with ultrasound guidance to the more solid areas of the tumor and/or a biopsy of a metastatic lesion. Complete resection is crucial and most neoplasms are treated according to the embryonal sarcoma regimens for other pediatric soft

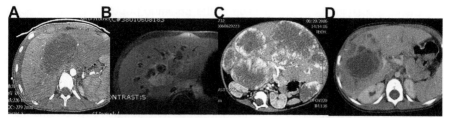

Fig. 5. Radiographic appearance of pediatric liver tumors. (*A*) Undifferentiated embryonal sarcoma (UESL) with a mixture of cystic/myxoid and solid components. (*B*) Biliary rhabdomyosarcoma, presentation with biliary tract obstruction is common. (*C*) Multifocal or diffuse subtype of infantile hepatic hemangioma can involve the entire liver with significant hepatomegaly. (*D*) Mesenchymal hamartoma presents as a multicystic mass with thick vascular sepatae.

tissue sarcoma anatomic sites. Response to multimodal therapy has improved and the overall survival rate is now about 70%.[67–69]

- *Biliary rhabdomyosarcoma.* Biliary rhabdomyosarcoma accounts for less than 1% of rhabdomyosarcoma in children; the median age at diagnosis is 3 years.[71] The typical presentation is with jaundice and biliary obstruction, occasionally cholangitis.[71] Imaging shows hypoechoic intraductal or periductal cystic solid mass with dilation of a partially obstructed biliary tract (**Fig. 5**B). Often, imaging is misdiagnosed as a choledochal cyst.[72] Biopsy can be either percutaneously or by endoscopic retrograde cholangiopancreatography.[73] Neoadjuvant chemotherapy and radiation therapy will decrease the mass effect and improve the biliary obstruction. Most tumors are localized and hence resectable, but complete resection can be challenging when located in the hilum. The reported 5-year survival for patients with local–regional disease is 50% to 78%. Metastatic disease is often fatal.[74]

- *Angiosarcoma.* A handful of pediatric cases have been reported, some of which seemed to be a malignant transformation of infantile hepatic hemangioma.[75–77] Infantile hepatic hemangioma and angiosarcoma can both have positive GLUT-1; hence, it is difficult to determine if angiosarcoma emerged from the infantile hepatic hemangioma or in association with the infantile hepatic hemangioma.[77] Refractory metastatic disease is common and the prognosis is poor, with a median survival of 14 to 18 months and an overall survival at 5 years of 20% to 35%.[75–77]

- *Malignant rhabdoid tumor of the liver.* Rhabdoid tumors are aggressive with poor survival. The typical age at diagnosis is 0 to 3 years and, although most common in the kidney, they can occur anywhere in the body; the liver is the fourth most common site. Some patients with an AFP of less than 100 in older HB trials may have been malignant rhabdoid tumors of the liver, which would explain their poor survival.[78] Malignant rhabdoid tumors of the liver are defined by lack of INI-1 tumor suppressor gene; therefore, the diagnosis requires immunohistochemistry.[79–82] Treatment is with aggressive chemotherapy combined with complete resection, but these are often metastatic neoplasms with a poor survival.[80–84]

- *Other malignant liver tumors in children.* A nested stromal epithelial tumor is a recently described rare neoplasm showing nests of spindled epithelioid cells with a potential for calcification.[83,84] Surgical resection is the treatment of choice, after which Cushing syndrome, when present, will resolve.

Cholangiocarcinoma is rarely seen in the pediatric population. If diagnosed before adulthood, it can be associated with choledochal cysts, primary sclerosing cholangitis, biliary atresia and other biliary anomalies, human immunodeficiency virus infection, and radiation therapy.[85,86] A primary yolk sac tumor of the liver is extremely rare, but has been reported in young children. It is easily confused with HB owing to age and high AFP so histologic examination is essential for diagnosis.[87] A primary hepatic lymphoma is a lymphoproliferative disorder confined to the liver, whereas non-Hodgkin's lymphoma may involve the liver as a secondary manifestation. The liver is the third most common abdominal organ with lymphoma involvement.[88] Liver disease may be focal, but more commonly shows multiple small ultrasound hypoechoic nodules.[89] Hepatomegaly is a common presentation in many pediatric hematologic malignancies including hemophagocytic lymphohistiocytosis, Langerhans cell histiocytosis, and acute megakaryoblastic leukemia. Many pediatric abdominal solid tumors can spread to the liver and metastatic liver tumors should always be considered in the differential diagnosis of any child with a neoplastic liver process. During the first year of life, liver metastases can be found in neuroblastoma. In older children, germ cell tumors, neuroendocrine pancreatic tumors, pancreatoblastoma, gastrointestinal stromal tumor, desmoplastic small round cell tumor, and Wilms' tumor can metastasize to the liver.[4]

Benign Liver Tumors in Children

- *Congenital hemangioma.* Congenital hemangiomas proliferate in utero and generally reach peak size before or at birth. Diagnosis may occur on prenatal imaging or through evaluation of a mass or heart failure in the newborn. Congenital hemangiomas are high-flow vascular lesions and may have intratumoral bleeding, thrombocytopenia, hypofibrinogenemia, and high-output cardiac failure. A newborn may present with significant anemia, thrombocytopenia, and mild hypofibrinogenemia. They are GLUT-1 negative and typically follow 1 of 3 clinical patterns: rapidly involuting congenital hemangioma), partially involuting congenital hemangioma, and noninvoluting congenital hemangioma.[90]
- *Infantile hemangioma.* Infantile hemangioma are GLUT-1 positive and continue to proliferate until approximately 6 to 12 months of age, with gradual involution until 3 to 9 years of age. Like congenital hemangiomas, they may be high flow, but the vascular symptoms will develop later during the postnatal proliferation period as shunting increases. Acquired consumptive hypothyroidism is specific for hepatic infantile hemangioma. Focal tumors may be silent clinically; however, multifocal or diffuse tumors may develop into abdominal compartment syndrome and failure to thrive.[90]
- *Multifocal or diffuse infantile hepatic hemangioma* (**Fig. 5**C). The treatment of symptomatic diffuse lesions is in conjunction with a multidisciplinary team well-versed in the natural history of these lesions and familiar with the medical treatment and percutaneous embolization approaches in children.[91]
- *Focal nodular hyperplasia.* These neoplasms are uncommon in children, but can occur in specific subgroups of patients with abnormal hepatic circulation, patients with a history of chemotherapy for a nonliver malignancy, and adolescent females.[92] MRI can be diagnostic showing isointense to hypointense on T1-weightged imaging, and isointense to mildly hyperintense on T2-weighted sequences.[93,94] In equivocal cases, a biopsy may be needed.[92]
- *Mesenchymal hamartoma.* These tumors, usually in a preschool age child, tend to be large with multiloculated cysts separated by thick vascularized septae[95,96]

(**Fig. 5**D). The differential diagnosis is sometimes challenging and includes UESL, simple hepatic cysts, teratoma, ciliated foregut cysts, echinococcal abscess, and purulent abscess. Occasionally, the AFP may be elevated.[97] Treatment usually consists of complete surgical resection with negative margins given a genetic association with UESL.[98,99]

- *Hepatocellular adenoma.* In children, the mean age of diagnosis is 14 years with rare cases in younger children.[100] Usually, they are solitary, although multiple adenomas may be seen in children with predisposing conditions such as glycogen storage disease. Apart from the special circumstance of glycogen storage disease, surgical excision has been recommended for lesions greater than 5 cm, dysplastic foci, enlarging size, features of malignant change on imaging, β-catenin activation, or male gender.[101]
- *Rare benign tumors.* Rare benign tumors include inflammatory myofibroblastic tumor,[102] teratoma,[103] intrahepatic bile duct adenoma,[104] and macroregenerative nodules.[105]

SUMMARY, DISCUSSION, AND FUTURE DIRECTIONS

The survival of children with liver tumors, especially HB, has improved significantly after the introduction of effective chemotherapeutic regimens and appropriate surgical approaches, including liver transplantation, resulting in an increase in the number of patients undergoing definitive tumor resection and a decrease in the incidence of postsurgical recurrences. With improvements in survival, decreasing late effects such as ototoxicity, secondary malignancies, and the long-term complications of transplantation should be an increased focus of our research effort. Future trials should investigate risk-based strategies for management of metastatic and refractory disease and minimizing treatment-related complications and long-term toxicities. Moreover, further histologic and biological studies are necessary in moving toward the individualization of therapy.

CLINICS CARE POINTS

- Screening of a palpable abdominal mass in a child is with ultrasound. When ultrasound shows liver mass in a young child diagnosis of HB includes elevated AFP, contrast-enhanced CT scan or MRI of the liver, and a chest CT scan.
- Radiographic staging of the pretreatment extent of the tumor (PRETEXT) includes PRETEXT group (I, II, III, and IV), depending on number of anatomic liver sections free of tumor, and PRETEXT annotation factors (VPEFRM), which denote extent of major vessel involvement and extraparenchymal tumor extension (see **Fig. 2**).
- Treatment protocols for HB depend on the PRETEXT group (I, II, III, or IV), PRETEXT annotations factors (VPEFR), metastasis (M), patient age, and AFP level (see **Fig. 3**).
- The survival of children with HB has improved significantly after the introduction of cisplatin-based chemotherapeutic regimens, which resulted in an increase in the number of patients ultimately undergoing complete tumor resection and a decrease in the incidence of postsurgical recurrences.
- Complete tumor resection remains the cornerstone of curative therapy for both HB and HCC.
- New developments in HB include the international collaborative multicenter trial (PHITT), sodium thiosulfate to protect against cisplatin ototoxicity, ICG navigation surgery, and increasing identification of biologic markers for prognosis.

- Long-term follow-up after treatment for HB is needed for late effects of therapy, such as ototoxicity, cardiotoxicity, renal toxicity, growth delay, and secondary malignancies.

FUNDING

The PHITT study is supported by SIOPEL's European Union's Horizon 2020 research and innovation programme CHILTERN grant agreement No. 668596, by COG's NIH/NCI grant U10CA180886 and by JCCG's AMED grants 19ck0106332h and 19lk0201066h.

DISCLOSURE

The authors have nothing to disclose.

REFERENCES

1. Lopez-Terrada D, Alaggio R, DeDavila MT, et al. Towards an international pediatric liver tumor consensus classification: proceedings of the Los Angeles COG International Pathology Pediatric Liver Tumors Symposium. Mod Pathol 2014;26:19–28.
2. Darbari A, Sabin KM, Shapiro CN, et al. Epidemiology of primary hepatic malignancies in US children. Hepatology 2003;38:560–6.
3. Allan BJ, Parikh PP, Diaz S, et al. Predictors of survival and incidence of hepatoblastoma in the pediatric population. HPB (Oxford) 2013;15:741–6.
4. Aronson DC, Meyers RL. Malignant tumors of the liver in children. Semin Pediatr Surg 2016;25:265–75.
5. Czauderna P, Haeberle B, Hiyama E, et al. The Children's Hepatic tumors International Collaboration (CHIC): novel global rare tumor database yields new prognostic factors in hepatoblastoma. Eur J Cancer 2016;52:92–101.
6. Rojas Y, Guillerman RP, Zhang W, et al. Relapse surveillance in AFP-positive hepatoblastoma: re-evaluating the role of imaging. Pediatr Radiol 2014;44(10):1275–80.
7. Powers JM, Pacheco MM, Wickiser JE. Addition of vincristine and irinotecan to standard therapy in a patient with refractory high-risk hepatoblastoma achieving long-term relapse-free survival. J Pediatr Hematol Oncol 2019;41(3):e171–3.
8. Semeraro M, Branchereau S, Maibach R, et al. Relapses in hepatoblastoma patients: clinical characteristics and outcome—experience of the International childhood liver tumor strategy group SIOPEL. Eur J Cancer 2013;49:915–22.
9. Trobaugh-Lotrario AD, Tomlinson GE, Finegold MJ, et al. Small cell undifferentiated variant of hepatoblastoma: adverse clinical and molecular features similar to rhabdoid tumors. Pediatr Blood Cancer 2009;52:328–34.
10. Meyers RL, Maibach R, Hiyama E, et al. Risk stratified staging in paediatric hepatoblastoma: a unified analysis from the Children's Hepatic tumor International Collaboration (CHIC). Lancet Oncol 2017;18(1):122–31.
11. Czauderna P, Lopez-Terrada D, Hiyama E, et al. Hepatoblastoma state of the art: pathology, genetics, risk stratification, and chemotherapy. Curr Opin Pediatr 2014;26:19–28.
12. Towbin AJ, Meyers RL, Woodley H, et al. PRETEXT 2017: radiologic staging system for primary hepatic malignancies of childhood revised for the Paediatric Hepatic International Tumour Trial (PHITT). Pediatr Radiol 2018;48:536–54.
13. Roebuck DJ, Aronson D, Clapuyt P, et al. 2005 PRETEXT: a revised staging system for primary malignant liver tumours of childhood developed by the SIOPEL group. Pediatr Radiol 2007;37:123–32, 1096–1100.

14. Weldon CB, Madenci AL, Tiao GM, et al. Evaluation of the diagnostic biopsy approach for children with hepatoblastoma: a report from the Children's Oncology Group AHEP0731 Liver Tumor Committee. J Pediatr Surg 2019;11. S0022-3468(19)30347.

15. Hawkins MC, Towbin AJ, Roebuck DJ, et al. Role of Interventional Radiology in managing pediatric liver tumors part two: endovascular interventions. Pediatr Radiol 2018;48:565.

16. Fuchs J, Rydzynski J, vonSchweinitz D, et al. Pretreatment prognostic factors and treatment results in children with hepatoblastoma: a report from the German Cooperative Pediatric Liver Tumor Study HB94. Cancer 2002;95:172–82.

17. Aronson DC, Schnater JM, Staalman CR, et al. Predictive value of the Pretreatment extent of disease system in hepatoblastoma: results from the international society of pediatric oncology liver tumor study group SIOPEL-1 study. J Clin Oncol 2005;23:1245–52.

18. Meyers RL, Rowland JH, Krailo M, et al. Pretreatment prognostic factors in hepatoblastoma: a report of the Children's Oncology Group. Pediatr Blood Cancer 2009;53:1016–22.

19. Maibach R, Roebuck D, Brugieres L, et al. Prognostic stratification for children with hepatoblastoma: the SIOPEL experience. Eur J Cancer 2012;48:1543–9.

20. Häberle B, Rangaswami A, Krailo M, et al. The importance of age as a prognostic factor for the outcome of patients with hepatoblastoma: analysis from the Children's Hepatic tumors International Collaboration (CHIC) database. Pediatr Blood Cancer 2020;67(8):e28350.

21. Mascarenhas L, Malvar J, Stein J, et al. Independent validation of the Children's Hepatic tumors International Collaboration (CHIC) risk stratification for hepatoblastoma. Liver tumors session, 50th Annual Meeting SIOP 2018, Kyoto Japan, November 18, 2018.

22. Perilongo G, Malogoloowkin M, Feusner J. Hepatoblastoma clinical research: lessons learned and future challenges. Pediatr Blood Cancer 2012;59:818–21.

23. Meyers RL, Tiao G, de ville de Goyet, et al. Hepatoblastoma state of the art: PRETEXT, surgical resection guidelines and the role of liver transplantation. Curr Opin Pediatr 2014;26:29–36.

24. Haeberle B, Maxwell R, vonSchweinitz D, et al. High dose chemotherapy with autologous stem cell transplantation in hepatoblastoma does not improve outcome. Results of the GPOH study HB99. Klin Padiatr 2019;231(6):283–90.

25. Katzenstein HM, Langham MR, Malogolowkin MH, et al. Minimal adjuvant chemotherapy for children with hepatoblastoma resected at diagnosis (AHEP0731): a Children's Oncology Group, multicentre, phase 3 trial. Lancet Oncol 2019;20:719–27.

26. Lim IIP, Bondoc AJ, Geller JI, et al. Hepatoblastoma-the evolution of biology, surgery, and transplantation. Children (Basel) 2018;6(1):1.

27. Aronson DC, Czauderna P, Maibach R, et al. The treatment of hepatoblastoma: its evolution and the current status as per the SIOPEL trials. J Indian Assoc Pediatr Surg 2014;19(4):201–7.

28. Lovorn HN, Hilmes M, Ayres D, et al. Defining hepatoblastoma responsiveness to neoadjuvant therapy as measured by tumor volume and serum alpha-fetoprotein kinetics. J Pediatr Surg 2010;45:121–8.

29. Lake CM, Tiao GM, Bondoc AJ. Surgical management of locally advanced and metastatic hepatoblastoma. Semin Pediatr Surg 2019;28:150856.

30. Fuchs J, Cavdar S, Blumenstock G, et al. POST-TEXT III and IV hepatoblastoma: extended hepatic resection avoids liver transplantation in selected cases. Ann Surg 2016;266:318–23.

31. Uchida H, Sakamoto S, Sasaki K, et al. Surgical treatment strategy for advanced hepatoblastoma: resection versus transplantation. Pediatr Blood Cancer 2018; 65:e27383.

32. Aronson DC, Weeda VB, Maibach R, et al. Microscopically positive resection margin after hepatoblastoma resection: what is the impact on prognosis? A Childhood Liver Tumors Strategy Group (SIOPEL) report. Eur J Cancer 2019; 106:126–32.

33. Meyers RL, Katzenstein HM, Krailo M, et al. Surgical resection of pulmonary metastatic lesions in hepatoblastoma. J Pediatr Surg 2007;42:2050–6.

34. O'Neill AF, Towbin AJ, Krailo MD, et al. Characterization of pulmonary metastases in children with hepatoblastoma treated on Children's Oncology Group protocol AHEP 0731 (The treatment of children with all stages of hepatoblastoma): a report from the Children's Oncology Group. J Clin Oncol 2017;35:3465–73.

35. Hishiki T, Watanabe K, Ida K, et al. The role of pulmonary metastasectomy for hepatoblastoma in children with metastasis at diagnosis: results from the JPLT-2 study. J Pediatr Surg 2017;52:2051–5.

36. Shi Y, Geller JI, Ma IT, et al. Relapsed hepatoblastoma confined to the lung is effectively treated with pulmonary metastasecotmy. J Pediatr Surg 2016;51(4): 525–9.

37. Kitagawa N, Shinkai M, Mochizuki K, et al. Navigation using indocyanine green fluorescence imaging for hepatoblastoma pulmonary metastases surgery. Pediatr Surg Int 2015;31(4):407–11.

38. Bondoc A, Dasgupta R, Tiao G, et al. ICG navigation Surgery for metastatic Hepatoblastoma. Boston: Abstract American Pediatric Surgical Association; 2019.

39. Lundgren MP, Towbin AJ, Roebuck DJ, et al. Role of interventional radiology in managing pediatric liver tumors part two: percutaneous interventions. Pediatr Radiol 2018;48:555–64.

40. Aguado A, Dunn SP, Averill LW, et al. Successful use of transarterial radioembolization with yttrium-90 (TARE-Y90) in two children with hepatoblastoma. Pediatr Blood Cancer 2020;67(9):e28421.

41. Brock PR, Maibach R, Childs M, et al. Sodium thiosulfate for protection from cisplatin induced hearing loss. N Engl J Med 2018;25:2376–85.

42. Zsiros J, Brugieres L, Brock P, et al. Dose-dense cisplatin-based chemotherapy and surgery for children with high risk hepatoblastoma (SIOPEL 4): a prospective, single-arm, feasibility study. Lancet Oncol 2013;14:834–42.

43. Meyers RL, Malogolowkin MH, Krailo M, et al. Doxorubicin in combination with cisplatin/5-flourouracil/vincristine is feasible and effective in unresectable hepatoblastoma: a report from the Children's Oncology Group (COG) AHEP0731 Study Committee. Presented High Impact Clinical Trials Session, SIOP 2017,Societe Internationale Oncologie Pediatriqe, October 22, 2016, Dublin, Ireland.

44. Katzenstein HM, Furman WL, Malogolowkin MH, et al. Upfront window vincristine/irinotecan treatment of high risk hepatoblastoma: a report from the children's oncology group AHEP 0731 study committee. Cancer 2017;123:2360–7.

45. Hiyama E, Hishiki T, Watanabe K, et al. Outcome and late complications of hepatoblastomas treated using the Japanese Study Group for Pediatric Liver Tumor 2 Protocol. J Clin Oncol 2020;38:2488–98.

46. Prokurat A, Kluge P, Kosciesza A, et al. Transitional liver cell tumors (TLCT) in older children and adolescents: a novel group of aggressive hepatic tumors expressing beta-catenin. Med Pediatr Oncol 2002;39:510–8.
47. Zhou S, Venkatramani R, Gupta S, et al. Hepatocellular malignant neoplasm-not otherwise specified (HEMNOS): a clinicopathological study of 11 cases from a single institution. Histopathology 2017;71:813–22.
48. Armengol C, Cairo S. Identification of theranostic biomarkers to improve the stratification of patients with pediatric liver cancer: opportunities and challenges. Hepatology 2018;68:10–2.
49. Sumazin P, Chen Y, Trevino LR, et al. Genomic analysis of hepatoblastoma identifies distinct molecular and prognostic subgroups. Hepatology 2017;65(1): 104–21.
50. Buendia MA, Armengol C, Cairo S. Molecular classification of hepatoblastoma and prognostic value of the HB 16 gene signature. Hepatology 2017;66:1351–2.
51. Czauderna P, MacKinley G, Perilongo G, et al. Hepatocellular carcinoma in children: results of the first prospective study of the international society of pediatric oncology group. J Clin Oncol 2002;20:2798–804.
52. Murawski M, Weeda VB, Maibach R, et al. Hepatocellular carcinoma in children: does modified platinum-and doxorubicin based chemotherapy increase tumor resectability and change outcome: lessons learned from the SIOPEL 2 and 3 studies. J Clin Oncol 2016;34:1050–6.
53. Weeda VB, Aronson DC, Verheij J, et al. Is hepatocellular carcinoma the same disease in children and adults? Comparison of histology, molecular background, and treatment in pediatric and adult patients. Pediatr Blood Cancer 2019;66:e274–5.
54. Kelly D, Sharif K, Brown RM, et al. Hepatocellular carcinoma in children. Clin Liver Dis 2015;19:433–47.
55. McAteer JP, Goldin AB, Healey PJ, et al. Surgical treatment of primary liver tumors in children: outcomes analysis of resection and transplantation in the SEER database. Pediatr Transpl 2013;17:744–50.
56. De Ville de Goyet J, Meyers RL, Tiao GM, et al. Beyond the Milan criteria for liver transplantation in children with hepatic tumours. Lancet Gastroenterol Hepatol 2017;2:456–62.
57. Ziogas IA, Ye F, Zhao Z, et al. Population-based analysis of hepatocellular carcinoma in children: identifying optimal surgical treatment. J Am Coll Surg 2020; 230:1035–44.
58. Ismail H, Broniszcak D, Kalicinski P, et al. Liver transplant in children with HCC: do Milan criteria apply to pediatric patients? Pediatr Transpl 2009;13:682–92.
59. Schmid I, Haberle B, Albert MH, et al. Sorafanib and cisplatin/doxorubicin (PLADO) in pediatric hepatocellular carcinoma. Pediatr Blood Cancer 2012; 58:539–44.
60. Katzenstein HM, Krailo MD, Malogolowkin MH, et al. Hepatocellular carcinoma in children and adolescents: results from the Pediatric Oncology Group and the Children's Cancer Group Study. J Clin Oncol 2002;29:2980–97.
61. Akinwande O, Kim D, Edwards J, et al. Is radioembolization (90Y) better than doxorubicin drug eluting beads (DEBOX) for hepatocellular carcinoma with portal vein thrombosis? Surg Oncol 2015 Sep;24(3):270–5.
62. Aguado A, Ristagno R, Towbin AJ, et al. Transarterial radioembolization with yttrium-90 of unresectable primary hepatic malignancy in children. Pediatr Blood Cancer 2019;66(7):e27510.

63. Eggert T, McGlynn KA, Duffy A, et al. Fibrolamellar hepatocellular carcinoma in the USA, 2000-2010: a detailed report on frequency, treatment and outcome based on the Surveillance, Epidemiology, and End Results database. United Eur Gastroenterol J 2013;1:351–7.

64. Katzenstein HM, Krailo MD, Malogolowkin MH, et al. Fibrolamellar hepatocellular carcinoma in children and adolescents. Cancer 2003;97:2006–12.

65. Weeda VB, Murawski M, McCabe AJ, et al. Fibrolamellar variant of hepatocellular carcinoma does not have a better survival than conventional hepatocellular carcinoma in children: results and treatment recommendations for the Childhood Liver Tumor Strategy Group (SIOPEL) experience. Eur J Cancer 2013; 49:2698–704.

66. Honeyman JN, Simon EP, Robine N, et al. Detection of a recurrent DNAJB1-PRKACA chimeric transcript in fibrolamellar hepatocellular carcinoma. Science 2014;343(6174):1010–4.

67. Techavichit P, Masand PM, Himes RW, et al. Undifferentiated embryonal sarcoma of the liver (UESL): a single center experience and review of the literature. J Pediatr Hematol Oncol 2016;38(4):261–8.

68. Shi Y, Rojas Y, Zhang W, et al. Characteristics and outcomes in children with undifferentiated embryonal sarcoma of the liver. A report from the National Cancer Database. Pediatr Blood Cancer 2017;64:e26272.

69. Murawski M, Scheer M, Leuschner I, et al. Undifferentiated sarcoma of the liver: multicenter international experience of the cooperative soft-tissue sarcoma group and Polish Paediatric Solid Tumor Group. Pediatr Blood Cancer 2020;e28598. https://doi.org/10.1002/pbc.28598.

70. Shehata BM, Gupta NA, Katzenstein HM, et al. Undifferentiated embryonal sarcoma of the liver is associated with mesenchymal hamartoma and multiple chromosomal abnormalities: a review of eleven cases. Pediatr Dev Pathol 2011; 14(2):111–6.

71. Malkan AD, Fernandez-Pineda I. The evolution of diagnosis and management of pediatric biliary tract rhabdomyosarcoma. Curr Pediatr Rev 2016 Jan 17.

72. Elwahab MA, Hamed H, Shehta A, et al. Hepatobiliary rhabdomyosarcoma mimicking choledochal cyst: lessons learned. Int J Surg Case Rep 2014;5: 196–9.

73. Scottoni F, DeAngelis P, Dall'Oglio L, et al. ERCP with intracholedocal biopsy for the diagnosis of biliary tract rhabdomyosarcoma in children. Pediatr Surg Int 2013;29:659–62.

74. Perruccio K, Cecinati V, Scagnellato A, et al. Biliary tract rhabdomyosarcoma: a report from the soft tissue sarcoma committee of the associazione Italiana Ematologia Oncologia Pediatrica. Tumori 2018;104(3):232–7.

75. Potanos KM, Hodgkinson N, Fullington NM, et al. Long term survival in pediatric hepatic angiosarcoma (PHAS): a case report and review of the literature. J Pediatr Surg Case Rep 2015;3:410–3.

76. Jeng MR, Fuh B, Blatt J, et al. Malignant transformation of infantile hemangioma to angiosarcoma: response to chemotherapy with bevacizumab. Pediatr Blood Cancer 2014;61:2115–7.

77. Grassia KL, Peterman CM, Iacobas I, et al. Clinical case series of pediatric hepatic angiosarcoma. Pediatr Blood Cancer 2017;64. Epub 2017 May 18. PMID: 28521077.

78. Trobaugh-Lotrario AD, Finegold MJ, Feusner JH. Rhabdoid tumors of the liver: rare, aggressive, and poorly responsive to standard cytotoxic chemotherapy. Pediatr Blood Cancer 2011;57:423–8.

79. Brennan B, Stiller C, Bourdeaut F. Extracranial rhabdoid tumors: what we have learned so far and future directions. Lancet Oncol 2013;14(8):e329–36.
80. Eaton KW1, Tooke LS, Wainwright LM, et al. Spectrum of SMARCB1/INI1 mutations in familial and sporadic rhabdoid tumors. Pediatr Blood Cancer 2011; 56:7–15.
81. Cornet M, DeLambert B, Pariente D, et al. Rhabdoid tumor of the liver: report of pediatric cases treated at a single institute. J Pediatr Surg 2018;53:567–71.
82. Oita S, Terui K, Komatsu S, et al. Malignant rhabdoid tumor of the liver: a case report and literature review. Pediatr Rep 2015;7:5578.
83. Rod A, Voicu M, Chiche L, et al. Cushing's syndrome associated with a nested stromal epithelial tumor of the liver: hormonal, immunohistochemical, and molecular studies. Eur J Endocrinol 2009;161:805–10.
84. Weeda VB, DeReuver P, Bras H, et al. Cushing syndrome presenting symptom of calcifying nested stromal epithelial tumor of the liver in an adolescent male: a case report. J Med Case Rep 2016;10:160–3.
85. Liu R, Cox K, Guthery SL, et al. Cholangiocarcinoma and high-grade dysplasia in young patients with primary sclerosing cholangitis. Dig Dis Sci 2014;59(9): 2320–4.
86. Madadi-Sanjani O, Wirth TC, Kuebler JF, et al. Choledochal cyst and malignancy: plea for lifelong followup. Eur J Pediatr Surg 2017. https://doi.org/10. 1055/s0037-1615275.
87. Littooij AS, McHugh K, McCarville MB, et al. Yolk sac tumour: a rare cause of raised serum alpha-foetoprotein in a young child with a large liver mass. Pediatr Radiol 2014;44(1):18–22.
88. Wu CH, Chiu NC, Yeh YC, et al. Uncommon liver tumors: case report and literature review. Medicine 2016;95:e4952.
89. Lu Q, Zhang H, Wang WP, et al. Primary non–Hodgkins lymphoma of the liver: sonographic and CT findings. Hepatobiliary Pancreat Dis Int 2015;14:75–81.
90. Iacobas I, Phung TL, Adams DM, et al. Guidance document for hepatic hemangioma (infantile and congenital) evaluation and monitoring. J Pediatr 2018;203: 294–300.e2.
91. Hoeger P, Harper J, Baselga E, et al. Treatment of infantile haemangiomas: recommendations of a European expert group. Eur J Pediatr 2015;174:855–65.
92. Ma IT, Rojas Y, Masand PM, et al. Focal nodular hyperplasia in children. J Pediatr Surg 2015;50:382–7.
93. Towbin AJ, Luo GG, Yin H, et al. Focal nodular hyperplasia in children, adolescents, and young adults. Pediatr Radiol 2011;41:341–9.
94. Valentino PL, Ling SC, Ng VL, et al. The role of diagnostic imaging and liver biopsy in the diagnosis of focal nodular hyperplasia in children. Liver Int 2014; 34(2):227–34.
95. Stringer MD, Alizai NK. Mesenchymal hamartoma of the liver: a systematic review. J Pediatr Surg 2005;40:1681–90.
96. Wildhaber B, Montaruli E, Guerin F, et al. Mesenchymal hamartoma or embryonal sarcoma of the liver in childhood: a difficult diagnosis before complete surgical excision. J Pediatr Surg 2014;49:1372–7.
97. Abrahao-Machado L, de Macedo F, Dalence C, et al. Mesenchymal hamartoma of the liver in an infant with Beckwith-Wiedemann syndrome: a rare condition mimicking hepatoblastoma. ACG Case Rep J 2015;2:258–60.
98. Mathews J, Duncavage E, Pfeifer J. Characterization of translocation in mesenchymal hamartoma and undifferentiated embryonal sarcoma of the liver. Exp Mol Pathol 2013;95:319–24.

99. Chiorean L, Cui XW, Tannapfel A, et al. Benign liver tumors in pediatric patients: review with emphasis on imaging features. World J Gastroenterol 2015;21: 8541–61.

100. Raft MD, Jorgensen EN, Vainer B. Gene mutations in hepatocellular adenomas. Histopathology 2015;66:910–21.

101. Liau SS, Qureshi MS, Prasseedom R, et al. Molecular pathogenesis of hepatic adenomas and its implications for surgical management. J Gastrointest Surg 2013;17(10):1869–82.

102. Durmus T, Kamphues C, Blaeker H, et al. Inflammatory myofibroblastic tumor of the liver mimicking an infiltrative malignancy in computed tomography and magnetic resonance imaging with Gd-EOB. Acta Radiol Short Rep 2014;3(7). 2047981614544404.

103. Karlo C, Leschka S, Dettmer M, et al. Hepatic teratoma and peritoneal gliomatosis: a case report. Cases J 2009;2:9302.

104. Hasebe T, Sakamoto M, Mukai K, et al. Cholangiocarcinoma arising in bile duct adenoma with focal area of bile duct hamartoma. Virchows Arch 1995;426: 209–13.

105. Citak EC, Karadenia C, Oquz A, et al. Nodular regenerative hyperplasia and focal nodular hyperplasia of the liver mimicking hepatic metastasis in children with solid tumors and a review of the literature. Pediatr Hematol Oncol 2007; 24:281–9.

106. Ortega JA, Douglass EC, Feusner JH, et al. Randomized comparison of cisplatin/vincristine/5-fluorouracil and cisplatin/doxorubicin for the treatment of pediatric hepatoblastoma (HB): a report from the Children's Cancer Group and the Pediatric Oncology Group. J Clin Oncol 2000;18:2665–75.

Management of Adrenal Tumors in Pediatric Patients

Simone de Campos Vieira Abib, MD, PhD[a], Christopher B. Weldon, MD, PhD[b],*

KEYWORDS

- Pediatric • Adrenal • Neoplasm • Cancer • Tumor • Child

KEY POINTS

- Adrenal tumors in children can be benign, malignant, or pseudotumors.
- Adrenal tumors are considered rare, frequently have a genetic underpinning, and are often hormone producing.
- Diagnostic algorithms depend on history, physical findings, biochemical testing, and radiologic analyses.
- Regardless of tumor type, surgery plays an essential role in their treatment, and surgical principles should be followed in order to avoid complications and contribute to better cure and survival rates.
- Ongoing surveillance after treatment is mandated in almost all cases.

INTRODUCTION

Adrenal tumors in children are caused by a wide variety of conditions and may be diagnosed from the fetal stage onwards.[1–4] From an embryologic perspective, the adrenal fetal cortex and medulla are formed by 7 weeks' gestation. The cortex comes from the mesoderm, whereas the medulla is derived from the ectoderm/neural crest. As such, adrenal tumors identified within the gland have different histopathologic origins and resultant symptoms. Neoplasms of the adrenal gland are classified and discussed here in an anatomic framework.

PRIMARY TUMORS
Cortex

Adrenocortical tumors (ACTs) are rare but aggressive endocrine neoplasms when carcinomas, comprising 0.2% of all pediatric malignancies.[5] Only 10% to 20% of pediatric cases are benign adenomas. The estimated worldwide incidence is about 0.3 new cases per million individuals per year.[6] However, in the south and southeast regions of

a Federal University of São Paulo (UNIFESP) – Paulista School of Medicine, Pediatric Oncology Institute – GRAACC/UNIFESP; b Departments of Surgery, Anesthesiology, & Pediatric Oncology, Boston Children's Hospital, Dana-Farber Cancer Institute, Harvard Medical School, 300 Longwood Ave, Fegan 3, Boston, MA 02115, USA
* Corresponding author.
E-mail address: Christopher.weldon@childrens.harvard.edu

Surg Oncol Clin N Am 30 (2021) 275–290
https://doi.org/10.1016/j.soc.2020.11.012
surgonc.theclinics.com

Brazil, ACT incidence rates are 15 to 20 times higher than those described in other countries. This ACT cluster in Brazil is caused by the presence of a founder TP53 mutation in this population.[7,8] Germline TP53 mutations are present in more than 80% of ACTs in children, and they underlie signaling abnormalities that are strongly associated with ACT. ACTs are also the most frequent neoplasms identified in families afflicted with Li-Fraumeni syndrome. De novo TP53 mutations are also observed, and relatives of children with ACT may have a higher incidence of cancer.[9] In North American children, the spectrum of germline TP53 mutations and the mechanisms and types of functional loss of heterozygosity in ACT are diverse, although germline mutations occur primarily in the TP53 DNA-binding domains (exons 4–8).[9] By contrast, in the Brazilian cases, the patients' families do not have a high incidence of cancer, and a single mutation in exon 10 of the TP53 gene is consistently observed.[9] The penetrance of this mutation is low (only 10%–15% of carriers develop ACT), and it seems not to predispose carriers to other malignancies later in life.[9] Therefore, additional genetic alterations may be necessary for malignant transformation. The early age of onset and the distinctive clinical features of childhood ACT suggest that they arise in the fetal zone of the adrenal cortex.[9] The fetal zone occupies 85% of the adrenal cortex during embryonic development and is oriented toward dehydroepiandrosterone production. A constitutional TP53 mutation may increase the risk of neoplastic transformation in the fetal adrenal cortex but not in the definitive adrenal cortex. The adrenal cortex is composed of 3 functional areas, defined as the glomerulosa, reticularis, and fasciculata zones. Complete differentiation of these areas occurs by the age of 3 years. Tumors can arise from all 3 zones, be benign (adenoma) or malignant (adenocarcinoma), and be hormone secreting. Neoplasms arising from the adrenal cortex are predominantly hormone secreting and can express mixed patterns of hormone production, which is explained by the embryologic zones of origin (aldosterone, granulosa; glucocorticoids, fasciculata; reticular, glucocorticoids and sex hormones). As such, ACT may present with virilization (precocious puberty, deepening voice, pubic and axillary hair, acne, genital growth), Cushing syndrome (hypertension, central obesity, buffalo pump, moon face, stretch marks), signs of hyperaldosteronism, or may be asymptomatic depending on the quantity of hormone produced. Because hormone-related symptoms generally are readily apparent, most patients in these situations have small, nonpalpable adrenal masses.

Therefore, the diagnosis of ACT is generally straightforward. Clinical presentation includes virilization and hypertension, and surgeons must be aware of the disease in order to make an early diagnosis. Because most patients have an endocrine syndrome, increased blood or urine concentrations of adrenocortical hormones and a suprarenal mass usually suggest a preoperative diagnosis of ACT. Imaging studies are necessary for adequate staging and surgery planning. Magnetic resonance (MR) and computed tomography (CT) of the primary site are necessary to detect invasion of adjacent structures, lymph node enlargement, and tumor thrombus in the venous drainage, all of which may require resection during the curative procedure. The tumors characteristically have a thin pseudocapsule and areas of calcification and necrosis. Vascular extension occurs in 20% of cases, and patients should be examined for intracaval tumor thrombus.[10] Some cases are diagnosed incidentally by imaging studies performed for other purposes. Distant metastases usually involve the liver, lungs, kidneys, and bone, and, hence, dedicated radiologic studies are required to evaluate these anatomic areas. In general, PET with concurrent diagnostic CT is warranted for evaluating for distant metastases.

The need for tumor biopsy is not indicated unless there is a question of the diagnosis or if the tumor is unresectable. Hence, surgical dictum recommends primary resection to prevent unnecessary tumor rupture, complete tumor staging with concurrent ipsilateral lymph node dissection, and tumor extirpation to control the overproduction of hormones. Hence, the authors strongly recommend that surgical excision should be done upfront whenever possible and that biopsies should be avoided.

Surgery is the only curative treatment modality in ACT, and, as such, it is the cornerstone of treatment. The goal in all cases is complete resection, including en bloc (partial) removal of adjacent organs if needed to achieve negative margins. The driving force behind this recommendation is the fact that patients with microscopic or macroscopic residual disease or metastatic disease have a dismal prognosis (**Fig. 1**). Before surgery, it is essential that the patients are properly prepared to avoid adrenal insufficiency in the perioperative period. As such, corticosteroids directed to both glucocorticoid and mineralocorticoid function are mandated. The reason for this recommendation is that, with the abrupt decrease in hormone production with surgical resection of the ipsilateral tumor (and if the adrenalytic agent mitotane is used in the adjuvant setting), the need for steroid supplementation in the perioperative and postoperative settings is absolute.

Meticulous and precise surgical technique is advised in all patients having resection of ACT and should include a complete discussion with the patient. A major concern is inadvertent tumor spillage because it increases the rate of recurrence and worsens prognosis by upstaging the patient and increasing therapy in the adjuvant setting, as shown in **Fig. 1**.

Known anatomic considerations and concerns need to be well understood and acknowledged by the surgeon too, because these issues can increase the risk of rupture.[11] ACT can present with a very thin capsule and be composed of gelatinous contents from intratumoral necrosis, which may also increase the risk of rupture and must be taken into account by the surgeon (**Figs. 2 and 3**A and B).

The decision on the type of surgery (open or closed) to perform in ACT is surgeon and case dependent. For smaller lesions, those with benign characteristics, those relegated to the gland, and in those without concern for spill, a closed or minimally

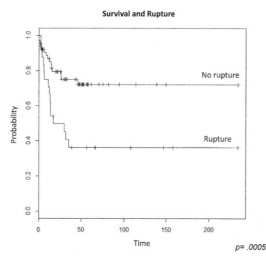

Fig. 1. Brazilian Pediatric ACT Cohort showing impact of tumor rupture on survival. Data analyzed on 151 Brazilian children diagnosed with ACT showed a statistically significant ($P<.0005$) reduction in survival when tumors were ruptured at surgery.

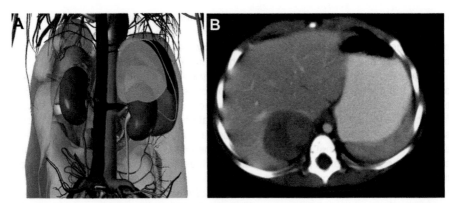

Fig. 2. Anatomic position of the right adrenal gland and the liver (*A*) and CT (*B*) showing the posterior view of the interface of the right adrenal gland with the liver with the right adrenal firmly adherent to the liver by fibrous union of the capsules, making it easier for the tumor rupture to occur.

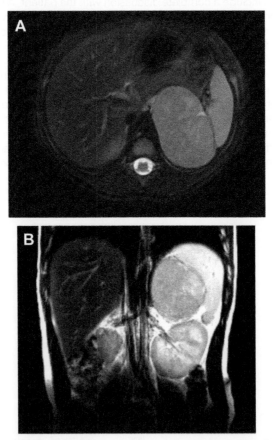

Fig. 3. Imaging comparison of 2 different ACT tumor consistencies. Radiologic comparison between 2 different tumor consistencies with the upper axial and coronal MRI (*A*) showing a homogeneous and solid lesion, whereas the lower images (*B*) shows a heterogeneous pattern and likely tenuous tissue consistency more prone to rupture.

invasive approach can be considered. The pros and cons of open and minimally invasive access (minimally invasive surgery [MIS]) are well known, but the surgeon must keep in mind that patients with ACT have inferior outcomes with higher relapse rates after MIS approaches, especially in large tumors. Thus, although feasible and tempting in many cases, the authors strongly recommend that laparoscopic resections should be carefully considered and performed in pediatric ACT in centers with experienced surgeons, high case volumes, and in patients with small tumors.

In larger tumors, tumors invading other organs, concern for intraoperative tumor rupture or spill, and tumors expected to be malignant ACT regardless of size and any sign of vascular involvement, an open approach should be prioritized. The open surgical approach can be done by laparotomy or a thoracoabdominal approach. A thoracoabdominal approach (**Fig. 4**) is recommended to decrease the risk of rupture and hemorrhage by widely opening the involved operative field and allowing access to the posterior structures of the retroperitoneum and body wall where perforation may be likely to occur, especially the large tumors that grow behind the liver. This approach is recommended for small tumors in this site as well, because the adrenal and liver capsules may be densely adherent and rupture can easily occur. Self-retaining liver retractors can be important tools to facilitate access and extirpation. In order to reach the adrenal glands, the surgeon must perform an ipsilateral (possibly bilateral) medial visceral rotation maneuver to mobilize the associated adjacent and overlying structures (surgeons also need to be able to mobilize the liver and the left and right triangular, falciform, and caudate ligaments) fully as well, so as to gain access to the right (or even left) adrenal gland. These maneuvers also allow access to the aorta, the vena cava, and their branches so as to achieve vascular control if required.

However, regardless of the technique used for the resection, the surgeon must be able to perform an ipsilateral retroperitoneal lymph node dissection (RPLND) as well for proper and complete staging of these tumors. Evidence of lymph node metastases (radiographically occult or not) upstages patients and intensifies adjuvant therapy. Because RPLND is a standard oncological principle, a careful understanding of the anatomic boundaries for this procedure need to be recognized and acted on. An RPLND should be performed to ensure adequate histopathologic staging. The lymphatic drainage of the adrenal gland includes the lymph node basins of the ipsilateral suprarenal space, kidney, and periaortic and paracaval regions, and these regions

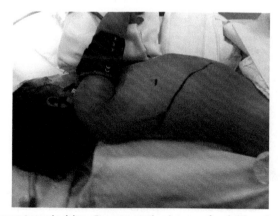

Fig. 4. Thoracolaparotomy incision. Representative image of a child undergoing open right adrenalectomy via a thoracolaparotomy incision.

should be included in a dissection. In order to determine the necessity of an RPLND as a formal component of treatment, the recently completed Children's Oncology Group (COG) ARAR0332 prospective trial is attempting to evaluate the necessity and results of RPLND in low-stage ACT. However, preliminary results have been inconclusive.[12]

Vascular extension is another surgical issue in ACT, because it is related to very poor prognosis and changes the surgical strategy considerably.[10] In some cases, cardiac bypass may be needed to achieve complete resection in those cases where the tumor thrombus ascends the vena cava to the level of the hepatic veins or more cephalad into the right atrium. It is important to evaluate this condition preoperatively with dedicated vascular imaging to assess the extent of the tumor thrombus. The tumor thrombus of ACT is also distinctive (**Fig. 5**), and **Table 1** outlines the qualitative differences between tumor thromboses in nephroblastoma and ACT. Considering the difficulties in resection that these features add, surgeons must be prepared to deal with these risks.

The benefit of primary tumor resection or debulking in general is yet to be defined in pediatric patients with metastatic ACT. In some cases, it may be indicated because of refractory hypertension and/or to relieve other symptoms of hormone overproduction. Aggressive locoregional debulking, including peritonectomy and metastasectomy, alone or in combination with hyperthermic intraperitoneal chemotherapy (HIPEC), is another consideration, but adequate data are lacking. Furthermore, pulmonary metastasectomy has been reported to have benefit, but the exact indications and in which patients (especially in children) have not been defined.[13]

Pathologically, small tumors can behave aggressively, suggesting that more specific prognostic factors should be considered other than simply tumor size. On histology, ACTs are classified as adenoma, indeterminate, or carcinoma.[14] Adenomas are associated with excellent prognosis because they are benign, but only about 20% of pediatric ACTs are classified as such.[9] However, the distinction between adenoma and carcinoma histopathologically is difficult,[15–18] and many times tumors are considered of indeterminate histology. If there is evidence of metastases and/or recurrence, then a diagnosis of carcinoma is obvious. To better define the malignant potential of ACT, a study is needed to quantitate markers of angiogenesis and lymphangiogenesis in ACT and controls.[19,20] From the angiogenic perspective, combined levels of vascular endothelial growth factor, endoglin, intratumoral microvessel density (MVD), and cluster of differentiation 34 (CD34) MVD were better able to predict prognosis in patients with indeterminate tumor histology. Inclusion of these components in the pathologic analysis of ACT may refine the classification in pediatric ACT.[19] No association was noted

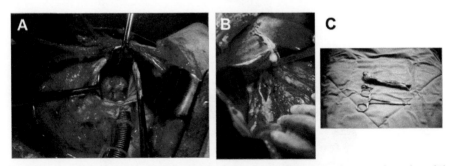

Fig. 5. Tumor thrombus in ACT and nephroblastoma. (*A–C*) Intracaval tumor thrombus. (*A*) The ACT tumor thrombus is a distinct mass and friable, whereas in nephroblastoma it is a plaquelike lesion adherent to the vessel wall. (*B*) Nephroblastoma in vivo, cavotomy; (*C*) ex vivo.

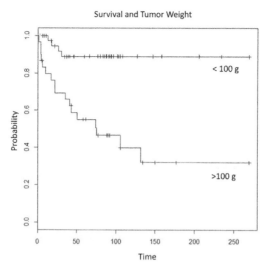

Survival and Tumor Weight

< 100 g

>100 g

Fig. 6. Brazilian Pediatric ACT Cohort showing impact of tumor weight on survival. Data analyzed on 151 Brazilian children diagnosed with ACT showed a statistically significant (*P* = .004) reduction in survival with larger tumors.

between positive lymph nodes and relapsed disease. In contrast, the lymphatic vessel density was inversely associated with local relapse, indicating that pediatric adrenocortical carcinoma (ACC) may not disseminate through lymphatic vessels.[20]

Staging of ACT combines several components, including tumor size (**Fig. 6**), evidence of local-regional extra-adrenal disease, and metastases. Complete staging necessitates both radiologic and anatomic considerations. An ACT staging system[21] used in the most recent COG ARAR0332 is provided in **Table 2**. At present, tumor size and disease stage remain the primary prognostic factors of this disease,[15–18,21] because other prognostic factors have not been firmly established for pediatric ACT.

Based on staging, the treatment proposed by the recently completed COG ARAR0332 protocol is shown in **Table 3**. Multimodal therapies are recommended, including surgery, cytotoxic chemotherapy, and the primary adrenalytic agent

Table 1
Qualitative differences between tumor thromboses in nephroblastoma and adrenocortical tumors

	WT Thrombus	ACT Thrombus
Consistency	Firm	Friable
Thrombus Regression	Possible	Unlikely
Stage	No change	Changes staging (spillage)
Oncological Prognosis	No change	Very poor
Constitution (Viable Tumor Cells)	Skeleton with/without tumor cells	Tumor cells
Embolism	Possible	Likely
Surgical Complications	Rare	More often

Abbreviation: WT, wilms tumor (nephroblastoma).

Table 2
Adrenocortical tumor staging per Children's Oncology Group ARAR0332

Stage	Definition
I	Completely resected, small tumors (<100 g and <200 cm³), with normal postoperative hormone levels
II	Completely resected, large tumors (>100 g and >200 cm³), with normal postoperative hormone levels
III	Unresectable gross or microscopic disease Tumor spillage Patients with stage I and II tumors who fail to normalize hormone levels after surgery Patients with lymph node involvement
IV	Presence of distant metastases

mitotane. Outcomes for children with malignant stage I ACT are excellent with surgery only.[9,12] However, failure rates for patients with localized large tumors (stage II) remain high after surgery. Hence, systemic therapy should be considered for this group of patients after careful multidisciplinary review. Patients with stage III ACC have an acceptable outcome combining surgery and standard chemotherapy regimens. Unfortunately, patients with stage IV ACT continue to have poor outcomes and new treatments need to be developed for this high-risk group (**Fig. 7**). The combination of mitotane and chemotherapy as prescribed in COG ARAR0332 resulted in significant toxicity in an initial review, with one-third of patients being unable to complete the scheduled treatment.[12]

Treatment in high-volume specialized centers is advised because of the complex nature of this tumor. The authors recommend enrollment of children with ACT in clinical trials and research studies directed at the delineation of ACT biology and genetic profiles so as to guide future treatment initiatives.

Medulla

Pheochromocytoma(Pheo)/paraganglioma (PGL) (PP) are a constellation of neuroendocrine tumors defined by their anatomic location (adrenal vs extra-adrenal) and that trace their common cell of origin to the catecholamine-secreting enterochromaffin cell. These tumors originate in either the adrenal gland (Pheo) or in extra-adrenal organs (PGL) such as the sympathetic ganglia, carotid body, organ of Zuckerkandl, bladder,

Table 3
Treatment by adrenocortical tumor stage per Children's Oncology Group ARAR0332

Stage	Treatment
I	Surgery alone
II	Surgery + RPLND
III	Mitotane CDDP/ETO/DOX Surgery + RPLND
IV	Mitotane CDDP/ETO/DOX Surgery + RPLND

Abbreviations: CDDP, cisplatin; DOX, doxorubicin; ETO, etoposide.

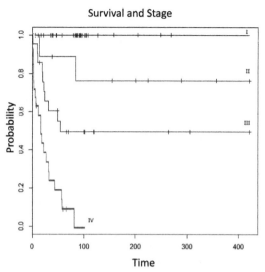

Fig. 7. Brazilian Pediatric ACT Cohort showing impact of tumor stage on survival. Data analyzed on 151 Brazilian children diagnosed with ACT showed a statistically significant ($P = .0174$) reduction in survival with increasing tumor stage.

or other locations as classified by the World Health Organization in 2017.[22] Some 85% are found in the adrenal medulla, and extrarenal sites account for the remainder.[23] They can also be sympathetic or parasympathetic, with the latter group being identified in the head and cervical regions primarily and being biochemically silent.[24] PP are rare, with an incidence of 0.6 per 100,000 person-years,[25] with approximately 10% occurring in children younger than 14 years, male individuals being affected at twice the rate as female, and extra-adrenal sites accounting for up to one-third of all pediatric cases.[26–29]

Regardless of the epidemiologic observations in these tumors, their genetic origins are traced to some 20 germline and/or somatic mutations that drive their oncogenesis in 3 distinct pathways: pseudohypoxic, kinase dependent, and Wnt-signaling clusters.[30] The pseudohypoxic pathway interferes with the normal regulation of hypoxia-inducible factor (HIF) signaling, whereby hypoxia is not the prime driver of the molecular events, but other components of the cellular milieu that mimic an oxygen-starved state. The genetic mutations found in this cohort include hypoxia-inducible factor 2-alpha (*HIF2a*), von Hippel-Lindau tumor suppressor (*vHL* [von Hippel-Lindau syndrome]), and Krebs cycle pathway components (eg, succinyl dehydrogenase [Carney triad, Carney-Stratakis syndrome], fumarate hydratase, malate dehydrogenase 2.) The kinase-dependent cluster involves the dysregulation of the phosphoinositide 3-kinase (PI3K)/mammalian target of rapamycin (mTOR) cell survival pathway by inducing cell growth and subverting apoptotic regulation via a mitogen-activated protein kinase (MAPK)–dependent mechanism via mutations in *RET*, *NF1* (neurofibromatosis 1 syndrome), *H-RAS*, *K-RAS*, *MAX*, *ATRX*, and several others. The Wnt group of mutations includes *MAML3* and *CSDE1*, which exploit the processes of cell development, motility, and differentiation to promote cell growth and tumorigenesis. No matter the selective genetic perturbation involved, these 3 common pathways serve as a foundation for both diagnostic and therapeutic interventions with significant clinical impact regardless of age or clinical presentation.

Patient presentation can span the spectrum from incidentally found lesions in asymptomatic children to expected masses identified in genetically predisposed patients. Symptoms can include some combination of sweating, pallor, nausea, flushing, anxiety, weight loss/failure to thrive, headaches, dizziness, and/or urinary symptoms (proteinuria, hematuria, polyuria), but there is no one pattern or symptom identified as dominant save sustained hypertension, which is found in most.[28] However, adults have a classic pattern of paroxysmal hypertension that is not found in children.[24] These symptoms are secondary to catecholamine excess, and, depending on the organ in which the tumor arises, the biochemical profile is different. Only in the adrenal medulla can norepinephrine be converted to the epinephrine secondary to the action of phenylethanolamine N-methyltransferase (PNMT),[31] and, as such, identification of increased levels of epinephrine (or its metabolites) in the serum and urine indicate an adrenal origin of the tumor. In contradistinction, isolated, increased levels of epinephrine's precursors (norepinephrine and especially dopamine)indicate an extra-adrenal origin. However, dopaminergic tumors are generally physiologically silent, and hence they may grow unnoticed until physical signs or symptoms develop secondary to mass effect on adjacent structures.[32]

PP diagnosis begins with a thorough history and physical examination focusing on the symptoms. Documenting each symptom's severity, change over time, and duration is critical to establish a differential diagnosis. A complete examination (including serial vital sign measurements) is critical to identify subtle findings (papilledema, bruits, or subtle fullness) that may be present but overlooked in the setting of more obvious issues, such as hypertension and hematuria. Baseline laboratory testing is warranted, including urinary and plasma free metanephrines (metanephrine and nor-metanephrine),[33] methoxytyramine (for dopaminergic tumors),[32] and chromogranin A levels (especially with succinate dehydrogenase [SDH]–deficient tumors and tumor syndromes).[34] The degree of increase in some of these values can also be diagnostically significant; there are reports of levels of plasma free and urine metabolites greater than 4-fold greater than baseline being highly suggestive of a lesion.[35] Imaging begins with dedicated plain radiographs of the involved area of concern, in addition to dedicated ultrasonography. Identification of masses or lesions in specific locations is both possible and probable depending on the anatomic location of the mass (paraspinous, adrenal, cervical, and so forth), in addition to identifying other organ involvement (liver, lung, lymph nodes, and so forth). If ultrasonography or plain radiographs identify a suspected mass, or if there is a high index of suspicion, then a dedicated CT or MR study can be undertaken. MR and CT have both shown a high sensitivity for identifying these tumors (90%),[36] but MRI is the preferred modality in children secondary to absence of ionizing radiation and risk of second malignancies.[37] Even in children with a known genetic predisposition syndrome (NF1, vHL, SDH mutations) who may undergo surveillance via whole-body MR to identify occult tumors at regular intervals, a dedicated MR scan of the involved area of concern is likely to be needed to better characterize the tumor. PP can also be characterized and identified by various nuclear medicine studies (alone or in conjunction with MR or CT), including PET scanning with various moieties (fluorodopamine, fluorodeoxyglucose), ^{123}I-MIBG (meta-iodobenzyl-guanidine), or DOTA (dodecane tetraacetic acid) peptides. These nuclear medicine studies can identify the focal lesion in question, in addition to metastatic foci.

Treatment of PP, once identified, is surgery in almost all cases. Before any anesthetic, patients require the combined care of providers who understand the metabolic demands and hormonal effects of PP. Coordination between surgeon, endocrinologist, oncologist, and anesthesiologist is critical to appropriately initiate and escalate perioperative blockade before surgery. Preoperative assessment with an electrocardiogram and echocardiogram is also important to show any effects on the heart (ventricular hypertrophy, conduction abnormalities) from long-standing tachycardia and hypertension.[38] The following protocol is used at this author's (C.B.W.) institution and has been found to be effective; however, there are many different drugs available. As such, the following discussion is simply one reference, and any institution of a treatment plan must include a multidisciplinary team well versed in these drugs because they can have profound sequelae if not managed properly. A goal reduction in the patient's blood pressure to less than 50% of expected for height, weight, and age is generally a recommend goal.[24] The optimization period begins with hyperhydration (1.5 times maintenance of fluid intake per day) and a high-salt diet (6–10 g/d) so as to assist in the prevention of postural hypotension in the setting of alpha blockade. Once fluid and dietary modifications have been established for 24 to 48 hours, alpha blockade is begun. Although many agents may be used, twice-daily doxazosin beginning at 1 mg per dose and escalated by 0.5 mg per dose per day over the course of a week to the point of development of orthostasis has proved to be effective, as previously reported.[28] Once postural hypotension is documented, assessment of the resting heart rate must occur, and the patient must be cautioned regarding sudden positional changes that may result in dizziness and subsequent inadvertent traumatic injury from falling. Beta blockade is initiated roughly 24 hours after optimal alpha blockade has been established, and ideally within 3 days of the proposed surgery date. A beta-1 selective agent (atenolol) is used, and a standing dosage established (0.5 mg/kg/d divided twice daily) and escalated (1 mg/kg/d) to keep the heart rate less than 100beats/min.[39] Approximately 24 hours before surgery, the child is admitted, begun on 1.5 times maintenance of 0.9% normal saline, while continuing all previously described components. If for any reason the blockade is not thought to be adequate, then careful escalation can be performed under the medical providers' care, possibly requiring admission to the intensive care unit. During surgery, parenteral alpha-antagonists and beta-antagonists are commenced using short-acting formulations and agents, in addition to having alpha-agonists and beta-agonists also available to support the patient with profound hypotension once the baseline circulating catecholamine production has ceased on tumor extirpation. These hypertensive medications (norepinephrine, epinephrine continuous infusions) may be required days to weeks postoperatively, and these patients require careful and ongoing observation and management in the immediate and longer-term perioperative periods secondary to the risk of cardiovascular and neurovascular sequelae.[40]

Whether attempted by open or closed techniques, the surgical principles are the same: complete extirpation of the tumor without damage to surrounding structures and assessment for any evidence of regional disease if indicated by preoperative evaluation or intraoperative assessment. Details regarding the nuances and technical steps for an open adrenalectomy are discussed earlier in this article. For a minimally invasive approach, appropriate port placement is critical. In general, 4 ports are required, with 2 being used by the surgeon to perform the dissection and resection, whereas the other 2 are used by the assistant to retract adjacent organs (liver, spleen, stomach, bowel) and operate the camera (transumbilical port site) (**Fig. 8**). These 4 ports are generally placed around the umbilicus, but they may be positioned anywhere on the anterior abdominal wall per surgeon's preference. Whether the patient is placed supine or on a small, ipsilateral flank roll is also a surgeon-specific decision. Furthermore, care should be taken to carefully and deliberately ligate (sutures, clips, fulguration, or a combination of techniques depending on the size of the vessel) the adrenal vein before extensive gland manipulation or dissection if possible, so as to minimize the uncontrolled release of catecholamines intraoperatively. For smaller tumors, bilateral tumors, or unilateral tumors

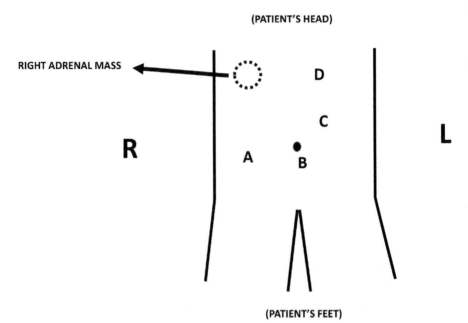

Fig. 8. Port placement for right adrenalectomy. The patient has a right adrenal mass, and the proposed port placement locations are shown for the primary surgeon (A and C) and the assistant (B). D, transumbilical port.

in children with known genetic predisposition syndromes where partial, cortical-sparing adrenalectomies are required when feasible, or if there is a question about the exact location of the mass within the adrenal and to ensure the mass is completely resected, intraoperative ultrasonography is an excellent adjuvant to define the anatomy and associated structures The results with this technique are excellent, with documented shorter operative times, less pain in the postoperative period, and a decreased length of stay in the hospital compared with open procedures.[41,42]

Treatment of nonmetastatic PP postoperatively requires primarily surveillance only, especially in patients with genetic predisposition syndromes who may develop other PP elsewhere over the course of time. Furthermore, any patient with a PP may have recurrence and/or metachronous metastases.[43,44] This surveillance is generally a combination of examinations, laboratory testing (urine and plasma catecholamine metabolites, chromogranin A levels, methoxytyramine levels) and radiological evaluations (whole-body MRI). There is no one regimen accepted or proposed in all cases, but those patients with genetic predisposition syndromes require lifelong surveillance.[27] Those nonsyndromic children require 10 years of observation postprocedure.[45]

The determination of malignancy in this disease cannot be made histopathologically despite several attempts to identify negative prognostic factors.[15,46,47] The definitive means of determining malignancy in PP is evidence of non–neural crest cell disease deposits, and malignancy is only identified in a minority (10%) of cases.[48] Treatment in metastatic PP involves a combination of catecholamine-induced symptom control, tumor debulking/destruction (surgical, percutaneous image guided, or both), cytotoxic chemotherapy, and radiopharmaceutical interventions.[49] When adjuvant therapies are required, referral to a dedicated, multidisciplinary care team is recommended.

PSEUDOTUMORS, MIMICS, AND THE UNEXPECTED

The adrenal gland is anatomically nestled in the retroperitoneum adjacent to and surrounded by several other organs from which tumors may arise and cause confusion about the origin of the neoplasm.[50] The kidney, pancreas, spleen, liver, stomach, sympathetic chain (schwannoma, paraganglioma, neuroblastic tumors, neurofibroma), and even the peritoneum (primary peritoneal cysts, inflammatory myofibroblastic tumors) and retroperitoneum (germ cell tumors, sarcomas [Ewing, liposarcoma, leiomyosarcoma], lymphomas, lipomas, fibrous tumors, echinococcus cysts, granulomatosis, xanthomatosis) may all serve as the originating organ from which a tumor may arise that compresses or interferes with identifying the adrenal gland as an uninvolved adjacent organ.[50–52]

In addition, a word of caution is needed when lesions are found incidentally antenatally or postnatally in any pediatric patient or any age. Clinicians must account for the identified lesion possibly being a focus of an ectopic organ from disordered embryogenesis (lung [pulmonary sequestrations, bronchogenic cysts], enteric duplications),[53] inborn errors of adrenal hormone synthesis (congenital adrenal hyperplasia),[54] or an adrenal hemorrhage[55] in evolution. These masses may be cystic, solid, or both, may be bilateral, may have characteristic echo or cross-sectional imaging features, and/or may have expected vascular inflow and outflow patterns that may help with the diagnosis. Hence, age may serve as a necessary component in the construction of a diagnostic algorithm.

SUMMARY

Pediatric adrenal neoplasms, although rare, span a broad differential from pseudotumors to frank malignancies. Considering the bivariate embryogenesis of the organ and its anatomic location, careful, multimodality diagnostic plans must be enacted to ensure the proper course of therapy is undertaken. Surgery is invariably required for both treatment of the benign entities and cure of the malignant tumors, and these children generally require fastidious and ongoing surveillance.

ACKNOWLEDGMENTS

The authors would like to recognize the following clinicians who provided valuable information and data in the construction of **Figs. 1**, **6**, and **7** representing the Brazilian Cohort of pediatric ACT. They are Eliana Caran, Fernanda Souza, Alexandre Alberto Barros Duarte, Denise Bousfield da Silva, José Antônio de Souza, Walberto de Azevedo Souza Júnior, Rodrigo Chaves Ribeiro, Vilani Kremer, Carmem M.C. M Fiori, Augusto del Arcos Carneiro Francisco, Lauro José Gregianin, Ísis Quezado, Acimar Gonçalves, Melissa Ferreira Macedo, Maurício Macedo, Ângela Rech Cagol, Eduardo Araujo, Ana Helena Dutra, and Carolina Prieto.

DISCLOSURE

The authors have no disclosures to make of any kind.

CLINICS CARE POINTS

- As these tumors frequently produce hormones, careful biochemical evaluation and chemical manipulation and/or supplementation may be required in the preoperative, perioperative or postoperative periods.

- Adrenal tumors in children can be benign or malignant and hormone-secreting or not. Although adrenal tumors are considered rare, it is of essence to perform the right diagnosis to guide treatment.
- Adrenocortical tumors are more common in the Southeast of Brazil.
- Surgical principles for each type of tumor should be followed in order to avoid complications and contribute to better cure and survival rates.

REFERENCES

1. Carsote M, Ghemigian A, Terzea D, et al. Cystic adrenal lesions: focus on pediatric population (a review). Clujul Med 2017;90(1):5–12.
2. Słapa RZ, Jakubowski WS, Dobruch-Sobczak K, et al. Standards of ultrasound imaging of the adrenal glands. J Ultrason 2015;15(63):377–87.
3. Quinn E, McGee R, Nuccio R, et al. Genetic predisposition to neonatal tumors. Curr Pediatr Rev 2015;11(3):164–78.
4. Baudin E. Endocrine tumor board of gustave roussy. Adrenocortical carcinoma. Endocrinol Metab Clin North Am 2015;44(2):411–34.
5. Liou LS, Kay R. Adrenocortical carcinoma in children. Review and recent innovations. Urol Clin North Am 2000;27(3):403–21.
6. Ribeiro RC, Michalkiewicz EL, Figueiredo BC, et al. Adrenocortical tumors in children. Braz J Med Biol Res 2000;33(10):1225–34.
7. Ribeiro RC, Sandrini F, Figueiredo B, et al. An inherited p53 mutation that contributes in a tissue-specific manner to pediatric adrenal cortical carcinoma. Proc Natl Acad Sci U S A 2001;98(16):9330–5.
8. Pinto EM, Billerbeck AEC, Villares MCBF, et al. Founder effect for the highly prevalent R337H mutation of tumor suppressor p53 in Brazilian patients with adrenocortical tumors. Arq Bras Endocrinol Metabol 2004;48(5):647–50.
9. Rodriguez-Galindo C, Figueiredo BC, Zambetti GP, et al. Biology, clinical characteristics, and management of adrenocortical tumors in children. Pediatr Blood Cancer 2005;45(3):265–73.
10. Ribeiro RC, Schettini ST, Abib S de CV, et al. Cavectomy for the treatment of Wilms tumor with vascular extension. J Urol 2006;176(1):279–83 [discussion 283–84].
11. Donnellan WL. Surgical anatomy of adrenal glands. Ann Surg 1961;154(Suppl 6): 298–305.
12. Rodriguez-Galindo C, Pappo AS, Krailo MD, et al. Treatment of childhood adrenocortical carcinoma (ACC) with surgery plus retroperitoneal lymph node dissection (RPLND) and multiagent chemotherapy: Results of the Children's Oncology Group ARAR0332 protocol. J Clin Oncol 2016;34(15_suppl):10515.
13. Kemp CD, Ripley RT, Mathur A, et al. Pulmonary resection for metastatic adrenocortical carcinoma: the National cancer institute experience. Ann Thorac Surg 2011;92(4):1195–200.
14. Teinturier C, Pauchard MS, Brugières L, et al. Clinical and prognostic aspects of adrenocortical neoplasms in childhood. Med Pediatr Oncol 1999;32(2):106–11.
15. Hanna AM, Pham TH, Askegard-Giesmann JR, et al. Outcome of adrenocortical tumors in children. J Pediatr Surg 2008;43(5):843–9.
16. Klein JD, Turner CG, Gray FL, et al. Adrenal cortical tumors in children: factors associated with poor outcome. J Pediatr Surg 2011;46(6):1201–7.
17. Aubert S, Wacrenier A, Leroy X, et al. Weiss system revisited: a clinicopathologic and immunohistochemical study of 49 adrenocortical tumors. Am J Surg Pathol 2002;26(12):1612–9.

18. Wieneke JA, Thompson LDR, Heffess CS. Adrenal cortical neoplasms in the pediatric population: a clinicopathologic and immunophenotypic analysis of 83 patients. Am J Surg Pathol 2003;27(7):867–81.
19. Dias AIB dos S, Fachin CG, Avó LRS, et al. Correlation between selected angiogenic markers and prognosis in pediatric adrenocortical tumors: Angiogenic markers and prognosis in pediatric ACTs. J Pediatr Surg 2015;50(8):1323–8.
20. Fachin CG, Bradley Santos Dias AI, Schettini ST, et al. Lymphangiogenesis in pediatric adrenocortical tumors. Pediatr Blood Cancer 2012;59(6):1071.
21. Ribeiro RC, Pinto EM, Zambetti GP, et al. The international pediatric adrenocortical tumor registry initiative: contributions to clinical, biological, and treatment advances in pediatric adrenocortical tumors. Mol Cell Endocrinol 2012;351:37–43.
22. Weltgesundheitsorganisation, Lloyd RV, Osamura RY, et al, editors. WHO classification of tumours of endocrine organs. 4th edition. Lyon (France): International Agency for Research on Cancer; 2017.
23. Lenders JWM, Eisenhofer G, Mannelli M, et al. Phaeochromocytoma. Lancet 2005;366(9486):665–75.
24. Bholah R, Bunchman TE. Review of pediatric pheochromocytoma and paraganglioma. Front Pediatr 2017;5:155.
25. Berends AMA, Buitenwerf E, de Krijger RR, et al. Incidence of pheochromocytoma and sympathetic paraganglioma in the Netherlands: a nationwide study and systematic review. Eur J Intern Med 2018;51:68–73.
26. Fonkalsrud EW. Pheochromocytoma in childhood. Prog Pediatr Surg 1991;26: 103–11.
27. Bausch B, Wellner U, Bausch D, et al. Long-term prognosis of patients with pediatric pheochromocytoma. Endocr Relat Cancer 2014;21(1):17–25.
28. Beltsevich DG, Kuznetsov NS, Kazaryan AM, et al. Pheochromocytoma surgery: epidemiologic peculiarities in children. World J Surg 2004;28(6):592 6.
29. Hodgkinson DJ, Telander RL, Sheps SG, et al. Extra-adrenal intrathoracic functioning paraganglioma (pheochromocytoma) in childhood. Mayo Clin Proc 1980;55(4):271–6.
30. Jochmanova I, Pacak K. Genomic landscape of pheochromocytoma and paraganglioma. Trends Cancer 2018;4(1):6–9.
31. Dobri GA, Bravo E, Hamrahian AH. Pheochromocytoma: pitfalls in the biochemical evaluation. Expert Rev Endocrinol Metab 2014;9(2):123–35.
32. Eisenhofer G, Goldstein DS, Sullivan P, et al. Biochemical and clinical manifestations of dopamine-producing paragangliomas: utility of plasma methoxytyramine. J Clin Endocrinol Metab 2005;90(4):2068–75.
33. Lenders JWM, Pacak K, Walther MM, et al. Biochemical diagnosis of pheochromocytoma: which test is best? JAMA 2002;287(11):1427–34.
34. Zuber S, Wesley R, Prodanov T, et al. Clinical utility of chromogranin A in SDHx-related paragangliomas. Eur J Clin Invest 2014;44(4):365–71.
35. Eisenhofer G, Goldstein DS, Walther MM, et al. Biochemical diagnosis of pheochromocytoma: how to distinguish true- from false-positive test results. J Clin Endocrinol Metab 2003;88(6):2656–66.
36. Ilias I, Pacak K. Current approaches and recommended algorithm for the diagnostic localization of pheochromocytoma. J Clin Endocrinol Metab 2004;89(2): 479–91.
37. Brenner D, Elliston C, Hall E, et al. Estimated risks of radiation-induced fatal cancer from pediatric CT. AJR Am J Roentgenol 2001;176(2):289–96.
38. Turner MC, Lieberman E, DeQuattro V. The perioperative management of pheochromocytoma in children. Clin Pediatr (Phila) 1992;31(10):583–9.

39. Romero M, Kapur G, Baracco R, et al. Treatment of hypertension in children with catecholamine-secreting tumors: a systematic approach. J Clin Hypertens (Greenwich) 2015;17(9):720–5.

40. Mamilla D, Araque KA, Brofferio A, et al. Postoperative management in patients with pheochromocytoma and paraganglioma. Cancers (Basel) 2019;11(7). https://doi.org/10.3390/cancers11070936.

41. Miller KA, Albanese C, Harrison M, et al. Experience with laparoscopic adrenalectomy in pediatric patients. J Pediatr Surg 2002;37(7):979–82 [discussion 979–82].

42. Vargas HI, Kavoussi LR, Bartlett DL, et al. Laparoscopic adrenalectomy: a new standard of care. Urology 1997;49(5):673–8.

43. Plouin PF, Amar L, Dekkers OM, et al. European society of endocrinology clinical practice guideline for long-term follow-up of patients operated on for a phaeochromocytoma or a paraganglioma. Eur J Endocrinol 2016;174(5):G1–10.

44. Lam AK-Y. Update on adrenal tumours in 2017 world health organization (WHO) of endocrine tumours. Endocr Pathol 2017;28(3):213–27.

45. Lenders JWM, Duh Q-Y, Eisenhofer G, et al. Pheochromocytoma and paraganglioma: an endocrine society clinical practice guideline. J Clin Endocrinol Metab 2014;99(6):1915–42.

46. Kimura N, Takayanagi R, Takizawa N, et al. Pathological grading for predicting metastasis in phaeochromocytoma and paraganglioma. Endocr Relat Cancer 2014;21(3):405–14.

47. Kimura N, Takekoshi K, Naruse M. Risk stratification on pheochromocytoma and paraganglioma from laboratory and clinical medicine. J Clin Med 2018;7(9). https://doi.org/10.3390/jcm7090242.

48. Edström Elder E, Hjelm Skog A-L, Höög A, et al. The management of benign and malignant pheochromocytoma and abdominal paraganglioma. Eur J Surg Oncol 2003;29(3):278–83.

49. Nölting S, Ullrich M, Pietzsch J, et al. Current management of pheochromocytoma/paraganglioma: a guide for the practicing clinician in the era of precision medicine. Cancers (Basel) 2019;11(10). https://doi.org/10.3390/cancers11101505.

50. Frey S, Caillard C, Toulgoat F, et al. Non-adrenal tumors of the adrenal area; what are the pitfalls? J Visc Surg 2020;157(3):217–30.

51. Shaikh F, Murray MJ, Amatruda JF, et al. Paediatric extracranial germ-cell tumours. Lancet Oncol 2016;17(4):e149–62.

52. Rashidi A, Fisher SI. Primary adrenal lymphoma: a systematic review. Ann Hematol 2013;92(12):1583–93.

53. White J, Chan YF, Neuberger S, et al. Prenatal sonographic detection of intraabdominal extralobar pulmonary sequestration: report of three cases and literature review. Prenat Diagn 1994;14(8):653–8.

54. Bittman ME, Lee EY, Restrepo R, et al. Focal adrenal lesions in pediatric patients. Am J Roentgenol 2013;200(6):W542–56.

55. Velaphi SC, Perlman JM. Neonatal adrenal hemorrhage: clinical and abdominal sonographic findings. Clin Pediatr (Phila) 2001;40(10):545–8.

Management of Neuroblastoma in Pediatric Patients

Nikke Croteau, MD[a], Jed Nuchtern, MD[b],
Michael P. LaQuaglia, MD[a,*]

KEYWORDS

- Neuroblastoma • Pediatric surgery • Risk status • Resection • Treatment • Staging
- Survival • Local control

KEY POINTS

- Assessment of neuroblastoma risk is paramount.
- Thorough resection of high-risk tumors improves local control.
- Incomplete resection or even observation alone may be the optimal treatment of specific risk types of neuroblastoma.
- Image-defined risk factors, the International Neuroblastoma Pathology Classification, and biological factors have replaced anatomic staging based on resection status.
- Antibody therapy has made a major impact on outcomes for patients with high-risk neuroblastoma.

INTRODUCTION

Neuroblastoma is characterized by great heterogeneity and is the third most common solid tumor and the most common abdominal tumor in childhood. High-risk neuroblastoma still is associated with a poor prognosis, with 5-year event-free survival in the 50% to 60% range. Additionally, overall survival follows the event-free survival curves, indicating relapse often cannot be treated successfully. Major advances have been made, however, based on a more thorough understanding of underlying biology, which may translate into more accurate risk stratification. This is true for both treatment intensification and deintensification. For instance, prospective (but not randomized) cooperative group data now are available from both the North American and European organizations supporting extensive tumor debulking in high-risk

[a] Department of Surgery, Pediatric Service, Memorial Sloan Kettering Cancer Center, 1275 York Avenue, New York, NY 10065, USA; [b] Department of Surgery, Baylor College of Medicine, 6701 Fannin Street, Houston, TX 77030, USA
* Corresponding author.
E-mail address: laquaglm@mskcc.org

Surg Oncol Clin N Am 30 (2021) 291–304
https://doi.org/10.1016/j.soc.2020.11.010

disease. In contrast, external beam radiotherapy has all but been eliminated for patients with intermediate-risk neuroblastoma, and neonatal tumors now can be observed safely thanks to a pioneering surgeon-led study.

Furthermore, systemic therapies have improved and include the routine incorporation of antineuroblastoma monoclonal antibodies, which have a particular activity against bone marrow metastases. This makes surgical efforts and other locoregional control more effective.

This article describes a brief history of neuroblastoma therapy, current staging and risk status, and the role of the surgeon in the various risk groups.

HISTORICAL ASPECTS

The first description of neuroblastoma is ascribed to Rudolf Virchow who called it an abdominal glioma.[1] Felix Marchand first connected these tumors with the autonomic nervous system, including the adrenal medulla, whereas William Pepper was the first to describe the clinical pattern now designated MS disease in infants (low amount of bone marrow, liver, and skin metastases but no cortical bone involvement).[2] James Homer Wright[3] was the first to describe the pseudorosettes still used diagnostically by pathologists. Karl Herxheimer used silver staining to visualize the tumors in 1914, and Harvey Cushing and S. Burt Wolbach showed that spontaneous regression was possible in some neuroblastomas, a first hint that risk assessment would be of great importance in this disease.[3,4] Robert Gross and C. Everett Koop were pioneers in neuroblastoma surgery in the United States.[5,6] Finally, neuroblastoma is the first cancer for which *MYCN* amplification has been used to assess risk.

CLINICAL PRESENTATION

Clinical presentation of neuroblastoma depends on the anatomic location of the primary tumor, stage or extent of disease and risk status. Patients with cervical primaries that are thought to arise from the stellate ganglion may present with Horner syndrome, which may be subtle at times. Parents may note that the affected side is dry and more flushed during exercise. The pupillary constriction may be difficult to appreciate in dark-eyed children, and the lid droop can be minimal. Tumors in the chest may be asymptomatic and grow to great size until dyspnea initiates a work-up. Abdominal and pelvic tumors also may reach great size and may be asymptomatic and incidentally discovered by palpation of a mass. The presence of metastases actually may be the first clinical indication of neuroblastoma. The most frequent site of metastases is the cortical bone and bone marrow. Both sites can give rise to bone pain, which causes limping or refusal to walk if it involves the lower extremity or pelvis. When the spine is involved, compression fractures can occur. Neuroblastoma may invade through the spinal foramina into the epidural space, and paraparesis, or Frank's paraplegia, may be the result. Bone metastases to the orbits can cause hemorrhage within the orbit and subsequent periorbital ecchymoses, colloquially referred to as raccoon eyes. Tumors arising in the pelvis from the sympathetic chains, or organ of Zuckerkandl, may affect the sacrum and pelvic nerves, causing a neurogenic bladder. Physical impingement may cause a partial rectal obstruction with severe constipation.

DIAGNOSTIC AND STAGING STUDIES
Laboratory Findings

Lactate dehydrogenase (LDH), ferritin, and catecholamine metabolites and urinary catecholamines often are checked when neuroblastoma is suspected. LDH is nonspecific; however, high serum levels can be caused by large tumor burden or high proliferative activity; levels higher than 1500 IU/L seem to be associated with a poor prognosis.[7–9] Ferritin levels greater than 150 ng/mL also can result from a large tumor burden or rapid progression; it often is seen in advanced neuroblastoma and, like elevated LDH, indicates a poor prognosis.[7,9] Serum ferritin often decreases to normal when patients are in clinical remission. Elevated urinary catecholamines are present in greater than 90% of patients with neuroblastoma.[10] These laboratory tests also can be used to monitor a patients' disease progression.

DIAGNOSTIC IMAGING
Radiographs

A posterior mediastinal mass, observed most commonly in the thoracic region, can be seen on a chest radiograph.[11] Abdominal radiography is not the standard for initial assessment of abdominal neuroblastomas. As many as half of these tumors, however, can be seen as a mass with fine calcifications.[7]

Ultrasonography

Ultrasonography (US) is the most common initial imaging modality used to assess a suspected abdominal mass. When a mass has been confirmed, computed tomography (CT) or magnetic resonance imaging (MRI) is used for further assessment, because these modalities are more sensitive and accurate than US.[12]

Computed Tomography and Magnetic Resonance Imaging

The accuracy of contrast-enhanced CT in defining the extent of neuroblastoma is 82% and increases to 97% when performed with technetium 99m bone scintigraphy.[13] Although some believe MRI has replaced CT, others consider CT the gold standard imaging modality when combined with bone scintigraphy.[14] Intraspinal tumor extension and metastases to the bone and bone marrow, however, are seen better on MRI.[15] The definition of encasement of major vessels also is observed better with MRI, especially with angiography.[15] A CT scan of a left adrenal neuroblastoma is depicted in **Fig. 1.**

Metaiodobenzylguanidine Imaging

Metaiodobenzylguanidine (MIBG) imaging is used to assess the bone and bone marrow for involvement by neuroblastoma. MIBG is transported to and stored in the chromaffin cells in the same way as norepinephrine.[7] The sensitivity and specificity

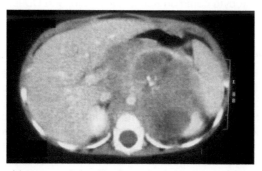

Fig. 1. A large neuroblastoma originating from the left adrenal gland.

of MIBG in detecting neuroblastoma with metastases to the bone and bone marrow are 82% and 91%, respectively. MIBG imaging largely has replaced technitium 99m bone scintigraphy for those patients whose tumors take up MIBG.

Image Defined Risk Factors

In the past 10 years, there has been a realization that staging and risk assessment based on radiographic imaging before therapy have many advantages, not the least of which is a uniform, preoperative approach agreed to by multiple pediatric cooperative groups. The list of image-defined risk factors (IDRFs) is lengthy but easily understood as a factor that complicates surgical resection in an anatomic site. For instance, a solitary, small adrenal mass does not have IDRFs. When that has metastasized to regional lymph nodes. However, the celiac axis can have many IDRFs. For blood vessels and peripheral nerves, the encasement must be greater than 50% of the vessel or nerve circumference to count. Neural foraminal involvement extending through the foramen or into the epidural space also an is IDRF. Using this logic, a staging system was devised. L1 tumors are localized and lack IDRFs. L2 tumors are localized but have IDRFs. M tumors have distant metastases. The stage assigned to metastatic neuroblastoma in children under 1 year of age with favorable biological factors (MS) is a special category (discussed later). Tumors with heavy regional lymph node involvement are considered localized unless distant nodes (>2 nodal echelons removed from the primary tumor) are positive for neuroblastoma.

PATHOLOGY

As discussed previously, neuroblastoma is a tumor of cells derived from the neural crest and can originate anywhere neural crest cells migrate, such as the adrenal medulla, paraspinal sympathetic ganglia, and the organ of Zuckerkandl.[7] Neuroblastoma is a small, round, blue cell tumor, which (especially when undifferentiated) must be distinguished from other tumors that fall into the small, round, blue cell group, such as Ewing sarcoma, non-Hodgkin lymphoma, and rhabdomyosarcoma. Histologically, neuroblastoma is distinguished by the presence of neuritic processes (neuropil) and Homer Wright rosettes (neuroblasts surrounding eosinophilic neuropil). Tumor cells can vary from undifferentiated cells to fully mature ganglion cells, and the tumors can have variable degrees of schwannian cell stroma intermixed as wavy bundles and sheets of spindle cells that produce factors important for neuronal differentiation.[16,17] Immunohistochemical analysis reveals positive staining when using antibodies to neuroblastoma-specific antigens, such as synaptophysin, neuron-specific enolase, and chromogranin; staining is negative when using antibodies to actin, desmin, cytokeratin, leukocyte common antigen, vimentin, and CD99.

TUMOR BIOLOGY
Histopathologic Classification

The first classification system was developed by Shimada and colleagues in 1984[18]; it was an age-linked classification system based on tumor morphology. Neuroblastomas were separated into 2 prognostic groups, favorable histology and unfavorable histology.[18] The International Neuroblastoma Pathology Classification was developed in 1999 and modified in 2003. It is adapted from the original Shimada system, and it remains an age-linked system, depending on the differentiation grade of the neuroblasts, the mitosis-karyorrhexis index (MKI), and the presence or absence of schwannian stroma.[19,20]

DNA Content

Although normal human cells have 2 copies of each of 23 chromosomes (46 chromosomes = diploid cells), a majority (55%) of primary neuroblastomas are triploid or near-triploid/hyperdiploid, containing between 58 and 80 chromosomes. The rest (45%) are near-diploid (35–57 chromosomes) or near-tetraploid (81–103 chromosomes).[7,21] The DNA index is the ratio of the number of chromosomes present to a diploid number of chromosomes (46). Therefore, diploid cells have a DNA index of 1.0, and near-triploid cells have a DNA index ranging from 1.26 to 1.76. Patients with near-diploid or near-tetraploid tumors usually have unfavorable clinical and biologic prognostic factors and poor survival rates compared with those patients who have near-triploid tumors.[22]

Amplification of MYCN

In the developing nervous system and other tissues, MYCN encodes a nuclear phosphoprotein that forms a transcriptional complex by associating with other nuclear proteins.[23] The expression of MYCN increases the rate of DNA synthesis and cell proliferation and can function as a classic dominant oncogene, cooperating with activated ras to transform normal cells.[24,25] MYCN amplification is present in 25% of primary neuroblastomas; the presence in advanced disease is 40%, whereas the presence in low-stage disease is only 5% to 10%.[26] Amplification of MYCN is an important prognostic indicator, because it is associated with advanced stages of disease, rapid tumor progression, and poor outcomes.[26,27]

RISK STATUS

Risk status in neuroblastoma depends on patient age and clinical factors, including stage, MYCN amplification, histopathology, segmental chromosomal aberrations, and ploidy. Age at diagnosis is the primary patient-related characteristic, and analyses have shown that children diagnosed before 18 months have a lower risk.[28] Diagnosis after 18 months of age is associated with a worsened event-free survival.

MYCN amplification is present in 25% to 35% of high-stage tumors but only 5% of low-stage tumors. It is an indicator of high biological risk except in the rare instance of a small, isolated, completely excised neuroblastoma. Diploid tumors are associated with worse outcomes than aneuploid or polyploid tumors in children under 18 months of age. Finally, there is a type of neuroblastoma grading system that stratifies tumors into favorable or unfavorable categories based on their MKI. In addition to these factors, many molecular findings have been associated with increased risk. These include 17q gain and loss of chromosome 1p or 11q.

The algorithms that use these factors to determine risk are complex and change slightly based on new knowledge. It is recommended that the most recent schema be consulted when determining the risk status for patients. It also is recommended that all neuroblastoma cases be discussed at a multidisciplinary tumor board to assess risk.

In 1993, The Children's Oncology Group (COG) and cooperative groups in Europe and Japan adopted the International Neuroblastoma Staging System (INSS).[29,30] This system emphasizes the extent of the primary tumor, presence and location of positive lymph nodes, and metastasis as means of categorizing patients into stages 1, 2 A/2B, 3, and 4/4S.[30] This staging system, along with tumor biology, was the basis of COG risk stratification prior to 2010. This system divides patients into low-risk, intermediate-risk, and high-risk groups to guide treatment.[30] In the early 2000s, the International Neuroblastoma Risk Group Staging System (INRGSS) began to replace the INSS.[31] It currently is the staging system used in ongoing COG studies. The advantage of the INRGSS is that it is not dependent on a resection variable but rather on pretreatment imaging combined with age and biological variables like *MYCN* amplification. According to the INRGSS system, tumors are assessed for surgical risk factors that predict unresectability using IDRFs and are separated into L1 (no IDRFs), L2 (at least 1 IDRF), M (metastatic), or MS (the equivalent of 4S in the INSS).[30] Based on this stage, along with age, histology, and tumor biology, patients are grouped into very-low-risk, low-risk, intermediate-risk, and high-risk groups. Regardless of which system is chosen, the stage and risk status of the patient have a great impact on treatment.

TREATMENT

Generally, small, localized, and easily removed lesions are considered low risk. The primary surgery for many of these tumors is resection. It is becoming more evident, however, that some of these patients can undergo observation alone.[32] Larger tumors with locoregional spread also are treated by resection, but some of these lesions can be quite extensive. Therefore, a course of neoadjuvant, multiagent chemotherapy may shrink the tumor and reduce vascularity, making resection easier. Also, the presence of IDRFs may dictate a course of chemotherapy. There is little evidence, however, that encased vessels are completely freed by this approach. Chemotherapy for intermediate-risk patients usually is given in a series of 2 cycles followed by radiologic assessment. If resection cannot be completed after 8 cycles (discussion about reducing the number of cycles is ongoing), observation often is performed, depending on the overall tumor response to chemotherapy and details of the biologic risk assignment. External beam radiotherapy is avoided with intermediate-risk tumors.

In summary, the current standard of treatment of children with neuroblastoma is based on stage as well as risk stratification; this takes into account clinical and biologic variables predictive of relapse.[7] The age at diagnosis (<18 months or ≥18 months) and stage at diagnosis are the most important clinical variables,[28,33,34] whereas *MYCN* amplification status and histopathologic classification are the most important biologic factors.[26,27,35]

VERY-LOW-RISK AND LOW-RISK GROUPS

The very-low-risk group exists only in the INRG risk group classification system and includes stage L1 without *MYCN* amplification and stage MS without *MYCN* amplification or 11q aberration. The low-risk group includes INSS stage 1, stage 2 A/2B without *MYCN* amplification and greater than 50% tumor resection, and stage 4S without *MYCN* amplification.[30] This group also includes INRG stage L1, stage L2 without *MYCN* amplification or 11q aberration, and stage M or MS without *MYCN* amplification or 11q aberration if the patient is less than 18 months old.[30]

The goal for this risk group is complete primary tumor resection, accurate staging by biopsy of nonadherent nodes, and adequate tissue sampling for molecular biologic studies.[30] As discussed previously, a significant portion of younger patients in this group can be treated with expectant observation.[30] Patients with low-risk disease over the age of 18 months have an overall survival of greater than 90%, with almost all patients receiving surgery alone.[36–38] Therefore, the standard treatment of patients with low-risk disease is surgery without chemotherapy or radiotherapy except for those in the observation arm.

INTERMEDIATE-RISK GROUP

The intermediate-risk group includes INRG stage L2 without *MYCN* amplification, but with 11q aberration or poorly differentiated histology, and stage M without *MYCN* amplification, but with diploid tumor and age less than 18 months.[30] This group also includes INSS stage 2 A/2B without *MYCN* amplification and less than 50% tumor resection, stage 3 without *MYCN* amplification, age less than 547 days with any histology or age greater than 547 days with favorable histology, and stage 4 or stage 4S without *MYCN* amplification and age less than 547 days.

The surgical goals for patients with intermediate-risk disease are to establish the diagnosis, resect as much of the primary tumor as safely as possible, accurately stage the disease through the sampling of nonadherent lymph nodes, and obtain an adequate amount of tissue for diagnostic studies.[30] Patients with unresectable tumors are treated with chemotherapy per COG guidelines. The most active agents against neuroblastoma are cyclophosphamide, doxorubicin, carboplatin, and etoposide.[7] Patients are monitored with CT or MRI after chemotherapy to assess response and resectability of the tumor.

HIGH-RISK GROUP

The high-risk group includes INRG stages L1 and L2 with *MYCN* amplification, stage M with *MYCN* amplification or age greater than 18 months, and stage MS with *MYCN* amplification or 11q aberration. This group also includes INSS stage 2 A/2B with *MYCN* amplification, stage 3 with *MYCN* amplification or without *MYCN* amplification but age greater than 547 days with unfavorable histology, stage 4 with *MYCN* amplification, or without *MYCN* amplification from ages 365 to 547 days with unfavorable histology, or age greater than 547 days regardless of tumor biology, and stage 4S with *MYCN* amplification.

The goal of surgery in patients with high-risk disease is an initial diagnostic biopsy to obtain an adequate amount of tissue for biologic studies. Treatment after diagnosis begins with neoadjuvant chemotherapy, followed by complete resection of the primary tumor.[30] High-risk patients also may receive myeloablative consolidation therapy with stem cell rescue and targeted therapy for any residual disease.[7] Immunotherapy with anti-GD2 antibodies has become standard treatment after consolidation therapy. Radiotherapy may be used for symptomatic residual disease and/or palliation.

The surgical approach to high-risk neuroblastoma has been influenced recently by the publication of cooperative group prospective (but not randomized) studies with a principal aim of assessing the impact of extent of resection on outcomes. Two studies, one from the COG and the other from SIOPEN, are consistent and show a distinct and independent effect of more extensive resection of primary loco-regional disease on the cumulative incidence of local progression.[39,40] The impact of more extensive resection on the cumulative incidence of local progression is shown in **Fig. 2**.

The SIOPEN study, which is larger with greater than 1500 patients, also showed that improved event-free and overall survival correlated with more extensive resection.[40] This is the first time such data have been available.

SURGICAL TECHNIQUES
Initial Biopsy

The goal of biopsy is to obtain an adequate amount of tissue for both diagnosis and clinically relevant molecular studies like *MYCN* amplification. Biopsy should take

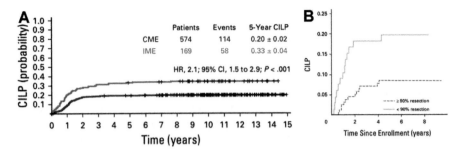

Fig. 2. (A) Shows the results of the High-Risk Neuroblastoma Study 1.8 (HR-NBL1)/SIOPEN study for cumulative incidence of local progression. (B) Shows the results from the COG A3973 trial. CILP, cartilage intermediate layer protein; HR, hazard ratio; IME, intermediate medical education.

into account each patient's overall status at the time of biopsy, because some patients may have breathing problems secondary to large abdominal or thoracic masses, bleeding and anemia from low platelets secondary to marrow infiltration, or severe bone pain because of osseous metastases. Laparoscopy, laparotomy, or percutaneous needle biopsy all are acceptable, as long as the diagnosis is obtained along with salient molecular studies. If a needle technique is used, the placement of a trocar to allow multiple needle passes as well as packing of the needle tract with hemostatic agents is preferred. For desperately ill patients, the finding of neuroblastoma cells in the bone marrow combined with a positive MIBG scan is considered adequate. The surgeon should ensure that an adequate biopsy has been obtained before leaving the operating room.

Cervical Lesion

Most primary cervical lesions occur in infants less than 1 year of age and have favorable biologic features. The approach to remove these lesions typically is a transverse neck incision followed by dissection of the carotid sheath contents.[30] Large lesions may require division of the sternocleidomastoid muscle for adequate exposure. In cases of grossly positive lymph nodes, a formal lymphadenectomy with a modified neck dissection technique should be performed.[30] The approach is depicted in **Fig. 3**.

Cervicothoracic Lesions

Primary cervical lesions may extend into the chest through the thoracic inlet. Adequate exposure is integral to achieving gross total resection of these tumors.[30] This usually can be achieved using a trap-door thoracotomy, which can be modified for lesions with a larger cervical component by extending the neck incision superior along the anterior border of the sternocleidomastoid.[30] Lesions that extend into both hemithoraces can be exposed reliably using a clamshell thoracotomy at the fifth interspace. Nerve stimulation often is 'used to monitor the vagus nerve and the brachial plexus.[30]

Mediastinal Lesions

The posterior mediastinum is the second most common primary site for neuroblastomas. Mediastinal lesions generally can be approached through a muscle-sparing posterolateral thoracotomy. Infiltration through spinal foramina may require foraminotomy.[30] This is depicted in **Fig. 4**. For L1 tumors, thoracoscopy is a reasonable alternative to thoracotomy.

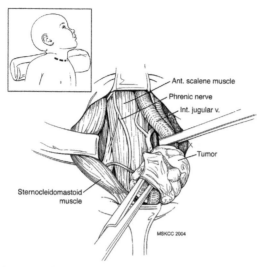

Fig. 3. Resection of a cervical neuroblastoma. ANT, anterior; INT, interior; v, vein.

Upper Abdominal and Retroperitoneal Lesions

A majority of neuroblastomas originate from the adrenal gland or sympathetic ganglia and are found in the upper abdomen. There is frequent involvement of regional lymph nodes in the ipsilateral paraaortic or the pericaval chains as well as interaortocaval

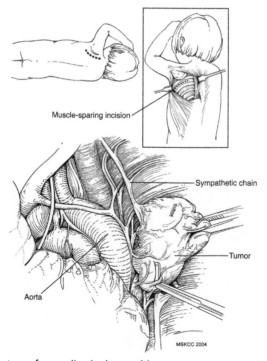

Fig. 4. Left thoracotomy for mediastinal neuroblastoma.

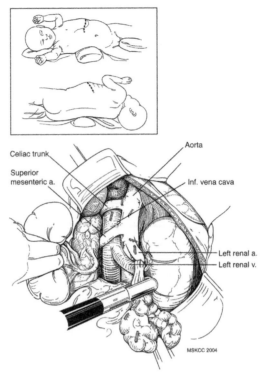

Fig. 5. Technique of left thoracoabdominal resection. Bivalving of the tumor is acceptable and necessary for neuroblastoma resection. A, artery; inf, inferior; v, valve.

lymph nodes. The primary tumor and involved lymph nodes often create a confluent mass that encases but does not invade the great vessels of the abdomen. For these tumors, a thoracoabdominal approach is ideal.[30] The surgical approach is depicted in **Fig. 5**, and the outcome of surgery in **Fig. 6**.

Pelvic Lesions

Pelvic tumors can be challenging to resect due to the encasement of iliac vessels and infiltration of the lumbosacral plexus. A midline incision extending from the umbilicus to the pubic symphysis provides good exposure of the pelvis and allows adequate

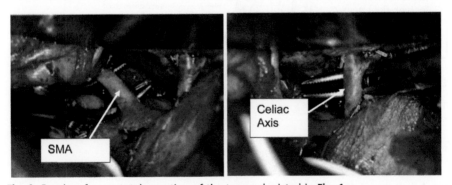

Fig. 6. Results of gross total resection of the tumor depicted in **Fig. 1**.

control of the distal aorta and vena cava.[30] Internal iliac vessels, if involved, may be ligated and resected without significant morbidity.

Surgical Complications and Mortality

Neuroblastomas that involve and/or encase major vascular and neural structures in their site of origin or surrounding nodes have a higher risk of surgical complications.[30] The most serious surgical complications include massive hemorrhage, major vascular injury, and respiratory failure requiring ventilatory support. The site of the tumor determines the possible surgical complications. Cervical and upper mediastinal resections can be associated with a permanent postoperative Horner syndrome. Paralysis can result from the excision of epidural tumors or tumors heavily involving spinal foramina.[41] Excision of retroperitoneal neuroblastomas can result in nephrectomy or renal infarction.[42] After the removal of pelvic tumors, there is increased frequency of complications, such as foot drop.[43] Despite the extent of these massive resections, operative mortality is rare. Complications after primary tumor resection in patients with high-risk tumors are reduced after initial treatment with neoadjuvant chemotherapy[44] that reduces tumor volume.[45,46]

SUMMARY

The key to effective neuroblastoma therapy is accurate risk stratification. This determines treatment, including surgical intervention. Resection alone is the standard of care for very-low-risk and low-risk neuroblastoma. Intermediate-risk tumors also may be treated with neoadjuvant chemotherapy and resection. A complete gross resection usually is not necessary for intermediate-risk neuroblastoma. Recent data indicate that a complete gross resection is a desired goal, if feasible, for high-risk neuroblastomas.

CLINICS CARE POINTS

- Realize that in neuroblastoma an R0 resection rarely is feasible.
- Resect or observe very-low-risk and low-risk tumors
- Resect intermediate-risk tumors either primarily, if feasible, or after neoadjuvant therapy. Complete gross (R1) resection is not necessary, although should be done if relatively straightforward.
- R1 resection of the primary tumor and regional involved lymph nodes is the goal of surgery for high-risk tumors if safe and feasible. This should be done after neoadjuvant therapy.
- In general, removal of normal organs (kidneys) should be avoided during neuroblastoma resection, if possible.

DISCLOSURE

This research was funded in part by the NIH/NCI Cancer Center Support Grant, P30 CA008748. The authors have no conflicts of interest.

REFERENCES

1. R V Hyperplasie der Zirbel und der Nebennieren. In: Die Krankhaften Geschwulste. Vol 2.1862:1864-1865.

2. F M. Beitrage zur Kentniss der normalen und pathologischen Anatomic der Glandula carotica und der Nebennieren. In: Festschrift fiir Rudolf Virchow. Vol 5. Berlin 1891:578.

3. Wright JH. Neurocytoma or neuroblastoma, a kind of tumor not generally recognized. J Exp Med 1910;12(4):556–61.

4. Cushing H, Wolbach SB. The Transformation of a Malignant Paravertebral Sympathicoblastoma into a Benign Ganglioneuroma. Am J Pathol 1927;3(3): 203–16, 207.

5. Gross RE, Farber S, Martin LW. Neuroblastoma sympatheticum; a study and report of 217 cases. Pediatrics 1959;23(6):1179–91.

6. Koop CE, Kiesewetter WB, Horn RC. Neuroblastoma in childhood; survival after major surgical insult to the tumor. Surgery 1955;38(1):272–8.

7. Davidoff AM. Neuroblastoma. In: Holcomb GJ, Murphy JP, Ostlie D, editors. Ashcraft's pediatric surgery. Philadelphia, PA: Elsevier; 2014.

8. Berthold F, Kassenbohmer R, Zieschang J. Multivariate evaluation of prognostic factors in localized neuroblastoma. Am J Pediatr Hematol Oncol 1994;16(2): 107–15.

9. Joshi VV, Cantor AB, Brodeur GM, et al. Correlation between morphologic and other prognostic markers of neuroblastoma. A study of histologic grade, DNA index, N-myc gene copy number, and lactic dehydrogenase in patients in the Pediatric Oncology Group. Cancer 1993;(71):3173–81.

10. Fitzgibbon MC, Tormey WP. Paediatric reference ranges for urinary catecholamines/metabolites and their relevance in neuroblastoma diagnosis. Ann Clin Biochem 1994;31(Pt 1):1–11.

11. Adams GA, Shochat SJ, Smith EI, et al. Thoracic neuroblastoma: a Pediatric Oncology Group study. J Pediatr Surg 1993;28(3):372–7 [discussion: 377–8].

12. Tanabe M, Yoshida H, Ohnuma N, et al. Imaging of neuroblastoma in patients identified by mass screening using urinary catecholamine metabolites. J Pediatr Surg 1993;28(4):617–21.

13. Stark DD, Moss AA, Brasch RC, et al. Neuroblastoma: diagnostic imaging and staging. Radiology 1983;148(1):101–5.

14. Cheung NK, Kushner BH. Should we replace bone scintigraphy plus CT with MR imaging for staging of neuroblastoma? Radiology 2003;226(1):286–7 [author reply: 287–8].

15. Siegel MJ, Ishwaran H, Fletcher BD, et al. Staging of neuroblastoma at imaging: report of the radiology diagnostic oncology group. Radiology 2002;223(1): 168–75.

16. Attiyeh EF, London WB, Mosse YP, et al. Chromosome 1p and 11q deletions and outcome in neuroblastoma. N Engl J Med 2005;353(21):2243–53.

17. Takayama H, Suzuki T, Mugishima H, et al. Deletion mapping of chromosomes 14q and 1p in human neuroblastoma. Oncogene 1992;7(6):1185–9.

18. Shimada H, Chatten J, Newton WA Jr, et al. Histopathologic prognostic factors in neuroblastic tumors: definition of subtypes of ganglioneuroblastoma and an age-linked classification of neuroblastomas. J Natl Cancer Inst 1984;73(2):405–16.

19. Shimada H, Ambros IM, Dehner LP, et al. Terminology and morphologic criteria of neuroblastic tumors: recommendations by the International Neuroblastoma Pathology Committee. Cancer 1999;86(2):349–63.

20. Peuchmaur M, d'Amore ES, Joshi VV, et al. Revision of the International Neuroblastoma Pathology Classification: confirmation of favorable and unfavorable prognostic subsets in ganglioneuroblastoma, nodular. Cancer 2003;98(10): 2274–81.

21. Kaneko Y, Kanda N, Maseki N, et al. Different karyotypic patterns in early and advanced stage neuroblastomas. Cancer Res 1987;47(1):311–8.
22. Look AT, Hayes FA, Nitschke R, et al. Cellular DNA content as a predictor of response to chemotherapy in infants with unresectable neuroblastoma. N Engl J Med 1984;311(4):231–5.
23. Kohl NE, Kanda N, Schreck RR, et al. Transposition and amplification of oncogene-related sequences in human neuroblastomas. Cell 1983;35(2 Pt 1): 359–67.
24. Lutz W, Stohr M, Schurmann J, et al. Conditional expression of N-myc in human neuroblastoma cells increases expression of alpha-prothymosin and ornithine decarboxylase and accelerates progression into S-phase early after mitogenic stimulation of quiescent cells. Oncogene 1996;13(4):803–12.
25. Yancopoulos GD, Nisen PD, Tesfaye A, et al. N-myc can cooperate with ras to transform normal cells in culture. Proc Natl Acad Sci U S A 1985;82(16):5455–9.
26. Brodeur GM, Seeger RC, Schwab M, et al. Amplification of N-myc in untreated human neuroblastomas correlates with advanced disease stage. Science 1984; 224(4653):1121–4.
27. Seeger RC, Brodeur GM, Sather H, et al. Association of multiple copies of the N-myc oncogene with rapid progression of neuroblastomas. N Engl J Med 1985;313(18):1111–6.
28. London WB, Castleberry RP, Matthay KK, et al. Evidence for an age cutoff greater than 365 days for neuroblastoma risk group stratification in the Children's Oncology Group. J Clin Oncol 2005;23(27):6459–65.
29. Brodeur GM, Pritchard J, Berthold F, et al. Revisions of the international criteria for neuroblastoma diagnosis, staging, and response to treatment. J Clin Oncol 1993; 11(8):1466–77.
30. Croteau NJ, Saltsman JA, LaQuaglia MP. Advances in Surgical Treatment of Neuroblastoma. In: Ray SK, editor. Neuroblastoma: molecular mechanisms and therapeutic interventions. Philadelphia, PA: Elsevier; 2019.
31. Cohn SL, Pearson AD, London WB, et al. The International Neuroblastoma Risk Group (INRG) classification system: an INRG Task Force report. J Clin Oncol 2009;27(2):289–97.
32. Nuchtern JG, London WB, Barnewolt CE, et al. A prospective study of expectant observation as primary therapy for neuroblastoma in young infants: a Children's Oncology Group study. Ann Surg 2012;256(4):573–80.
33. Moroz V, Machin D, Faldum A, et al. Changes over three decades in outcome and the prognostic influence of age-at-diagnosis in young patients with neuroblastoma: a report from the International Neuroblastoma Risk Group Project. Eur J Cancer 2011;47(4):561–71.
34. Evans AE, D'Angio GJ, Propert K, et al. Prognostic factor in neuroblastoma. Cancer 1987;59(11):1853–9.
35. Shimada H, Umehara S, Monobe Y, et al. International neuroblastoma pathology classification for prognostic evaluation of patients with peripheral neuroblastic tumors: a report from the Children's Cancer Group. Cancer 2001;92(9):2451–61.
36. Bernardi Bd, Conte M, Mancini A. Localized resectable neuroblastoma: results of the second study of the Italian Cooperative Group for Neuroblastoma. J Clin Oncol 1995;13:884–93.
37. Kushner BH, Cheung NK, LaQuaglia MP, et al. International neuroblastoma staging system stage 1 neuroblastoma: a prospective study and literature review. J Clin Oncol 1996;14(7):2174–80.

38. Evans AE, Silber JH, Shpilsky A, et al. Successful management of low-stage neuroblastoma without adjuvant therapies: a comparison of two decades, 1972 through 1981 and 1982 through 1992, in a single institution. J Clin Oncol 1996; 14(9):2504–10.
39. von Allmen D, Davidoff AM, London WB, et al. Impact of extent of resection on local control and survival in patients from the COG A3973 study with high-risk neuroblastoma. J Clin Oncol 2017;35(2):208–16.
40. Holmes K, Pötschger U, Pearson ADJ, et al. Influence of surgical excision on the survival of patients with stage 4 high-risk neuroblastoma: a report from the HR-NBL1/SIOPEN Study. J Clin Oncol 2020;38(25):2902–15.
41. Shimada Y, Sato K, Abe E, et al. Congenital dumbbell neuroblastoma. Spine (Phila Pa 1976) 1995;20(11):1295–300.
42. Shamberger RC, Smith EI, Joshi VV, et al. The risk of nephrectomy during local control in abdominal neuroblastoma. J Pediatr Surg 1998;33(2):161–4.
43. Cruccetti A, Kiely EM, Spitz L, et al. Pelvic neuroblastoma: low mortality and high morbidity. J Pediatr Surg 2000;35(5):724–8.
44. Shamberger RC, Allarde-Segundo A, Kozakewich HP, et al. Surgical management of stage III and IV neuroblastoma: resection before or after chemotherapy? J Pediatr Surg 1991;26(9):1113–7 [discussion: 1117–8].
45. La Quaglia MP. Surgical management of neuroblastoma. Semin Pediatr Surg 2001;10:132–9.
46. Medary I, Aronson D, Cheung NK, et al. Kinetics of primary tumor regression with chemotherapy: implications for the timing of surgery. Ann Surg Oncol 1996;3(6): 521–5.

Surgical Management of Wilms Tumor (Nephroblastoma) and Renal Cell Carcinoma in Children and Young Adults

Natalie M. Lopyan, MD[a], Peter F. Ehrlich, MD, MSc[b],*

KEYWORDS

- Pediatric Wilms tumor • Pediatric renal cell carcinoma
- Treatment and surgical management

KEY POINTS

- Well-designed surgical protocols exist that impact both event-free and overall survivals in children and young adults with renal tumors and should be followed in detail.
- Wilms tumor is the most common renal tumor in childhood and has an excellent survival rate.
- The treatment of Wilms tumor focuses both on oncologic cure and reduction of late effects of treatment.
- Renal cell carcinoma is the second most common pediatric renal malignancy.
- Renal cell carcinoma tends to present at advanced stages with poor outcomes in children and young adults.

INTRODUCTION

Renal tumors are the second most common abdominal tumor seen in infants and children, behind neuroblastoma, contributing to 7% of all newly diagnosed pediatric solid malignancy cases.[1,2] The most common renal tumor is a nephroblastoma or Wilms tumor (WT) accounting for 90% of solid renal tumors in children. Renal cell carcinoma (RCC) variants are the second most frequent. These are found more commonly in adolescents. Although surgery remains the mainstay of treatment, the management of renal tumors has evolved over the last 4 decades into a multimodal, risk-based

a C.S. Mott Children's Hospital Section of Pediatric Surgery, 1540 East Hospital Drive, Ann Arbor, MI 48109, USA; b University of Michigan, C.S. Mott Children's Hospital Section of Pediatric Surgery, 1540 East Hospital Drive, SPC 4811, Ann Arbor, MI 48109, USA
* Corresponding author.
E-mail address: pehrlich@umich.edu

Surg Oncol Clin N Am 30 (2021) 305–323
https://doi.org/10.1016/j.soc.2020.11.002
1055-3207/21/© 2020 Elsevier Inc. All rights reserved.

approach consisting of surgery, chemotherapy, and radiotherapy. Improved treatment is now focused on multiple risk factors in addition to pathology and stage, including age, response, and genetics. Staging and risk stratification have become more personalized and have helped improve overall survival and event-free survival.

WILMS TUMOR

WT is the most frequent tumor of the kidney in infants and children, with an incidence of 600 to 650 cases a year in North America. The mean age at diagnosis is 36 months, with the majority of children presenting between the ages of 12 and 48 months.[2] African American children are at greatest risk, followed by Caucasian and then East Asian populations. Most children present with unilateral tumors, although synchronous bilateral tumors occur in approximately 10% of patients. The frequency of bilateral disease is increased in familial cases, and such cases are often associated with an earlier age of onset. Nearly 10% of all WT cases arise in the setting of a well-described syndrome (eg, Beckwith–Wiedemann syndrome). WT represents one of the great success stories in modern medicine, with survival rates increasing from 5% in 1900 to more than 90% currently.[3] This increase reflects in large part the systematic data collection and analysis facilitated by multinational consortiums—the National Wilms Tumor Study Group, now a part of the Children's Oncology Group (COG) and the Société Internationale d'Oncologie Pédiatrique (SIOP)—which supported several large controlled trials in children with WT.

Clinical Presentation and Imaging

A renal tumor is often detected as an asymptomatic abdominal mass. Renal tumors a may present with hematuria—gross in 18.2% and microscopic in 24.5% of patients.[4] Overall, 20% to 25% of patients present with hypertension and 10% with fever. Rarely, a child may have abdominal trauma and demonstrate pain out of proportion to what is expected, and an abdominal mass is found that cannot be attributed to the trauma. Renal tumors can extend through the renal vein (11%), inferior vena cava (IVC) (4%), and right atrium (4%), or down through the ureter.[5] The common sites of metastatic spread include the lungs and the liver. Ultrasound examination is a good screening examination to determine if a mass is renal or extra renal in origin. A computed tomography (CT) scan of the abdomen or MRI will further define the tumor. Although there are no pathognomonic radiographic findings of a WT or other renal tumor. A "claw sign" is characteristic of a primary renal tumor (**Fig. 1**). In addition, WT tend to push other structures away whereas a neuroblastoma grows in and around structures. Vascular tumor extension is best detected by Doppler ultrasound examination or CT scan (**Fig. 2**).[6] A CT scan of the chest is the best method to detect the presence of pulmonary disease (**Fig. 3**).

Pathophysiology

Nephrogenesis in the normal kidney is usually complete by 34 to 36 weeks of gestation. The presence of nephrogenic rests (NRs)—persistent metanephric tissue in the kidney after the 36th week of gestation has been associated with the occurrence of WT. NRs are considered precursor lesions to WT. The presence of multiple or diffuse NRs is termed nephroblastomatosis. NRs may be further classified by their growth phase, which has been separated into 3 phases: (1) incipient or dormant, (2) hyperplastic NRs, which are composed of epithelial elements with nodular expansive growth, and (3) sclerosing rests, which consist of stromal and epithelial elements with few blastemal nephrogenic elements. Most NRs are dormant or in the sclerosing phase, and the majority will resolve

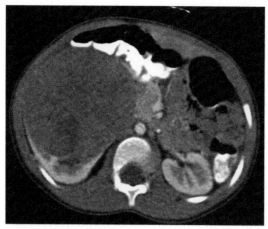

Fig. 1. CT scan showing the classic "claw" sign for a WT.

spontaneously. The pathologic distinction between NR and WT can be very difficult. In fact, it is impossible to distinguish a hyperplastic NR from a WT based on an incisional or needle biopsy specimen that does not include the margin between the NR and the remaining kidney.[7] Most hyperplastic nodules lack a pseudocapsule at their periphery, whereas most WTs will have one (**Fig. 4**). It is very difficult to diagnose NRs on imaging. Although MRI may be helpful, there is no gold standard.[8] Diffuse hyperplastic perilobar nephroblastomatosis is a unique category of nephroblastomatosis in which the rests form a thick rind around the periphery of the kidney (**Fig. 5**). Infants with diffuse hyperplastic perilobar

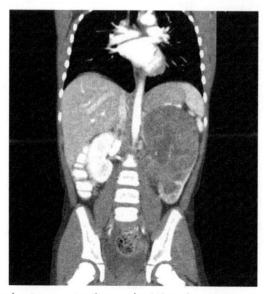

Fig. 2. CT scan showing tumor extension up the IVC to the atrium.

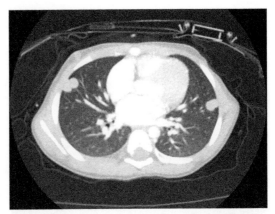

Fig. 3. CT scan of a pulmonary metastatic lesion in a patient with WT.

nephroblastomatosis may initially present with large unilateral or bilateral flank masses and are considered premalignant lesions.[9]

Staging and Prognostic Factors

Staging

WT staging occurs either at the time presentation (primary nephrectomy or biopsy) for children treated on COG protocols or after neoadjuvant therapy and nephrectomy on SIOP protocols (**Table 1**). Patients are given a local stage and a disease stage ranging from I to V for bilateral disease. The local stage defines the extent of abdominal disease, and the disease stage considers both the local extent of disease and distant metastasis. Both factors determine therapy. Therapeutic modalities can include

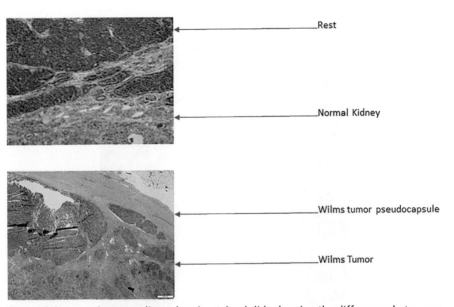

Fig. 4. High-power hematoxylin and eosin–stained slide showing the differences between a NR and a WT.

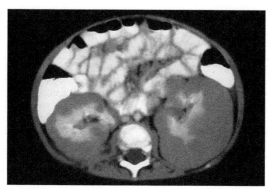

Fig. 5. CT scan of the abdomen demonstrating diffuse perilobar hyperplastic nephroblastomatosis.

surgery alone, chemotherapy regimens and/or radiation therapy to the flank, abdomen, or lungs.[10]

Prognostic factors

The current prognostic factors used in COG trials are histology, stage, age (<2 years), tumor weight (<550 g), response to therapy, and loss of heterozygosity (LOH) at 1p and 16q. The 2 most important factors continue to be the pathology and the stage of the tumor.[11,12] **Table 2** shows the risk stratification for the COG system. The SIOP risk classification was revised in 2010 based on a review of the histologic appearance of the tumors at resection (after neoadjuvant chemotherapy) and the corresponding outcomes[13] **(Table 3)**.

Pathology

WTs are classified as either favorable or unfavorable. Favorable histology comprises 90% of the tumors. These tumors are the classic WT consisting of 3 elements: blastemal, stromal, and epithelial tubules. The proportion of these 3 elements in WTs have been studied, but have not been shown to predict outcomes before neoadjuvant treatment. However, data from SIOP (where prenephrectomy chemotherapy is routinely is used) the amount of blastemal elements that remains is predictive of outcome. Blastemal predominant subtypes are considered high risk tumors.[14,15] Unfavorable tumors (unfavorable histology) are those with focal or diffuse anaplasia.[7,16] Anaplasia is defined by multipolar polyploid mitotic figures, marked nuclear enlargement (giant nuclei with diameters at least 3 times those of adjacent cells), and hyperchromasia.[17] Anaplasia can be either focal or diffuse.[11]

Molecular genetics

There are 3 major epigenetic and genetic changes observed in WT: (a) WT 1 loss, (b) WNT pathway activation, and (c) IGF2 overexpression (most common) without WT-1. The *WT1* gene, a tumor suppressor gene, was the first gene to be linked with WT development.[18,19] Wild-type *WT1* is involved in cell growth, differentiation, and apoptosis.[20] Patients heterozygous for *WT1* germline mutations are predisposed to WT, and *WT1* is inactivated in tumors (eg, WAGR). Based on this observation, it would be expected that many patients with sporadic WT would have a mutation in the *WT1* gene. Surprisingly, the incidence of mutations of *WT1* associated with WT in the sporadic form of the disease is low (10%–20%).[20,21]

Table 1
Comparison between the COG and the SIOP staging systems

Stage	COG	SIOP
I	The tumor is limited to the kidney and has been completely resected. The tumor was not ruptured or biopsied before removal. No penetration of the renal capsule or involvement of renal sinus vessels. Lymph node status is known and negative.	The tumor is limited to the kidney or surrounded with a fibrous pseudocapsule if outside the normal contours of the kidney; the renal capsule or pseudocapsule may be infiltrated with the tumor but it does not reach the outer surface, and it is completely resected. The tumor may be protruding (bulging) into the pelvic system and dipping into the ureter, but it is not infiltrating their walls. The vessels of the renal sinus are not involved. Intrarenal vessels may be involved.
II	The tumor extends beyond the capsule of the kidney but was not completely resected with no evidence of tumor at or beyond the margins of resection. There is penetration of the renal capsule. There is penetration of the renal sinus vessels. Lymph node status is known and negative.	The tumor extends beyond the kidney or penetrates through the renal capsule and/or fibrous pseudocapsule into the perirenal fat, but is completely resected. The tumor infiltrates the renal sinus and/or invades blood and lymphatic vessels outside the renal parenchyma, but it is completely resected. The tumor infiltrates adjacent organs or vena cava, but is completely resected. The tumor has been surgically biopsied (wedge biopsy) before preoperative chemotherapy or surgery.
III	Gross or microscopic residual tumor remains postoperatively including: inoperable tumors, positive surgical margins, tumor spillage surfaces, regional lymph node metastasis, positive peritoneal cytology or transected tumor thrombus. The tumor was ruptured or biopsied before removal.	Incomplete excision of the tumor, which extends beyond resection margins (gross or microscopic tumor remains postoperatively). Any abdominal lymph nodes are involved. Tumor rupture before or during surgery (irrespective of other criteria for staging). The tumor has penetrated the peritoneal surface. Tumor implants are found on the peritoneal surface. The tumor thrombi present at resection, margins of vessels or ureter transected or removed piecemeal by surgeon.
IV	Hematogenous metastases or lymph-node metastases outside the abdomen (eg, lung, liver, bone, brain).	Hematogenous metastases (lung, liver, bone, brain, etc.) or lymph node metastases outside the abdominopelvic region.
V	Bilateral renal tumors at diagnosis. Each side has to be substaged according to above classifications.	Bilateral renal tumors at diagnosis. Each side has to be substaged according to above classifications.

IGF2 (WT2) was the second set of genes to be associated with WT gene location was identified by linkage analysis in children with Beckwith–Wiedemann syndrome.[22] This site is not a single gene, but contains several genes that may play a role in tumor development. In patients with Beckwith–Wiedemann syndrome, it was found that the

Table 2
COG risk stratification for WTs

Age	Tumor Weight, g	Stage	LOH 1p and 16q	Rapid Response	Pathology	Risk Group
<2	<550	I	Any	N/A	FH	Very low
Any	≤550	I	None	N/A	FH	Low
≥2	Any	I	None	NA	FH	Low
Any	Any	II	None	N/A	FH	Low
≥2	Any	I	LOH +	N/A	FH	Standard
Any	≤550	I	LOH +	N/A	FH	Standard
Any	Any	II	LOH+	N/A	FH	Standard
Any	Any	III	None	Any	FH	Standard
Any	Any	III	LOH +	Any	FH	Higher
Any	Any	IV	LOH +	Any	FH	Higher
Any	Any	IV	None	Yes	FH	Standard
Any	Any	IV	None	No	FH	Higher
Any	Any	1-IV	Any	Any	UH	Higher
Any	Any	V	Any	Any	FH/UH	Bilateral

Abbreviations: FH, favorable histology; UH, unfavorable histology.

maternal allele of 11p15 was uniformly lost.[23] The process that causes this loss is termed genomic imprinting, whereby 1 allele is imprinted, in a parental-specific manner, to be functionally inactive. Recent studies suggest the loss of imprinting caused by hypermethlyation leading to WT is primarily located in the IC1 gene.[24–26] A LOH at 1p and 16 is used to risk stratify patients. Event-free survival and overall survival in patients with WT tumor with LOH at 1p and 16q were noted to be lower than those without LOH.[27] Prospective studies showed that increasing therapy could reverse those differences in event-free survival and overall survival.[28] Despite these exciting improvements, LOH is found in only 5% of patients. Chromosome 1q gain is found in up to 30% of patients with WT.[29–31] Recent retrospective studies have shown that 1q gain is associated with inferior outcomes across all stages of favorable

Table 3
SIOP postchemotherapy risk stratification

Risk	Histology
Low	Completely necrotic Favorable histology
Intermediate	Nephroblastoma epithelial type Nephroblastoma stromal type Nephroblastoma mixed type Nephroblastoma regressive type Nephroblastoma focal anaplasia type
High	Nephroblastoma blastemal type Nephroblastoma diffuse anaplasia type

histology WT.[32,33] In the upcoming COG studies, the augmentation and reduction of therapy will be based on the presence or absence of a 1q gain.

Age and weight
The current prognostic factors used in COG trials are histology, stage, age (<2 years), tumor weight (<550 g), response to therapy, and LOH at 1p and 16q. The 2 most important factors continue to be the histology and the stage of the tumor.[11,12] Children less than 2 years of age and had tumors that weighed less than 550 g with a favorable histology can be treated by surgery alone.[34]

Rapid response
Rapid response to chemotherapy was recently tested on ARENO533, which evaluated children in whom CT evidence of pulmonary metastases resolved after 6 weeks. In these patients, it was shown to be safe to avoid pulmonary radiation.[35]

Renal cell carcinoma
RCC is the second most common renal malignancy diagnosed among pediatric and adolescent patients, accounting for 2% to 6% of renal cancers. In contrast with patients with WT, those with RCC are generally older, with a median age at diagnosis of 12.9 years. RCC associated with familial syndromes (eg, Von Hippel–Lindau disease) typically presents with a higher proportion of multifocality and bilaterality.[36] Syndrome-associated RCC often presents at a younger age. In an investigation by Selle and colleagues[37] of the German Childhood Cancer Registry, one-third of patients with RCC were found to have an underlying medical condition, such as tuberous sclerosis, or previous treatment (eg, chemotherapy). Although uncommon as a secondary malignancy, RCC has been reported in children diagnosed with other cancers, neuroblastoma in particular.[38] RCC in children displays gross and histologic features similar to those seen in adults. Subtypes of RCC include papillary, medullary, translocation cell, clear cell, chromophobe, collecting duct, multilocular cystic, and unclassified. In a report from the COG translocation, RCC was the most common form of RCC.[39] Staging of RCC combines the TMN classification as well as stages I to IV. The clinical stage at the time of diagnosis is the most important prognostic factor, and the identification of renal vascular invasion does not seem to be an adverse predictor in children with RCC. Radical nephrectomy and regional lymphadenectomy have been the primary modality for cure, and children with distant spread have a very poor prognosis. The overall survival is much worse than for WT, with the best prognosis for those with complete resection and no metastatic disease. RCC is remarkably resistant to chemotherapy, preventing cure in most children with metastatic disease. The recent use of monoclonal antibody therapy for metastatic disease has been promising.[40] The first prospective study of pediatric and adolescent RCC was performed by the COG between 2006 and 2012. Surgery was the main treatment for localized disease and the investigator could choose any neoadjuvant therapy. Sixty-eight patients were enrolled, and the event-free survival rate was 80.2%; the overall survival rate was 84.8% (stage I = 92, stage II = 100%, stage III = 79.5, and stage IV = 33.3%).[41]

There are some subtle differences between the surgical management of RCC in adults and children. First, there are fewer partial nephrectomies performed and that is because WT are far more common than RCC and a biopsy will upstage WT. Second in adults, lymph node disease is based on cross-sectional imaging and not pathologic confirmation. This approach is not supported in pediatric RCC. Lymph node disease is common and observed among patients with small primary tumors. Using a size cutoff of 1 cm, imaging detection of lymph node involvement had a sensitivity of 57.14% (20 of 35 cases; 95% confidence interval, 39.35%–73.68%) and a specificity of 94.59% (35 of 37 cases; 95% confidence interval, 81.81%–99.34%).[39] Owing to the relative frequency of translocation RCC and the poor outcomes in high stage disease in both adolescents and young adults, the National Institutes of Health sponsored a combined study between the COG and adult cancer groups comparing double mono-clonal antibody therapy in patients with translocation RCC.[42] That study is currently open and accruing.

Surgical management of renal tumors
The goals of primary surgery for unilateral renal tumors include clearance of all local disease, accurate nodal staging, and complete pathologic evaluation. While achieving these goals, the surgeon must avoid actions, that may require more inten-sive postoperative therapy, such as biopsy or tumor spillage, or that result in avoid-able complications, such as the unneeded resection of surrounding organs. Unilateral radical nephroureterectomy with lymph node sampling is the recommen-ded procedure and is supported by multiple cooperative trials.[43–45] In COG trials, a primary nephrectomy is preferred and in SIOP upfront neoadjuvant therapy is preferred for WT. In children less than 7 months of age who have a renal tumor, both cooperative groups agree that primary nephrectomy is associated with better outcomes.[46]

Preparing the child for the operating room
A complete blood count and typing is needed because children can have anemia at presentation. Coagulation studies are also important owing to the possibility of ac-quired von Willebrand disease. Acquired von Willebrand disease has been reported in patients with WT and other malignancies and has important implications for the sur-geon.[47,48] Initially thought to be clinically insignificant, recent reports of profuse intra-operative bleeding that only stopped after ligation of the renal vessels have contradicted this assumption. The mechanism of acquired von Willebrand disease in WT is unknown, but the initial sign was a prolonged prothrombin time and partial thromboplastin time. When found, acquired von Willebrand disease should mandate collecting a further history for bleeding and factor analysis. Although correction of fac-tor levels before surgery seems to help in most cases, it does not guarantee that sig-nificant intraoperative bleeding will not occur. Preoperative embolization should be considered as a management strategy.

Incision
A transabdominal or thoracoabdominal incision is used, because other incisions have been shown to increase the risk of tumor spillage and limit necessary staging evalua-tion. Complete peritoneal exploration and sampling of hilar and aortocaval nodes are mandatory. If preoperative imaging suggests any possibility of a contralateral lesion, the opposite kidney should be evaluated before nephrectomy.[43–45,49,50] The renal pelvis or ureter can be involved with the tumor and should be divided at the most distal level possible, with care taken to avoid tumor spillage.[51] The presence of hematuria may suggest involvement of the ureter and cystoscopy could be considered. The renal vein requires evaluation by palpation and/or intraoperative ultrasound examination to rule out tumor thrombus, which should be resected en bloc when present, avoiding spillage.[5]

WT can be adherent to, but rarely invades, the surrounding organs. Upfront hepa-tectomy or en bloc resection of the surrounding organs for metastasis or direct spread is unwarranted, because this practice increases complications and confers no benefit in survival.[43,44,49,52] Ipsilateral adrenalectomy, previously standard, is no longer recommended if the gland is easily separated from the tumor; a retrospective study showed tumor invasion in fewer than 5% of ipsilateral adrenal glands.[53] Resection of small portions of diaphragm or other nonvital structures to avoid rupture is recommended. Surgical treatment combined with imaging, pathologic, and biological data is used to assign the patient an appropriate local and disease stage. All the factors are then combined to determine the patient's risk group and subsequent therapy. The risk of long-term renal failure in unilateral WT and other renal tumors is less than 1% and does not justify nephron-sparing surgery.

There are a few indications when WT tumors are considered unresectable. These indications are (1) a solitary kidney, bilateral WT, or genetic risk factors for the development of bilateral WT; (2) pulmonary compromise owing to extensive pulmonary metastases; (3) a tumor with extension of the tumor thrombus into the IVC that extends to the level of the hepatic veins (owing to an associated 26% increase in massive bleeding[5]); and (4) contiguous structure involvement, whereby the only means of removing the kidney and tumor requires removal of the other structures (eg, spleen, pancreas, colon, but excluding the adrenal gland and diaphragm). Finally, should the surgeon or anesthesiologist feel that upfront resection would incur unnecessary morbidity or mortality, neoadjuvant chemotherapy with a reevaluation at 6 weeks is an option.[54] Neoadjuvant chemotherapy generally leads to regression tumor shrinkage in the situation of caval or atrial thrombus with a low risk of progression or embolism.[5,44,55]

In patients with a known or suspected diagnosis of RCC, a partial nephrectomy should be attempted if possible. Furthermore, effective cytoreductive therapy is not available for patients with RCC and therefore may require more aggressive surgery to remove the primary mass.

Specific Surgical Conditions

Vascular extension

Vascular extension of the tumor thrombus to the IVC has been reported in 6% to 10% of patients, with atrial extension in 1%[5] (**Fig. 6**). For patients with WT, the overall survival is comparable with similarly staged patients without vascular extension, and survival is comparable whether the thrombus is resected upfront or after initial chemotherapy.[5,55] Vascular extension above the hepatic veins increases the risk of bleeding complications, and neoadjuvant chemotherapy is currently recommended in cases where the thrombus extends into the retrohepatic cava.[5,43,44] CT scans and Doppler ultrasound examinations are equally useful for assessing vascular extension to inform presurgical planning,[6] but intraoperative IVC and/or renal vein palpation remains essential to avoid transecting an unidentified thrombus. Intraoperative ultrasound can also be used if preoperative imaging and intraoperative palpation is unclear at defining the presence or extension of intravascular disease. In the National Wilms Tumor Study-4, 87% of patients with IVC extension and 58% of patients with atrial extension had significant regression of their tumor thrombus with initial chemotherapy, and complications during neoadjuvant treatment were rare.[5] Excision of vascular extension of tumor requires proximal and distal control, which may require cardiopulmonary bypass in cases of persistent atrial thrombus. Intraoperative ultrasound examination and hepatic mobilization may help with mapping of the thrombus. Most often, the tumor thrombus can be gently delivered out of the affected vein, but venotomy and curettage may be necessary for large or adherent thrombi. Division of the tumor thrombus constitutes spillage and consequent upstaging to stage III, so all efforts should be made to resect it in continuity with the primary tumor.

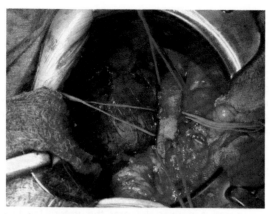

Fig. 6. Intraoperative photograph of a WT with IVC tumor.

Horseshoe kidney

WT or RCC presenting in a horseshoe kidney is rare. In patients with a renal tumor arising in a horseshoe kidney, care must be taken to identify anomalous vasculature, collecting system, and ureteral anatomy on preoperative imaging and at the time of surgical exploration. Complete resection of the affected renal moiety and the isthmus is recommended, and care should be taken to ensure hemostasis after division of the isthmus. As with all unilateral WT or RCC resections, complete resection, adequate nodal sampling, and avoidance of spillage are paramount. A horseshoe kidney does not increase the risk of having a bilateral tumor. This misconception is common, especially in children with WT.

Surgical Management of Wilms Tumor Metastases at the Time of Presentation

Intra-abdominal metastases

Peritoneal metastasis may be encountered in a patient with WT. Any suspicious site in the abdomen or liver should be biopsied or resected (if easily removed) at exploration to determine the nature of the mass, because it will affect tumor stage and therapy (particularly the extent of radiotherapy). The resection of liver masses or tumor that would require removal of intra-abdominal organs and bowel is not indicated as a primary procedure. If residual intra-abdominal metastatic disease remains at week 12 of chemotherapy, it should be resected only if complete resection is feasible. If complete resection is not feasible, then the residual disease should be reassessed for feasibility of resection at the completion of therapy.

Pulmonary metastasis

The lung is the most frequent site of metastatic disease. The treatment of pulmonary disease has changed. In the past, all patients with pulmonary disease received pulmonary radiation. However, the results of the ARENO533 study demonstrated that up to 40% of patients with pulmonary disease will completely respond to chemotherapy after 2 cycles and do not require pulmonary radiation. There are 3 situations in which a surgeon may be needed for the management of pulmonary metastases. First, if there is any doubt regarding the nature of the pulmonary nodule(s) at presentation, these nodules should be biopsied. As many as one-third of small (<1 cm) lesions may not be metastatic tumor. Second, if at the end of 2 cycles or 6 weeks of chemotherapy doubt remains about the nature of the pulmonary lesion, a biopsy should be performed before proceeding with pulmonary radiation. Third, if there are 3 or fewer lesions remaining on a single side that are able to be removed by thoracoscopic resection, this procedure should be performed. Depending on the pathology of these lesions, such patients may be spared pulmonary radiation. Note, however, that it is only for patients with local stage I and II tumors that it is critical to define the nature of small pulmonary lesions at diagnosis. Patients with stage III and IV disease will receive identical chemotherapy regimens for the first 6 weeks. Patients with residual pulmonary lesions and viable tumor at the 6-week time period will receive whole lung radiation and intensified chemotherapy. If pulmonary nodules remain after week 12 of chemotherapy and irradiation, they should be resected if complete resection is feasible. If complete resection is not feasible, then imaging studies should be repeated at the end of protocol therapy to reassess for the feasibility of resection.

Management of tumor extension in the ureter

Extension of WT into the ureter is a rare event and can be difficult to detect on preoperative imaging. In the National Wilms Tumor Study-5, the incidence of ureteral extension was 2% and preoperative imaging detected the ureteral involvement in only 30% of the cases. Clinical findings of ureteral involvement can include gross hematuria, passage of tissue per urethra, hydronephrosis, and a urethral mass. If these findings are encountered, ureteral involvement should be suspected. Cystoscopy with a retrograde ureterogram may aid in the preoperative evaluation. When encountered or suspected, the ureter with tumor extension should be resected with clear margins when possible.

Bilateral Wilms tumors

Bilateral WT occur in up to 13% of patient with WT .[56,57] In addition, there is a population of children with either genetic disorders or tumor-specific features that increase their risk for synchronous and metachronous tumors.[58] In these patients, nephron-sparing surgery is a goal along with oncologic cure. Historically, when compared with patients with unilateral WT, patients with bilateral WT have lower event-free survival and overall survival, higher rates of renal failure, and often undergo protracted courses of chemotherapy and radiotherapy. The 4 year event-free survival for all patients with bilateral WT on the National Wilms Tumor Study-5 was 56%. Recently, the first prospective trial of patients with bilateral WT and unilateral high-risk tumors was published and has greatly improved our understanding of bilateral WT. The primary aims related to patients with bilateral WT were to improve the 4-year event-free survival to 73%, to prevent complete removal of at least 1 kidney in 50% of patients by using a prenephrectomy 3-drug chemotherapy regimen (vincristine, dactinomycin and doxorubicin), and to perform definitive surgical treatment in 75% of children with bilateral WT by 12 weeks after the initiation of chemotherapy. For the 189 patients with bilateral WT enrolled on this study, the 4-year event-free survival and overall survival were 82% and 95%, respectively.[57] Sixty-one percent of the patients required complete nephrectomy of at least 1 kidney. Definitive surgical treatment (partial or complete nephrectomy, or wedge resection in at least 1 kidney) was achieved in 84% of patients by 12 weeks after the initiation of chemotherapy, meeting the goals of the study. A similar excellent result was obtained for those patients with unilateral tumors with a predisposition syndrome.[59]

Wilms tumors in adults

WTs occur rarely in adults and, in most cases, the diagnosis is made on pathology after nephrectomy for a presumed RCC.[60] The outcomes in adults have been mixed. For those patients treated on one of the standard stage risk-based pediatric protocols, the outcomes are equivalent to the pediatric population.[61,62] For those treated on individual plans, outcomes are poorer. In 2011, the SIOP and COG oncologist performed a systematic review and developed protocols for adults with WT.[60] Surgical recommendations are identical to those in the pediatric population, as are the chemotherapy regimens and radiation therapy recommendations. The major changes are to dosing, because the toxicity profiles are different in adults and children.

Treatment outcomes

The excellent 5-year event-free survival and overall survival for favorable histology WT have allowed for a decrease in the intensity of treatment, possibly mitigating late effects. Despite this progress, late effects are still noted. Renal failure, congestive heart failure, hypertension, pulmonary disease, pregnancy complications, and second malignancies are reported in survivors. At 25 years after therapy, a WT survivor's cumulative incidence of severe chronic health conditions is 65.4% compared with 24.2% of the general population.[63] The long-term risk of renal failure at 20 years after treatment among the standard, unilateral, nonsyndromic favorable histology WT patients is 0.6%. The major risk factors for renal failure were exposure to radiation, bilateral WT, and congenital syndromes. Congestive heart failure and hypertension are related to the cumulative doxorubicin dose ($P<.001$), lung irradiation ($P = .037$), and left abdominal irradiation ($P = .013$).[64,65] Nearly 15% of female survivors of WT who were treated with pulmonary radiation therapy developed invasive breast cancer by age 40 years. Pregnancy complicated by hypertension, premature labor, and malposition of the fetus were all statistically more frequent among irradiated women and were related to the radiation therapy dose.[66] The risk of second malignant neoplasms (leukemia and solid tumors) is 6.7% by age 40.[67]

Neoadjuvant Therapy for Wilms Tumor and Renal Cell Carcinoma

Chemotherapy

WT was the first malignant pediatric solid tumor with a demonstrated response to dactinomycin.[68] The current COG chemotherapeutic regimens for unilateral WT are presented in **Table 4**. Adjuvant therapy for RCC in the pediatric population has been varied and determined by the treating physician. Recently, the National Institutes of Health sponsored a pediatric and adult phase II trial for translocation RCC. Efficacy data for vascular endothelial growth factor receptor tyrosine kinase inhibitor (axitinib) and programmed death 1/programmed death ligand 1 targeted therapy (nivolumab), 2 key RCC therapeutic targets, will be assessed prospectively as a 2-arm randomized trial assessing axitinib and nivolumab in combination or nivolumab alone.[42]

Radiotherapy

The 3 principle fields for radiation therapy for renal tumors are whole abdominal, flank, and lung (metastatic lung disease). Favorable histology tumors are generally very radiosensitive. Current guidelines for radiation therapy for WT in the North American protocols are based on the results of prior cooperative group studies.[69,70] Abdominal radiation is used for stage III or higher disease. In most cases, flank radiation of 10 Gy is used. Currently, for favorable histology WT whole abdominal radiation is only used in (1) peritoneal seeding, (2) preoperative tumor rupture, and (3) an intraoperative spill that is widespread in the opinion of the operating surgeon. The role of radiation therapy has yet to be properly clarified for liver metastasis and a retrospective review showed that, for liver metastasis, some children did not receive radiation therapy, some received only flank radiation, and some received a radiation boost to the liver.[52] The treatment portal includes that portion of the liver involved on CT scan or MRI studies. The whole liver is treated in children with diffuse hepatic metastases. The

Table 4
Standard chemotherapy regimens for the COG WT

Regimen	Agents
VAD	Vincristine, dactinomycin, doxorubicin (maximum 12 wk)
EE-4A	vincristine and dactinomycin (19 wk)
DD-4A	Vincristine, dactinomycin, doxorubicin and radiation therapy (with or without radiation therapy) (25 wk)
Regimen I	Vincristine, dactinomycin, doxorubicin, cyclophosphamide, and etoposide, as well as radiation therapy (with or without radiation therapy) (28 wk)
Regimen M	Vincristine, dactinomycin, doxorubicin, etoposide and cyclophosphamide (31 wk) with or without radiation therapy
Regimen VI	Vincristine and Irinotican
UH-1/revised UH-1	Vincristine, dactinomycin, doxorubicin, cyclophosphamide carboplatin, etoposide and radiation (31 wk)

improvement in focal radiation therapy strategies are playing more important roles in treatment, because more precise targeting and sparing of uninvolved tissue is becoming a reality.[71,72]

The management of pulmonary disease in children with WT has become more complicated. Using CT scans results in several lung nodules being identified, not all of which may be WT.[73–76] Pulmonary radiation is used for lesions that do not completely disappear after 6 weeks of 3 drug chemotherapy.[77] To date there are no guidelines for the routine use of radiation therapy in patients with RCC.

CLINICS CARE POINTS

- Renal tumors in children although ofter large are easily resectable.
- Renal tumors in chilsren have both a local and disease stage that affects treatment and short and long term toxicities.
- Failure to sample lymph nodes is the most common mistake made by surgeons treating pediatric renal tumors.

DISCLOSURE

The authors have nothing to disclose.

REFERENCES

1. Howlander N, Noone A, Krapecho M. SEER cancer statistics review 1975-2008 2008. Available at: http://seer.cancer.gov/csr/1975_2008.

2. Breslow N, Olshan A, Beckwith JB, et al. Epidemiology of Wilms tumor. Med Pediatr Oncol 1993;21:172–81.

3. Dome JS, Perlman EJ, Ritchey ML, et al. Renal tumors. In: PA P, DG P, editors. Principles and practice of pediatric oncology. 7th edition. Philadelphia (PA): Lippincott Williams and Wilkins; 2015. p. 753–72.

4. Chu A, Heck JE, Ribeiro KB, et al. Wilms' tumour: a systematic review of risk factors and meta-analysis. Paediatr Perinat Epidemiol 2010;24(5):449–69.

5. Shamberger RC, Ritchey ML, Haase GM, et al. Intravascular extension of Wilms tumor. Ann Surg 2001;234(1):116–21.

6. Khanna G, Rosen N, Anderson JR, et al. Evaluation of diagnostic performance of CT for detection of tumor thrombus in children with Wilms tumor: a report from the Children's oncology group. Pediatr Blood Cancer 2012;58(4):551–5.

7. Perlman EJ. Pediatric renal tumors: practical updates for the pathologist. Pediatr Dev Pathol 2005;8(3):32–338.

8. Sandberg JK, Chi YY, Smith EA, et al. Imaging characteristics of nephrogenic rests versus small Wilms tumors: a report from the children's oncology group study AREN03B2. AJR Am J Roentgenol 2020;214(5):987–94.

9. EJ P, P F, A S, et al. Hyperplastic perilobar nephroblastomatosis: long term survival in 52 patients. Pediatr Blood Cancer 2006;46:203–21.

10. Grundy PE, D JS, Ehrlich PF, al e. Renal tumors classification, biology and banking studies. Available at: https://memberschildrensoncologygrouporg/Prot/AREN03B2/AREN03B2DOCpdf. 2016. p. 18–33.

11. Dome JS, Fernandez CV, Mullen EA, et al. Children's oncology group's 2013 blueprint for research: renal tumors. Pediatr Blood Cancer 2013;60(6):994–1000.

12. Dome JS, Graf N, Geller JI, et al. Advances in Wilms tumor treatment and biology: progress through international collaboration. J Clin Oncol 2015;33(27): 2999–3007.

13. Vujanic G, Sandstedt B. The pathology of Wilms' tumour (nephroblastoma): the International society of paediatric oncology approach. J Clin Pathol 2010;63: 102–9.

14. Reinhard H, Semler O, Bürger D. Results of the SIOP 93-01/GPOH trial and study for the treatment of patients with unilateral nonmetastatic Wilms Tumor. Klin Padiatr 2004;216(3):132–40.

15. Pasqualini C, Furtwangler R, van Tinteren H, et al. Outcome of patients with stage IV high-risk Wilms tumour treated according to the SIOP2001 protocol: a report of the SIOP renal tumour study group. Eur J Cancer 2020;128:38–46.

16. Scelo G, Hofmann JN, Banks RE, et al. International cancer seminars: a focus on kidney cancer. Ann Oncol 2016;27(8):1382–5.

17. Zuppan CW, Beckwith JB, Luckey DW. Anaplasia in unilateral Wilms tumor. A report from the National Wilms tumor study pathology center. Hum Path 1988; 19:1199–209.

18. van den Heuvel-Eibrink MM. Wilms tumor. Brisbane (Australia): Codon; 2016.

19. Yang Y, Han Y, Sauez Saiz F, et al. A tumor suppressor and oncogene: the WT1 story. Leukemia 2007;21(868):876.

20. Deng C, Dai R, Li X, et al. Genetic variation frequencies in Wilms' tumor: a meta-analysis and systematic review. Cancer Sci 2016;107(5):690–9.

21. Huff V. Wilms' tumours: about tumour suppressor genes, an oncogene and a chameleon gene. Nat Rev Cancer 2011;11(2):111–21.

22. Ping AJ, Reeve AE, Law DJ, et al. Genetic linkage of Beckwith-Wiedemann syndrome to 11p15. Am J Hum Genet 1989;44(5):720–3.

23. Riccio A, Sparago A, Verde G, et al. Inherited and sporadic epimutations at the IGF2-H19 locus in Beckwith-Wiedemann syndrome and Wilms' tumor. Endocr Dev 2009;14:1–9.

24. DeBaun MR, Niemitz EL, McNeil DE, et al. Epigenetic alterations of H19 and LIT1 distinguish patients with Beckwith-Wiedemann syndrome with cancer and birth defects. Am J Hum Genet 2002;70(3):604–11.

25. Alexandrescu S, Akhavanfard S, Harris MH, et al. Clinical, pathologic, and genetic features of Wilms tumors with WTX gene mutation. Pediatr Dev Pathol 2017;20(2):105–11.

26. Carraro DM, Ramalho RF, Maschietto M. Gene expression in Wilms tumor: disturbance of the Wnt signaling pathway and MicroRNA biogenesis. In: van den Heuvel-Eibrink MM, editor. Wilms tumor. Codon Publications: Brisbane (AU). 2016.Chapter-10.p.150-162.

27. Grundy PE, Breslow N, Li S, et al. Loss of heterozygosity for chromosomes 1p and 16q is an adverse prognostic factor in favorable-histology Wilms tumor: a report from the National Wilms tumor study group. J Clin Oncol 2005;23(29): 7312–21.

28. Dix DB, Fernandez CV, Chi YY, et al. Augmentation of therapy for favorable-histology Wilms tumor with combined loss of heterozygosity of chromosomes 1p and 16q: a report from the Children's Oncology Group studies AREN0532 and AREN0533. J Clin Oncol 2015;33(15 supplement):10009.

29. Bown N, Cotterill SJ, Roberts P, et al. Cytogenetic abnormalities and clinical outcome in Wilms tumor: a study by the U.K. cancer cytogenetics group and the U.K. Children's cancer study group. Med Pediatr Oncol 2002;38(1):11–21.

30. Segers H, van den Heuvel-Eibrink MM, Williams RD, et al. Gain of 1q is a marker of poor prognosis in Wilms' tumors. Genes Chromosomes Cancer 2013;52(11): 1065–74.

31. Chagtai T, Zill C, Dainese L, et al. Gain of 1q as a prognostic biomarker in Wilms tumors (WTs) treated with preoperative chemotherapy in the international society of paediatric oncology (SIOP) WT 2001 trial: a SIOP renal tumours biology consortium study. J Clin Oncol 2016;34(26):3195–203.

32. Gratias EJ, Dome JS, Jennings LJ, et al. Association of chromosome 1q Gain with inferior survival in favorable-histology Wilms tumor: a report from the children's oncology group. J Clin Oncol 2016;34(26):3189–94.

33. Gratias EJ, Jennings LJ, Anderson JR, et al. Gain of 1q is associated with inferior event-free and overall survival in patients with favorable histology Wilms tumor: a report from the Children's oncology group. Cancer 2013;119(21):3887–94.

34. Shamberger RC, Anderson JR, Breslow N, et al. Long-term outcomes for infants with very low risk Wilms tumor treated with surgery alone in National Wilms tumor study-5. Ann Surg 2010;251(3):555–8.

35. Verschuur A, Van Tinteren H, Graf N, et al. Treatment of pulmonary metastases in children with stage IV nephroblastoma with risk-based use of pulmonary radiotherapy. J Clin Oncol 2012;30(28):3533–9.

36. van der Beek JN, Geller JI, de Krijger RR, et al. Characteristics and outcome of children with renal cell carcinoma: a narrative review. Cancers (Basel) 2020; 12(7):1776.

37. Selle B, Furtwangler R, Graf N, et al. Population-based study of renal cell carcinoma in children in Germany, 1980-2005: more frequently localized tumors and underlying disorders compared with adult counterparts. Cancer 2006;107(12): 2906–14.

38. Gupta S, Vanderbilt CM, Leibovich BC, et al. Secondary renal neoplasia following chemotherapy or radiation in pediatric patients. Hum Pathol 2020. https://doi.org/10.1016/j.humpath.2020.07.014.

39. Geller JI, Ehrlich PF, Cost NG, et al. Characterization of adolescent and pediatric renal cell carcinoma: a report from the Children's oncology group study AREN03B2. Cancer 2015;121(14):2457–64.

40. Lalani AA, Li H, Heng DYC, et al. First-line sunitinib or pazopanib in metastatic renal cell carcinoma: the Canadian experience. Can Urol Assoc J 2017; 11(3–4):112–7.

41. Geller J, Cost NG, Chi YY, et al. A prospective study of pediatric and adolescent renal cell carcinoma: a report from the children's oncology group (COG) study AREN0321. Cancer 2020;26(23):5156–64.

42. Geller JI, Cost NG, Dome JS, et al A Randomized Phase 2 Trial of Axitinib/Nivolumab combination therapy vs single agent Nivolumab for the treatment of TFE/ Translocation Renal Cell Carcinoma across all age groups. 2020.

43. Ritchey ML, Kelalis PP, Breslow N, et al. Surgical complications after nephrectomy for Wilms' tumor. Surg Gynecol Obstet 1992;175(6):507–14.

44. Ritchey ML, Shamberger RC, Haase G, et al. Surgical complications after primary nephrectomy for Wilms' tumor: report from the National Wilms' Tumor study group. J Am Coll Surg 2001;192(1):63–8 [quiz 146].

45. Ehrlich PF, Anderson JR, Ritchey ML, et al. Clinicopathologic findings predictive of relapse in children with stage III favorable-histology Wilms tumor. J Clin Oncol 2013;31(9):1196–201.

46. van den Heuvel-Eibrink MM, Paul G, Norbert G. Characteristics and survival of 750 children diagnosed with a renal tumor in the first seven months of life: a collaborative study by the SIOP/GPOH/SFOP, NWTSG, and UKCCSG Wilms tumor study groups. Pediatr Blood Cancer 2008;50(6):1130–4.

47. Baxter PA, Nutchtern JG, Guillerman RP, et al. Acquired von Willebrand syndrome and Wilms tumor: not always benign. Pediatr Blood Cancer 2009;52: 392–428.

48. Coppes MJ, Zandvoort SW, Sparling CR. Acquired von Willebrand disease in Wilms' tumor patients. J Clin Oncol 1992;10(3):422–7.

49. Shamberger RC, Guthrie KA, Ritchey ML, et al. Surgery-related factors and local recurrence of Wilms tumor in National Wilms Tumor Study 4. Ann Surg 1999; 229(2):292–7.

50. Ehrlich PF, Ritchey ML, Hamilton TE, et al. Quality assessment for Wilms' tumor: a report from the National Wilms' Tumor Study-5. J Pediatr Surg 2005;40(1):208–12.

51. Ritchey M, Daley S, Shamberger RC, et al. Ureteral extension in Wilms' tumor: a report from the National Wilms' tumor study group (NWTSG). J Pediatr Surg 2008; 43(9):1625–9.

52. Ehrlich PF, Ferrer FA, Ritchey ML, et al. Hepatic metastasis at diagnosis in patients with Wilms tumor is not an independent adverse prognostic factor for stage IV Wilms tumor: a report from the Children's oncology group/national Wilms tumor study group. Ann Surg 2009;250(4):642–8.

53. Kieran K, Anderson JR, Dome JS, et al. Is adrenalectomy necessary during unilateral nephrectomy for Wilms Tumor? A report from the Children's oncology group. J Pediatr Surg 2013;48(7):1598–603.

54. Kieran K, Ehrlich PF. Current surgical standards of care in Wilms tumor. Urol Oncol 2016;34(1):13–23.

55. Nakayama DK, Norkool P, deLorimier AA, et al. Intracardiac extension of Wilms' tumor. A report of the National Wilms' tumor study. Ann Surg 1986;204(6):693–7.

56. Coppes MJ, de Kraker J, van Dijken PJ. Bilateral Wilms' tumor: long-term survival and some epidemiological features. J Clin Oncol 1989;7(3):310–5.

57. Ehrlich P, Chi YY, Chintagumpala MM, et al. Results of the first prospective multi-institutional treatment study in children with bilateral Wilms tumor (AREN0534): a report from the children's oncology group. Ann Surg 2017;266(3):470–8.

58. Coppes MJ, Beckwith JB, Ritchey ML, et al. Factors affecting the risk of contra-lateral Wilms tumor development (a report from the national Wilms tumor study group). Cancer 1999;85(7):1616–25.

59. Ehrlich PF, Chi YY, Chintagumpala MM, et al. Results of treatment for patients with multicentric or bilaterally predisposed unilateral Wilms tumor (AREN0534): a report from the children's oncology group. Cancer 2020;126(15):3516–25.

60. Segers H, van den Heuvel-Eibrink MM, Pritchard-Jones K, et al. Management of adults with Wilms' tumor: recommendations based on international consensus. Expert Rev Anticancer Ther 2011;11(7):1105–13.

61. Kalapurakal JA, Nan B, Norkool P, et al. Treatment outcomes in adults with favor-able histologic type Wilms tumor-an update from the National Wilms Tumor Study Group. Int J Radiat Oncol Biol Phys 2004;60(5):1379–84.

62. Reinhard H, Aliani S, Ruebe C. Wilms' tumor in adults: results of the society of pe-diatric oncology (SIOP) 93-01/society for pediatric oncology and hematology (GPOH) study. J Clin Oncol 2004;22(22):4500–6.

63. Termuhlen AM, Tersak JM, Liu Q, et al. Twenty-five year follow-up of childhood Wilms tumor: a report from the childhood cancer survivor study. Pediatr Blood Cancer 2011;57(7):1210–6.

64. Green DM, Grigoriev YA, Nan B, et al. Congestive heart failure after treatment for Wilms' tumor: a report from the National Wilms' Tumor Study group. J Clin Oncol 2001;19(7):1926–34.

65. Green DM, Grigoriev YA, Nan B, et al. Correction to "Congestive heart failure after treatment for Wilms' tumor". J Clin Oncol 2003;21(12):2447–8.

66. Green DM, Lange JM, Peabody EM. Pregnancy outcome after treatment for Wilms tumor: a report from the national Wilms tumor long-term follow-up study. J Clin Oncol 2010;28(17):2824–30.

67. Breslow N, Lange JM, Friedma n DL, et al. Secondary malignant neoplasms after Wilms tumor: an international collaborative study. Int J Cancer 2009;127:657–66.

68. Farber S. Chemotherapy in the treatment of leukemia and Wilms' tumor. JAMA 1966;198:826–36.

69. D'Angio GJ, Evans AE, Breslow N, et al. The treatment of Wilms' tumor: results of the National Wilms' tumor study. Cancer 1976;38:633–46.

70. D'Angio GJ, Tefft M, Breslow N, et al. Radiation therapy of Wilms' tumor: results according to dose, field, post-operative timing and histology. Int J Radiat Oncol Biol Phys 1978;4:769–80.

71. Kalapurakal JA, Pokhrel D, Gopalakrishnan M, et al. Advantages of whole-liver in-tensity modulated radiation therapy in children with Wilms tumor and liver metas-tasis. Int J Radiat Oncol Biol Phys 2013;85(3):754–60.

72. Choi M, Hayes JP, Mehta MP, et al. Using intensity-modulated radiotherapy to spare the kidney in a patient with seminoma and a solitary kidney: a case report. Tumori 2013;99(2):e38–42.

73. Green DM. Use of chest computed tomography for staging and treatment of Wilms' tumor in children. J Clin Oncol 2002;20(12):2763–4.

74. Ehrlich PF, Hamilton TE, Grundy PE, et al. The value of surgery in directing ther-apy of Wilms tumor patients with pulmonary disease. a report from the national Wilms tumor study group (NWTS -5). J Pediatr Surg 2006;41(1):162–7.

75. Lange JM, Takashima JR, Peterson SM, et al. Breast cancer in female survivors of Wilms tumor: a report from the national Wilms tumor late effects study. Cancer 2014;120(23):3722–30.

76. Green DM, Lange JM, Qu A, et al. Pulmonary disease after treatment for Wilms tumor: a report from the national Wilms tumor long-term follow-up study. Pediatr Blood Cancer 2013;60(10):1721–6.
77. Kalapurakal JA, Li SM, Breslow N, et al. Influence of radiation therapy delay on abdominal tumor recurrence in patients with favorable histology Wilms' tumor treated on NWTS-3 and NWTS-4: a report from the National Wilms' Tumor Study Group. Int J Radiat Oncol Biol Phys 2003;57:495–9.

Management of Germ Cell Tumors in Pediatric Patients

Brent R. Weil, MD, MPH[a],*, Deborah F. Billmire, MD[b]

KEYWORDS

- Germ cell tumor • Pediatric • Adolescent • Teratoma • Surgery

KEY POINTS

- Optimal surgical treatment for germ cell tumors involves intact resection of the tumor without rupture or spillage while sparing vital structures whenever possible.
- If upfront surgical resection is not possible, would require resection of adjacent organs, and/or would result in unacceptable morbidity, biopsy and chemotherapy should be pursued as an initial strategy.
- Appropriate staging involves both radiographic and intraoperative assessment and is critical for determining needed treatment.
- Platinum-based chemotherapy is used for all malignant germ cell tumors, except for stage I ovarian or testicular germ cell tumors, for which a strategy of observation may be undertaken.
- Future efforts will focus on how to safely decrease the intensity of therapy for low-risk tumors and improving surveillance and treatment for relapsed or refractory disease.

INTRODUCTION

Germ cell tumors (GCT) arise from primordial germ cells and vary widely in their clinical behavior, histology, and locations. The majority of GCTs will develop in the gonads or along the midline structures of the body.[1] Genetic aberrations leading to disruption in the molecular signaling responsible for primordial germ cell migration early in development may provide rationale for why GCTs originate in extragonadal locations.[2]

Because GCTs are often managed by different specialists with outcomes heavily influenced by factors such as patient age and tumor location, variation in their management is common. Thus, establishing best practices for the treatment of pediatric GCTs remains an area of active investigation. Recent advances and current efforts have focused on limiting the toxicities of therapy, identifying new therapies for relapsed and refractory tumors, defining the best practices for surgical staging and

[a] Department of Pediatric Surgery, Boston Children's Hospital, 300 Longwood Avenue, Boston, MA 02115, USA; [b] Department of Pediatric Surgery, Riley Hospital for Children at Indiana University Health, 705 Riley Hospital Drive, Indianapolis, IN 46202, USA
* Corresponding author.
E-mail address: brent.weil@childrens.harvard.edu

Surg Oncol Clin N Am 30 (2021) 325–338
https://doi.org/10.1016/j.soc.2020.11.011
1055-3207/21/© 2020 Elsevier Inc. All rights reserved.

surgonc.theclinics.com

resection, and developing novel methods to monitor for disease relapse. Owing to the rarity of pediatric GCTs, the establishment of multidisciplinary, multi-institutional, and multinational collaboratives has been vital for the study of such efforts.[3]

Herein we review the current concepts that are essential for the successful management of extracranial GCTs developing in children and young adults. Areas of controversy, treatments remaining under active investigation, and scenarios where treatment may vary for children and young adults are highlighted.

EPIDEMIOLOGY

Pediatric GCTs are rare, with an estimated incidence of 11.7 and 6.7 per million among boys and girls, respectively.[4] Although uncommon, GCTs account for approximately 3% of tumors occurring in children under the age of 15, and approximately 14% of tumors among children and young adults ages 15 to 19 years.[2,5] Benign, mature teratomas (MT) represent the most common histology, with the incidence of malignant GCTs varying based on age, sex, and location.

Although most individuals developing GCTs have no known predisposing risk, several conditions associated with an increased risk have been identified. Males with cryptorchidism or Klinefelter's syndrome are at an increased risk for the development of testicular and mediastinal GCTs.[6] Females with Turner's syndrome carry an increased risk for development of ovarian GCTs.[7] Individuals with gonadal dysgenesis syndromes are also at an increased risk for developing GCTs, particularly gonadoblastoma, in streak gonads.[8] An increased incidence of GCTs observed to occur among some families also points to the possibility of heritable genetic risk factors, and the identification of these risk factors remains a subject of ongoing research.[9]

CLASSIFICATION

GCTs arise from pluripotent primordial germ cells. The extent and mode of cellular differentiation that has occurred at the point of tumorigenesis serves as the basis for the categorization of the various histologic subtypes (**Fig. 1**). For clinical purposes, GCTs are commonly classified according to **Box 1**.

MTs are characterized by the presence of well-differentiated tissue derived from ectodermal, mesodermal, and/or endodermal germ layers. The clinical behavior of MTs is generally benign, such that surgical extirpation is the only treatment required. Rare cases of malignant degeneration of tissues within MTs have been described in adults. Immature teratomas (IT) contain immature neuroepithelium and are graded

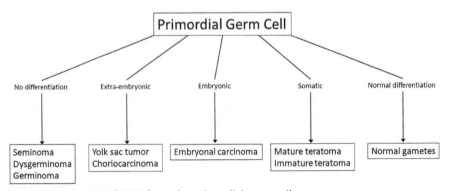

Fig. 1. Development of GCTs from the primordial germ cell.

Box 1
Classification of GCTs

Teratomas
  Mature
  Immature

Malignant GCTs
  Germinomatous GCTs
    Seminoma (testicle)
    Dysgerminoma (ovary)
    Germinoma (extragonadal)
  Nongerminomatous GCTs
    Yolk sac (endodermal sinus) tumor
    Choriocarcinoma
    Embryonal carcinoma
    Gonadoblastoma

Mixed GCTs   Different histologies present within the same tumor

as I, II, or III based on the degree of immaturity. Among adult practitioners, ITs are considered malignant owing to their propensity for local recurrence and local and distant spread.

Malignant GCTs are subdivided into germinomatous and nongerminomatous subtypes ("seminomatous" and "nonseminomatous" are synonymous). Germinomatous GCTs are rare in young children, but their incidence increase among teenagers and young adults. Nongerminomatous tumors, particularly yolk sac tumors, are the most common malignant GCTs occurring before puberty. Gonadoblastomas are rare and can transform to become GCTs of other histologies. They occur almost exclusively in the streak gonads of individuals with disorders of sexual development and such a disorder should be suspected when the diagnosis of gonadoblastoma is made.[8] It is common for tumors to exhibit mixed histologies, with more than 1 malignant GCT type present with or without the presence of a teratoma as well. Somatic malignancies can also develop from within a GCT and should be suspected when tumors are not responding to therapy as anticipated.

ROLE OF TUMOR MARKERS

GCTs secrete substances that are detectable in the systemic circulation, the 2 most relevant being alpha fetoprotein (AFP) and β-hCG (**Table 1**). AFP is elevated in the serum of an estimated 95% to 100% of patients with yolk sac tumors. The measurement of serum AFP is informative during the initial workup for a suspected GCT, for surveillance, and to assess the response to therapy.[10] One exception is in the context of a suspected GCT occurring in infants, for whom serum AFP levels are difficult to interpret because of the marked elevation from the time of birth until its eventual decrease to adult ranges throughout the first 2 to 3 years of life.[11] In addition to its role at diagnosis, the rate of AFP decline after the initiation of therapy is an important prognostic indicator and may provide guidance with respect to the need for therapeutic intensification.

β-hCG is a placental protein that can be elevated in the serum of patients with choriocarcinoma. It is more rarely, and less markedly, elevated in the context of embryonal and germinomatous tumors. It is also useful in the initial workup and surveillance of GCTs, and its rate of decline may hold prognostic value during the course

Table 1
Serum tumor marker levels for pediatric GCTs

GCT Type	AFP	β-hCG	LDH
MT	-	-	-
IT	+/−	-	+/−
Seminoma/dysgerminoma	-	-	+
Yolk sac tumor	+	-	-
Choriocarcinoma	-	+	-
Embryonal carcinoma	+	+	+/−

+ usually elevated; +/− may be elevated; - usually not elevated.

of treatment for germinomatous tumors in adults.[12] Last, lactate dehydrogenase, although less specific than either AFP or β-hCG, is also useful in the initial diagnosis and surveillance of GCTs, particularly germinomatous tumors.

STAGING AND RISK GROUPS

Pediatric GCTs are staged according to the Children's Oncology Group (COG) system (**Table 2**).[13] Distinct adult staging systems for gonadal GCTs also exist and include the International Federation of Gynecology and Obstetrics for ovarian malignancies, and the American Joint Committee on Cancer system for testicular malignancies.

Risk groups for pediatric GCTs have been developed based on factors known to influence outcomes. The current system was developed with international collaboration between COG and the UK Children's Cancer and Leukemia Group as a part of the Malignant Germ Cell International Collaborative (MaGIC) (**Table 3**).[14] The MaGIC risk stratification schema identifies which pediatric patients with GCT may be appropriate to receive reduced therapy and who may require an intensification of therapy based on historical outcomes. In this regard, it is expected to inform treatment recommendations for future clinical trials.

MEDICAL THERAPY

Platinum-based chemotherapy serves as the backbone for the medical treatment of pediatric and adult GCTs.[15] Bleomycin, etoposide, and cisplatin are administered as the standard regimen for adult GCTs. The regimen has been adapted for the treatment of pediatric GCTs by including a reduced dose of bleomycin and is commonly referred to as "PEb."[16] Owing to the pulmonary toxicity of bleomycin and ototoxicity and other toxicities of cisplatin, both adult and pediatric studies have examined the role of alternative agents and dose reduction strategies.[17] Recent experience in children suggests, for instance, that carboplatin may be substituted for cisplatin leading to reduced toxicity while maintaining similar event-free survival rates and overall survival rates.[18,19]

A recognition that most children with GCTs experience excellent overall survival has led to a decrease in the amount of chemotherapy given.[14] Historically, chemotherapy was recommended for all malignant GCTs. Studies have shown, however, that stage I gonadal GCTs can be successfully treated with surgery and observation alone, with many patients requiring no further therapy, and those experiencing relapse nearly always being successfully salvaged with chemotherapy.[20,21] As such, observation alone after complete surgical staging and resection may be appropriate for children with

Table 2
COG staging system for pediatric GCTs

Stage	Testis	Ovary	Extragonadal
I	Complete resection via orchiectomy. Lymph nodes negative.	Limited to ovary (with negative evaluation of peritoneum), no evidence of extraovarian disease	Complete resection at any site with negative margins (including coccygectomy for sacrococcygeal teratomas)
II	Trans-scrotal biopsy performed, microscopic disease in scrotum or cord, failure of tumor markers to normalize	Microscopic residual disease, peritoneal evaluation negative, failure of tumor markers to normalize	Microscopic residual disease with negative lymph nodes, failure of tumor markers to normalize
III	Retroperitoneal lymph node involvement without visceral or extra-abdominal involvement	Lymph node involvement, metastatic nodule, gross residual disease, or biopsy only, contiguous visceral involvement (omentum, bladder, intestine), peritoneal evaluation positive	Lymph node involvement, gross residual disease, biopsy only
IV	Distant metastases	Distant metastases	Distant metastases

Data from Rescorla F, Billmire D, Stolar C, et al. The effect of cisplatin dose and surgical resection in children with malignant germ cell tumors at the sacrococcygeal region: a pediatric intergroup trial (POG 9049/CCG 8882). *J Pediatr Surg.* 2001;36(1):12-17.

stage I malignant gonadal GCTs. Otherwise, PEb is recommended for intermediate and poor risk GCTs (stage I extragonadal outside of a clinical trial and all stage II–IV disease).

Medical therapy for IT is controversial. Platinum-based chemotherapy was historically administered, with early adult studies noting higher rates of relapse among women with grades 2 and 3 ovarian ITs who did not receive chemotherapy.[22] As such, the administration of bleomycin, etoposide, and cisplatin chemotherapy for all grades 2 and 3 IT is commonly recommended by adult practitioners. For children, it has long been recognized that outcomes for IT are excellent without chemotherapy.[23] Among pediatric practitioners, it is now generally accepted that ITs are largely unresponsive to chemotherapy and its use has fallen out of favor.[23,24]

GENERAL PRINCIPLES IN THE SURGICAL MANAGEMENT OF PEDIATRIC GERM CELL TUMORS

Surgery is a key component in both the treatment and staging of pediatric GCTs. During the initial workup, ultrasound examination, computed tomography (CT) scans, or MRI may be useful for imaging the primary tumor. Both cystic and solid components may be appreciated. CT scans or MRI are then generally necessary to evaluate the primary tumor. The presence of fat and calcium, often present in MTs and mixed GCTs, may be appreciated on CT scans and MRIs. It must be emphasized that, although the presence of cystic components, calcium, and fat are frequently identified on diagnostic imaging for MTs, these features can frequently be seen in mixed and other malignant GCTs, so the diagnosis of MT must not be assumed given these findings (**Fig. 2**).

As a part of the staging process for ovarian, testicular, sacrococcygeal, and retroperitoneal GCTs, abdominal and retroperitoneal imaging via CT scan or MRI is

Table 3
Proposed MaGIC pediatric GCT risk stratification system

Risk Group	Age (y)	Location	COG Stage	Survival (%)
Low	Any age	Testis	I	100
	Any age	Ovary	I	96
	Any age	Extragonadal	I	93
Standard	<11	Testis	II/III	99
	<11	Testis	IV	96
	≥11	Testis	II/III	93
	≥11	Testis	IV	83
	<11	Ovary	II/III	97
	<11	Ovary	IV	92
	≥11	Ovary	II/III	85
	<11	Extragonadal	II/III	91
	<11	Extragonadal	IV	79
Poor	≥11	Testis	IV	83
	≥11	Extragonadal	III	61
	≥11	Ovary	IV	60
	≥11	Extragonadal	IV	40

Adapted from Frazier AL, Hale JP, Rodriguez-Galindo C, et al. Revised risk classification for pediatric extracranial germ cell tumors based on 25 years of clinical trial data from the United Kingdom and United States. J Clin Oncol. 2015;33(2):195-201.

necessary to evaluate for signs of intraperitoneal spread and/or retroperitoneal lymphadenopathy. Chest imaging is indicated to rule out pulmonary metastases. When feasible and when the expected morbidity is minimal, upfront surgical resection for all GCTs is preferable. If a tumor is deemed unresectable or resection would be associated with unacceptable morbidity, a preoperative biopsy and the establishment of venous access for chemotherapy is most appropriate, followed by definitive surgical resection when appropriate.

SURGICAL MANAGEMENT OF PEDIATRIC OVARIAN GERM CELL TUMORS

The optimal operation for ovarian GCTs involves a complete resection of the tumor without rupture or spillage and performance of complete peritoneal staging.[20] Rupture or spillage will result in upstaging and may necessitate the addition of chemotherapy that might have otherwise been avoided. If complete resection of the tumor would require en bloc removal of any organ other than the ipsilateral ovary and fallopian tube, a biopsy should be performed and resection should be postponed until after the administration of neoadjuvant chemotherapy.

For suspected malignant GCTs, resection via ipsilateral oophorectomy is the operation of choice. If uninvolved, the fallopian tube can be preserved. If an MT is suspected in the setting of negative serum tumor markers, an ovarian-sparing approach should be pursued whenever possible. This factor is especially relevant, considering that the development of metachronous lesions on the contralateral ovary can occur in an estimated 8% to 10% of patients.[25] If an ovarian-sparing operation is performed and the diagnosis of IT is ultimately rendered, completion oophorectomy has traditionally been recommended, although some investigators would advocate instead for close surveillance.

The performance of complete intraperitoneal staging is of vital importance. Failure to do so may result in an inability to assign stage I and the need for chemotherapy

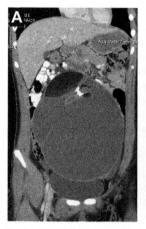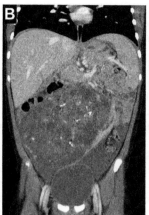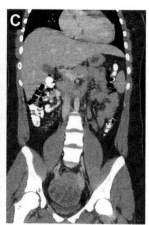

Fig. 2. Coronal CT images of ovarian GCTs. (*A*) Left ovarian MT in a 14-year-old girl. The tumor is mostly cystic with solid elements including calcium and fat noted in the most cephalad portion. (*B*) Left ovarian grade 3 IT in a 7-year-old girl. The tumor is complex with cystic and solid components including internal fat and calcifications noted. The fluid in the pelvis is worrisome for preoperative rupture. Rupture and diffuse nodularity of the peritoneal cavity was confirmed at laparotomy. Microscopic foci of yolk sac tumor were present throughout the mass on final pathology. (*C*) Right ovarian yolk sac tumor in a 15-year-old girl. The tumor is complex, also with cystic and solid components.

when it otherwise may have been omitted. Pelvic ascites and/or peritoneal washings should be sent for cytology. The uterus and contralateral adnexa should be examined with suspicious lesions biopsied. Biopsy of a normal-appearing ovary is not indicated. For bilateral tumors, resection can be pursued if ovarian parenchyma can be spared and the tumors fully resected. Otherwise, biopsy and neoadjuvant chemotherapy are recommended. The omentum should be examined with suspicious lesions biopsied or resected via omentectomy. Peritoneal surfaces should be inspected and masses or nodules resected or biopsied.[26] Finally, retroperitoneal lymph nodes should be visualized and palpated. Abnormal-appearing, firm, or enlarged nodes should be removed. Sampling of normal-appearing nodes is not indicated, a practice that differs from traditional Federation of Gynecology and Obstetrics guidelines, where routine pelvic and retroperitoneal lymph node dissection is recommended.[16]

With modern therapy, the overall survival for pediatric malignant ovarian GCTs is generally excellent. The initial COG experience with observation only for stage I GCTs revealed an event-free survival of just 52%, but nearly all patients who experienced relapse were later salvaged with chemotherapy for an overall survival of 96%.[27] For advanced stage ovarian malignant GCTs, the overall survival after surgery and platinum-based chemotherapy remains high, especially for prepubertal girls, with rates expected to be between 85% and 100%.[14] Stage IV ovarian GCTs, particularly girls older than age 11 who have an estimated overall survival of 60%, represent a more challenging scenario where better treatments are needed. Studies have also shown that fertility and ovarian function can be preserved successfully for most patients treated for ovarian GCTs and efforts to improve on this outcome continue.[28,29]

SURGICAL MANAGEMENT OF PEDIATRIC TESTICULAR GERM CELL TUMORS

Surgical treatment of malignant testicular GCTs involves radical orchiectomy with high ligation of the spermatic cord at the level of the internal inguinal ring via an inguinal incision. If an MT is suspected in a young child, a testicular sparing approach can be considered, but orchiectomy is still recommended for peripubertal and post-pubertal males. A scrotal approach to biopsy or resection is discouraged. Scrotal or-chiectomy, provided that intact resection of the tumor and testicle are accomplished, will not result in upstaging if the remainder of the spermatic cord is resected to the level of the internal inguinal ring during a subsequent procedure.[30] If there is tumor present in the latter specimen, the patient is upstaged to at least stage II. If a trans-scrotal biopsy is performed, the patient will be upstaged to at least stage II, and completion inguinal orchiectomy is recommended, although hemiscro-tectomy is not needed.

A CT scan or MRI of the abdomen and pelvis should be obtained to assess for retroperitoneal adenopathy and chest imaging obtained to assess for metastatic dis-ease. Nodes less than 1 cm in maximal diameter are considered negative. Nodes that are 2 cm or more are considered positive for metastatic disease, designating the patient as having at least stage III disease. Nodes that measure 1 cm to less than 2 cm are considered indeterminate and for a patient who would otherwise be classified as stage I, follow-up imaging in approximately 4 to 6 weeks is required. If these nodes are unchanged or enlarging, a biopsy is recommended. If the biopsies are negative, the patient can remain as stage I. If they are positive or a biopsy is not pursued, the patient is upstaged to stage III and should receive chemotherapy accordingly.

For most pediatric patients with testicular GCTs, lymph node metastases are effectively treated with standard chemotherapy.[31] For prepubertal boys (age <11) who have completed chemotherapy in whom (1) persistently elevated tumor markers with a residual mass, or (2) negative tumor markers and a mass 2 cm or more, or one that is growing 6 to 8 weeks after completing therapy is encountered, resection of the mass should be pursued. Formal retroperitoneal lymph node dissection is not needed.[30] It is recommended, however, that peripubertal or postpubertal males (≥11 years of age) with a residual mass in the retroperitoneum at the completion of chemotherapy, with or without persistently elevated tumor markers, undergo retroperitoneal lymph node dissection using a nerve-sparing template. These rec-ommendations differ from adult guidelines, where either prechemotherapy or postchemotherapy retroperitoneal lymph node dissection is more commonly performed.[32]

Outcomes for pediatric patients treated for malignant testicular GCTs are generally excellent. Observation alone after appropriate surgical resection of stage I testicular GCTs has been well-studied in the context of multiple trials, with event-free survival rates ranging from 48% to 95%.[21,30,33] Importantly, the overall survival after an initial period of postsurgical observation approaches 100%, indicating, as with ovarian GCTs, that patients experiencing relapse of their disease after surgery are highly salvageable with addition of platinum-based chemotherapy. Patients presenting with more advanced stage testicular GCT continue to have a quite good survival, with the overall survival raging between 83% and nearly 100%, depending on the stage and age of the patient.[16,17,31]

SURGICAL MANAGEMENT OF PEDIATRIC EXTRAGONADAL GERM CELL TUMORS
Sacrococcygeal Germ Cell Tumors

Sacrococcygeal GCTs presenting in the neonatal period are more likely to be tera-tomas and predominately external in location. Those occurring later in childhood are more likely to be intrapelvic and malignant. The optimal surgical treatment for neonatal sacrococcygeal GCTs involves intact removal of the tumor en bloc with the coccyx while avoiding injury or resection of adjacent organs, including pelvic floor musculature, so that future bowel, bladder, and reproductive functions are preserved and optimized.[34]

For suspected malignant sacrococcygeal GCTs, the primary tumor should be assessed with a CT scan or MRI to determine the feasibility of resection and the optimal operative approach. Should a peritoneal approach be used for resection, fluid and/or pelvic washings should be sent, and peritoneal surfaces and retroperitoneal lymph nodes assessed to evaluate for disease spread.[13] Preoperative imaging should be reviewed, and involvement of the tumor with surrounding structures, including the neural foramina, rectum, and/or genitourinary structures, assessed. Any suggestion that the tumor cannot be safely separated from vital structures should prompt a biopsy followed by the administration of neoadjuvant chemotherapy in lieu of upfront resection.[35] This point is particularly important in light of the fact that patients undergoing treatment for sacrococcygeal GCTs exhibit high rates of long-term bowel and bladder dysfunction.[36] The provision of neoadjuvant chemotherapy can facilitate eventual, less morbid surgical resection, with the expectation for similar overall survival compared with upfront resection.[13,35]

Mediastinal Germ Cell Tumors

Primary mediastinal GCTs are commonly large and involve critical structures. As with GCTs at other sites, the optimal surgical treatment involves complete resection of the tumor without rupture or spillage while preserving vital structures. The thymus is often involved and should be removed en bloc with the tumor. Large lesions with negative tumor markers and features consistent with an MT should be resected primarily. In asymptomatic or minimally symptomatic patients, this procedure can usually be done safely under general anesthesia via lateral thoracotomy or sternotomy. Lesions with elevated tumor markers that seem to be unresectable should be biopsied with chemotherapy administered if malignancy is confirmed.[37] An image-guided, percutaneous core needle biopsy is preferred. General anesthesia may be contraindicated in patients exhibiting findings of greater than 35 to 50% tracheal compression on CT scan or MRI, a peak expiratory flow rates of less than 50% predicted, or those with orthopnea.[38] These patients may require anesthetic strategies to allow for biopsy that do not risk airway collapse.

Germ Cell Tumors at Other Sites

Extracranial GCTs may also arise from the retroperitoneum, vagina, head and neck, and other sites. Cervical GCTs occurring in the neonatal period are often teratomas and require surgical resection for definitive management. Airway compromise is a critical concern and may require immediate postnatal securement of a safe airway and, in some cases, may necessitate in utero or extrapartum interventions. Malignant retroperitoneal GCTs may involve vital structures requiring an initial biopsy and the administration of neoadjuvant chemotherapy. At the time of eventual resection, intraperitoneal fluid and/or washings should be sent for cytology. Retroperitoneal lymph nodes and evidence of peritoneal spread should be assessed, and abnormal-appearing nodes or peritoneal implants should be removed or biopsied. Vaginal GCTs should be managed with the intent for vaginal preservation with neoadjuvant chemotherapy most commonly being given to facilitate a more limited, vagina-preserving resection.[39]

SURGICAL MANAGEMENT OF METASTATIC, REFRACTORY, AND RECURRENT DISEASE

Chemotherapy is administered when metastatic disease is diagnosed initially. Surgical resection should then be considered for the remaining residual masses that are more than 1 cm in size and/or when tumor markers remain elevated. Even in the context of metastatic disease, the administration of proper multimodality therapy, including surgical resection of distant metastases, is associated with long-term survival and is encouraged.[27]

Surgical resection must also be considered in the presence of recurrent or refractory disease.[40] Recurrent malignant GCTs may require salvage chemotherapy with consideration given to surgical resection of any residual mass.[41] Multiple regimens, including high-dose chemotherapy with stem cell rescue, have been used.[42] Biopsies revealing transformation to a somatic malignancy should be treated with therapy appropriate for that histology.[43] A teratoma without a malignant component is unlikely to respond to chemotherapy, and surgical resection for growing and/or symptomatic disease is warranted.

Growing teratoma syndrome describes a scenario in which local or distant metastases from a GCT continue to grow despite normalization of tumor markers with or without prior chemotherapy.[44] Given the lack of response to other therapies, surgical resection is warranted for lesions that are growing and/or causing symptoms. For cases where diffuse peritoneal studding is encountered, aggressive cytoreductive operations involving the stripping of peritoneal surfaces and the incorporation of hyperthermic intraperitoneal chemotherapy have been attempted and are commonly performed for adult ovarian carcinomatosis. The precise role of these treatments for pediatric GCTs is less clear.[45] There is little published information regarding outcomes for pediatric growing teratoma syndrome, although reports among adult patients indicate that, with surgical resection, outcomes are good with the majority of patients achieving long-term survival.[46,47]

FUTURE DIRECTIONS

Despite overall excellent outcomes associated with the majority of pediatric GCTs, several challenges remain. These issues include a need to identify areas where adult and pediatric providers can collaborate to study treatments and outcomes, fostering international collaborations to enroll more patients into clinical trials, improving outcomes for patients with stage III and IV disease, and decreasing the late effects associated with therapy. To this end, the ongoing COG AGCT 1531 trial will enroll children and young adults treated at both pediatric and adult centers and, in addition to North America, will enroll participants from multiple international centers. A commitment to international collaboration has been further established via the MaGIC consortium.

Additionally, targeted therapies have been evaluated for the treatment of otherwise medically refractory GCTs, with some success being reported for the tyrosine kinase inhibitor, sunitinib, and the cyclin-dependent kinase inhibitor, palbociclib.[48,49] Finally, given the limitations associated with the use of tumor markers, promising new methods including measurement of serum microRNA are being studied for the purposes of better monitoring disease burden, response to therapy and relapse.[50]

SUMMARY

Because they take their origin from migrating primordial germ cells, pediatric GCTs represent a vast array of histologies and occur in multiple locations. Overall, GCTs are quite responsive to treatment, including surgery and chemotherapy. Proper technique for surgical resection and staging is critical to ensure favorable outcomes and to ensure that patients can receive appropriate therapy without being exposed to the risks associated with overtreatment or undertreatment. International collaborations and collaboration with adult centers will be critical in the support of current and future efforts focused on safely reducing the toxicities and the late effects associated with therapy and improving outcomes for high-risk patients.

CLINICS CARE POINTS

- Serum alpha fetoprotein, beta human gonadotropin and lactate dehydrogenase levels can be elevated and should be measured prior to treatment whenever a germ cell tumor is suspected.
- Rupture of germ cell tumors results in upstaging and must be avoided during operative resection.
- Intraoperative staging at the time of ovarian germ cell tumor resection is critical to ensure that an appropriate stage is assigned to ensure the patient is not over- or under-treated.
- Orchiectomy with high ligation of the spermatic cord via an inguinal incision is the preferred surgical approach to testicular germ cell tumor resection. A transscrotal approach should be avoided.

DISCLOSURE

The authors have nothing to disclose.

REFERENCES

1. Dehner LP. Gonadal and extragonadal germ cell neoplasia of childhood. Hum Pathol 1983;14(6):493–511.
2. Shaikh F, Murray MJ, Amatruda JF, et al. Paediatric extracranial germ-cell tumours. Lancet Oncol 2016;17(4):e149–62.
3. Hurteau JA, Febbraro T. Germ cell tumors: treatment consensus across all age groups through MaGIC [Malignant Germ Cell International Collaborative]. Cancer 2016;122(2):181–3.
4. Ries LAG, Smith MA, Gurney JG, et al, editors. Cancer incidence and survival among children and adolescents: United States SEER program 1975-1995. Bethesda (MD): National Cancer Institute; 1999. SEER Program. NIH Pub. No. 99-4649. Available at: https://seer.cancer.gov/archive/publications/childhood/. Accessed June, 2020.
5. Poynter JN, Amatruda JF, Ross JA. Trends in incidence and survival of pediatric and adolescent patients with germ cell tumors in the United States, 1975 to 2006. Cancer 2010;116(20):4882–91.
6. Williams LA, Pankratz N, Lane J, et al. Klinefelter syndrome in males with germ cell tumors: a report from the Children's Oncology Group. Cancer 2018; 124(19):3900–8.
7. Tam YH, Wong YS, Pang KKY, et al. Tumor risk of children with 45,X/46,XY gonadal dysgenesis in relation to their clinical presentations: further insights into the gonadal management. J Pediatr Surg 2016;51(9):1462–6.
8. Dicken BJ, Billmire DF, Krailo M, et al. Gonadal dysgenesis is associated with worse outcomes in patients with ovarian nondysgerminomatous tumors: a report

of the Children's Oncology Group AGCT 0132 study. Pediatr Blood Cancer 2018; 65(4):10.

9. Poynter JN, Richardson M, Roesler M, et al. Family history of cancer in children and adolescents with germ cell tumours: a report from the Children's Oncology Group. Br J Cancer 2018;118(1):121–6.

10. O'Neill AF, Xia C, Krailo MD, et al. α-Fetoprotein as a predictor of outcome for children with germ cell tumors: a report from the Malignant Germ Cell International Consortium. Cancer 2019;125(20):3649–56.

11. Blohm ME, Vesterling-Hörner D, Calaminus G, et al. Alpha 1-fetoprotein (AFP) reference values in infants up to 2 years of age. Pediatr Hematol Oncol 1998; 15(2):135–42.

12. Mazumdar M, Bajorin DF, Bacik J, et al. Predicting outcome to chemotherapy in patients with germ cell tumors: the value of the rate of decline of human chorionic gonadotrophin and alpha-fetoprotein during therapy. J Clin Oncol 2001;19(9): 2534–41.

13. Rescorla F, Billmire D, Stolar C, et al. The effect of cisplatin dose and surgical resection in children with malignant germ cell tumors at the sacrococcygeal region: a pediatric intergroup trial (POG 9049/CCG 8882). J Pediatr Surg 2001; 36(1):12–7.

14. Frazier AL, Hale JP, Rodriguez-Galindo C, et al. Revised risk classification for pediatric extracranial germ cell tumors based on 25 years of clinical trial data from the United Kingdom and United States. J Clin Oncol 2015;33(2):195–201.

15. Einhorn LH, Donohue J. Cis-diamminedichloroplatinum, vinblastine, and bleomycin combination chemotherapy in disseminated testicular cancer. Ann Intern Med 1977;87(3):293–8.

16. Rogers PC, Olson TA, Cullen JW, et al. Treatment of children and adolescents with stage II testicular and stages I and II ovarian malignant germ cell tumors: a Pediatric Intergroup Study–Pediatric Oncology Group 9048 and Children's Cancer Group 8891. J Clin Oncol 2004;22(17):3563–9.

17. Cushing B, Giller R, Cullen JW, et al. Randomized comparison of combination chemotherapy with etoposide, bleomycin, and either high-dose or standard-dose cisplatin in children and adolescents with high-risk malignant germ cell tumors: a pediatric intergroup study–Pediatric Oncology Group 9049 and Children's Cancer Group 8882. J Clin Oncol 2004;22(13):2691–700.

18. Frazier AL, Stoneham S, Rodriguez-Galindo C, et al. Comparison of carboplatin versus cisplatin in the treatment of paediatric extracranial malignant germ cell tumours: a report of the Malignant Germ Cell International Consortium. Eur J Cancer 2018;98:30–7.

19. Mann JR, Raafat F, Robinson K, et al. The United Kingdom Children's Cancer Study Group's second germ cell tumor study: carboplatin, etoposide, and bleomycin are effective treatment for children with malignant extracranial germ cell tumors, with acceptable toxicity. J Clin Oncol 2000;18(22):3809–18.

20. Billmire DF, Cullen JW, Rescorla FJ, et al. Surveillance after initial surgery for pediatric and adolescent girls with stage I ovarian germ cell tumors: report from the Children's Oncology Group. J Clin Oncol 2014;32(5):465–70.

21. Rescorla FJ, Ross JH, Billmire DF, et al. Surveillance after initial surgery for Stage I pediatric and adolescent boys with malignant testicular germ cell tumors: report from the Children's Oncology Group. J Pediatr Surg 2015;50(6):1000–3.

22. Gershenson DM, del Junco G, Silva EG, et al. Immature teratoma of the ovary. Obstet Gynecol 1986;68(5):624–9.

23. Marina NM, Cushing B, Giller R, et al. Complete surgical excision is effective treatment for children with immature teratomas with or without malignant elements: a Pediatric Oncology Group/Children's Cancer Group Intergroup Study. J Clin Oncol 1999;17(7):2137–43.
24. Pashankar F, Hale JP, Dang H, et al. Is adjuvant chemotherapy indicated in ovarian immature teratomas? A combined data analysis from the Malignant Germ Cell Tumor International Collaborative. Cancer 2016;122(2):230–7.
25. CCLG Surgeons Collaborators, Braungart S, Craigie RJ, Farrelly P, et al. Ovarian tumors in children: how common are lesion recurrence and metachronous disease? A UK CCLG Surgeons Cancer Group nationwide study. J Pediatr Surg 2020;55(10):2026–9.
26. Billmire D, Vinocur C, Rescorla F, et al. Outcome and staging evaluation in malignant germ cell tumors of the ovary in children and adolescents: an intergroup study. J Pediatr Surg 2004;39(3):424–9.
27. Pfister D, Haidl F, Paffenholz P, et al. Metastatic surgery in testis cancer. Curr Opin Urol 2016;26(6):590–5.
28. Brewer M, Gershenson DM, Herzog CE, et al. Outcome and reproductive function after chemotherapy for ovarian dysgerminoma. J Clin Oncol 1999;17(9):2670–5.
29. Gershenson DM, Miller AM, Champion VL, et al. Reproductive and sexual function after platinum-based chemotherapy in long-term ovarian germ cell tumor survivors: a Gynecologic Oncology Group Study. J Clin Oncol 2007;25(19):2792–7.
30. Schlatter M, Rescorla F, Giller R, et al. Excellent outcome in patients with stage I germ cell tumors of the testes: a study of the Children's Cancer Group/Pediatric Oncology Group. J Pediatr Surg 2003;38(3):319–24.
31. Haas RJ, Schmidt P, Göbel U, et al. Treatment of malignant testicular tumors in childhood: results of the German National Study 1982-1992. Med Pediatr Oncol 1994;23(5):400–5.
32. Heidenreich A, Pfister D. Retroperitoneal lymphadenectomy and resection for testicular cancer: an update on best practice. Ther Adv Urol 2012;4(4):187–205.
33. Göbel U, Haas R, Calaminus G, et al. Testicular germ cell tumors in boys <10 years: results of the protocol MAHO 98 in respect to surgery and watch & wait strategy. Klin Padiatr 2013;225(6):296–302.
34. Rescorla FJ. Pediatric germ cell tumors. Semin Pediatr Surg 2012;21(1):51–60.
35. Göbel U, Schneider DT, Calaminus G, et al. Multimodal treatment of malignant sacrococcygeal germ cell tumors: a prospective analysis of 66 patients of the German cooperative protocols MAKEI 83/86 and 89. J Clin Oncol 2001;19(7):1943–50.
36. Hambraeus M, Hagander L, Stenström P, et al. Long-term outcome of sacrococcygeal teratoma: a controlled cohort study of urinary tract and bowel dysfunction and predictors of poor outcome. J Pediatr 2018;198:131–6.
37. Schneider DT, Calaminus G, Reinhard H, et al. Primary mediastinal germ cell tumors in children and adolescents: results of the German cooperative protocols MAKEI 83/86, 89, and 96. J Clin Oncol 2000;18(4):832–9.
38. Shamberger RC, Holzman RS, Griscom NT, et al. Prospective evaluation by computed tomography and pulmonary function tests of children with mediastinal masses. Surgery 1995;118(3):468–71.
39. Vural F, Vural B, Paksoy N. Vaginal teratoma: a case report and review of the literature. J Obstet Gynaecol 2015;35(7):757–8.
40. Allen JC, Kirschner A, Scarpato KR, et al. Current management of refractory germ cell tumors and future directions. Curr Oncol Rep 2017;19(2):8.

41. Dorff TB, Hu JS, Quinn DI. Salvage chemotherapy for refractory germ cell tumors. Oncol 2014;28(6):498–500.
42. Goldman S, Bouffet E, Fisher PG, et al. Phase II trial assessing the ability of neo-adjuvant chemotherapy with or without second-look surgery to eliminate measurable disease for nongerminomatous germ cell tumors: a children's oncology group study. J Clin Oncol 2015;33(22):2464–71.
43. Speir R, Cary C, Foster RS, et al. Management of patients with metastatic teratoma with malignant somatic transformation. Curr Opin Urol 2018;28(5):469–73.
44. Logothetis CJ, Samuels ML, Trindade A, et al. The growing teratoma syndrome. Cancer 1982;50(8):1629–35.
45. Hayes-Jordan A, Lopez C, Green HL, et al. Cytoreductive surgery (CRS) and hyperthermic intraperitoneal chemotherapy (HIPEC) in pediatric ovarian tumors: a novel treatment approach. Pediatr Surg Int 2016;32(1):71–3.
46. Bentivegna E, Azaïs H, Uzan C, et al. Surgical outcomes after debulking surgery for intraabdominal ovarian growing teratoma syndrome: analysis of 38 cases. Ann Surg Oncol 2015;22(Suppl 3):S964–70.
47. Vaughn DJ, Flaherty K, Lal P, et al. Treatment of growing teratoma syndrome. N Engl J Med 2009;360(4):423–4.
48. Oechsle K, Honecker F, Cheng T, et al. Preclinical and clinical activity of sunitinib in patients with cisplatin-refractory or multiply relapsed germ cell tumors: a Canadian Urologic Oncology Group/German Testicular Cancer Study Group cooperative study. Ann Oncol 2011;22(12):2654–60.
49. Vaughn DJ, Hwang W-T, Lal P, et al. Phase 2 trial of the cyclin-dependent kinase 4/6 inhibitor palbociclib in patients with retinoblastoma protein-expressing germ cell tumors. Cancer 2015;121(9):1463–8.
50. Dieckmann K-P, Radtke A, Geczi L, et al. Serum levels of MicroRNA-371a-3p (M371 test) as a new biomarker of testicular germ cell tumors: results of a prospective multicentric study. J Clin Oncol 2019;37(16):1412–23.

Management of Rhabdomyosarcoma in Pediatric Patients

Timothy N. Rogers, MBBCh, FCS(SA), FCS(paed), FRCS(paed)[a],[*],
Roshni Dasgupta, MD, MPH[b]

KEYWORDS

- Rhabdomyosarcoma • Pediatric • Soft tissue sarcoma • Surgery

KEY POINTS

- Rhabdomyosarcoma is the commonest soft tissue sarcoma in children, requiring clinician vigilance to recognize the multitude of site-specific presentations.
- Biopsy enables pathologic, genetic, and biological characterization of the tumor, and accurate staging with imaging and surgical sampling informs risk-based therapy.
- A specialist multidisciplinary team assigns each patient to a risk group with treatment delivered by a risk-based approach.
- Patients always require chemotherapy and usually a combination of complex, site-specific surgery and/or radiotherapy.
- Outcomes for localized rhabdomyosarcoma continue to improve but locoregional relapse remains a problem, as does metastatic/metastatic relapsed disease, so new treatment approaches are required.

BACKGROUND

Rhabdomyosarcoma (RMS) is the most common soft tissue sarcoma in children, accounting for 4.5% of all childhood cancers. It follows neuroblastoma and nephroblastoma as the third most common extracranial solid tumor of childhood.[1] The incidence is 4.5 cases per million children/adolescents per year.[2] It is rare in adults, with an incidence of 0.9 cases per million per year, where soft tissue sarcomas constitute less than 1% of all malignancies, and RMS accounts for only 3% of all soft tissue sarcomas.[3]

RMSs are malignant tumors of mesenchymal origin and can therefore occur at any anatomic site and often show cellular differentiation toward muscle tissue. RMSs have

[a] Department of Pediatric Surgery, University Hospitals Bristol NHS Foundation Trust, Bristol, UK; [b] Division of Pediatric General and Thoracic Surgery, Cincinnati Children's Hospital Medical Center, University of Cincinnati, 3333 Burnet Ave, Cincinnati, OH 45229, USA
* Corresponding author.
E-mail address: timothy.rogers@uhbristol.nhs.uk

Surg Oncol Clin N Am 30 (2021) 339–353
https://doi.org/10.1016/j.soc.2020.11.003
1055-3207/21/© 2020 Elsevier Inc. All rights reserved.

small round blue cells that usually mark positive immunohistochemically for the proteins desmin, vimentin, myoglobin, actin, and myoD.[4]

Childhood RMS is subdivided into 2 major subtypes, the commonest is PAX fusion–negative RMS (previously called embryonal RMS), occurring in 70%, and PAX fusion–positive RMS (previously called alveolar RMS). Spindle cell/sclerosing RMS is a third RMS subtype, whereas pleiomorphic RMS occurs exclusively in adults.[5,6] In adulthood, the distribution of subtypes differs, with most (65%) being adult-type RMS (pleiomorphic, spindle cell, and not otherwise specified).[3]

Most PAX fusion–negative RMSs show loss of heterozygosity at the 11p15 locus, the site of the IGF-II (insulin-like growth factor II) gene that has shown significant involvement in the pathogenesis of these tumors. PAX fusion–positive RMS is usually (80%) associated with one of several balanced chromosomal translocations, most commonly t(2;13) in approximately 60%, or t(1;13) in 20%, with the remaining 20% translocation negative. These chromosomal fusions result in expression of proteins (aberrant transcription factors) that induce cancer development.[7] PAX fusion-positive status in nonmetastatic disease is a poor prognostic marker (36.1% event-free survival [EFS] at 5 years); conversely, PAX fusion–negative status carries a better prognosis (70% EFS at 5 years).[8,9]

There are primary peaks of incidence in the 2-year-old to 6-year-old age group, with tumors generally within the head and neck and genitourinary tract, and in adolescents who present with extremity, truncal, or paratesticular tumors.

Outcomes in localized RMS have improved steadily and approach 80% survival; however, for patients who present with metastatic and relapsed disease, outcomes remain poor (<30%) and have not changed in several decades, prompting the need for new treatment approaches. Adult patients with RMS have a poorer overall survival than pediatric patients: 43% for localized RMS and 5% for metastatic RMS.[3,9–11]

PATIENT EVALUATION OVERVIEW

RMS occurs in multiple anatomic sites with the approximate distribution shown in **Table 1**.

Because of the variable sites of tumor origin, clinicians need vigilance to recognize patients with differing presenting signs and symptoms of RMS, as shown in **Table 2**.

Rarely (~5%), patients (PAX fusion negative) present with an underlying cancer-predisposition syndrome, such as neurofibromatosis, Li-Fraumeni syndrome, DICER1 syndrome, Rubinstein-Taybi syndrome, Gorlin basal cell nevus syndrome, Beckwith-Wiedemann syndrome, or Costello syndrome.[12,13] It is important to recognize any potential genetic predisposition to cancer so that genetic counseling, screening, surveillance, and timely treatment can be offered.[14]

Table 1 Distribution of rhabdomyosarcoma primary sites	
Primary Tumor Site	**Percentage**
Head and neck	40
Genitourinary	20
Extremities	20
Trunk	10
Other	10

Table 2
Common presenting signs and symptoms by primary site

Primary Site	Symptoms and Signs
Head and neck	Painless or painful swelling
	Proptosis
	Ptosis
	Ophthalmoplegia
	Headache
	Vomiting
	Cranial nerve palsy
	Other cranial nerve palsies
	Nasal discharge
	Nasal/sinus congestion
	Trismus
	Systemic hypertension
Limbs/trunk	Asymptomatic swelling
Genitourinary tract/pelvis	Painless scrotal lesions
	Hematuria
	Urinary retention/dribbling
	Vulval nodule
	Polypoid vaginal lesions
	Vaginal bleeding/discharge
	Constipation
Abdomen/liver/biliary	Asymptomatic swelling
	Abdominal pain
	Intestinal obstruction
	Jaundice
	Cholangitis
Metastatic disease (20% at diagnosis)	Otherwise unexplained:
• Bone	Poor feeding
• Bone marrow	Seizures
• Lung	Pain
• Lymph nodes	Irritability
	Pancytopenia

When RMS is suspected, the patient requires imaging and biopsy to confirm the diagnosis, followed by accurate staging and a treatment plan made by a specialist multidisciplinary team using a risk-based approach.

Imaging Studies

Initial ultrasonography of a suspicious lesion can be helpful to delineate whether the mass is solid or cystic and can also assess its vascular characteristics.

MRI is the optimal imaging modality to assess most primary lesions, with RMS usually, but not invariably, isointense to muscle on T1-weighted images, and intermediate to high intensity on T2-weighted images.[15] Computed tomography (CT) is excellent for assessing bone involvement, and can be performed when osseous invasion is suspected. Cross-sectional imaging of the primary tumor should include the regional draining lymph nodes for staging, and, in the case of extremity tumors, the entire limb (**Fig. 1**). Chest CT should be performed as part of staging for the detection of pulmonary metastases.

When available, either whole-body fluorodeoxyglucose (FDG) PET/CT or FDG-PET/MRI can be used for the assessment of disease burden, but these cannot be relied on

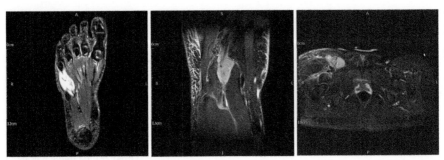

Fig. 1. MRI scans of a 15-year girl with a fusion-positive RMS of the right foot and lymph node metastases in the popliteal fossa and groin.

to give accurate representation of lymphatic metastasis.[16,17] Biopsy core needle or incisional biopsy should be the initial surgical procedure in all patients except when primary wide excision of the mass with adequate margins is possible without loss of function or excessive morbidity.[18,19] Fluorescence in situ hybridization (FISH) is performed on the biopsy tissue to detect the presence of a translocation and reverse transcription polymerase chain reaction (RT-PCR) is used to determine the specific fusion. Bone marrow biopsy should be performed in all intermediate-risk and high-risk patients to determine metastatic spread to the marrow.[20]

For parameningeal tumors, cerebrospinal fluid (CSF) cytology should be obtained to detect central nervous system involvement. Regional lymph nodes should be evaluated surgically in patients with tumors of the extremity, trunk, head and neck, perineal/perianal site, and patients more than 10 years old with paratesticular RMS, because lymph node involvement is more common at these sites and imaging is not able to reliably exclude lymph node metastases. Sentinel lymph node biopsy (SLNB) is more accurate than random lymph node sampling. Pathologic confirmation should be obtained for patients with abnormal lymph nodes (>1 cm in diameter), or they should be treated as having pathologic lymphadenopathy.

Staging and Risk Stratification

Staging and risk stratification in RMS is complex but important, because treatment intensity follows a risk-adapted approach.[21] Patients are assigned to a pretreatment stage using the tumor, node, metastasis (TNM) classification (**Table 3**) and to a surgicopathologic group using the Intergroup Rhabdomyosarcoma (IRS) group classification (**Table 4**). The IRS group is a prechemotherapy staging system determined by the extent of the initial surgical resection and the presence of pathologic lymph nodes and distant metastases. Factors that determine prognosis include tumor biology, including PAX fusion status; favorable or unfavorable tumor site (**Table 5**); lymph node status; patient age; tumor size; metastases; and IRS group (see **Table 4**).

Risk-group assignment incorporates pretreatment stage (**Table 6**), IRS group, tumor biology, and patient age.[22]

TREATMENT OPTIONS

Treatment of patients with RMS is multimodal, always includes chemotherapy, and usually includes a combination of radiotherapy (RT) and surgery.

Table 3	
Tumor, node, metastasis staging classification	
T1	Tumor confined to tissue of origin
T2	Tumor extends beyond tissue of origin
A	≤5 cm in maximum diameter
B	>5 cm in maximum diameter
N0	No nodal involvement
N1	Nodal involvement
NX	Regional lymph nodes not examined; no information
M0	No distant metastases
M1	Distant metastases

Chemotherapy

The intensity and duration of chemotherapy are increased according to risk-group assignment (**Tables 7** and **8**). The Children's Oncology Group (COG) and European Pediatric Soft Tissue Sarcoma Study Group (EpSSG) use chemotherapy backbone regimens that differ in that the alkylating agent is substituted, with cyclophosphamide used by COG and ifosfamide by EpSSG. Comparisons between these alkylating agents have shown no significant differences in outcome but each gives rise to different late effects: ifosfamide is more nephrotoxic and cyclophosphamide is more gonadotoxic.[23]

Adult patients are likely to benefit from entering clinical trials in common with pediatric patients and, when treated in line with pediatric treatment protocols, have had better outcomes.[24] However, pleiomorphic RMS is chemoresistant like other high-grade soft tissue sarcomas of adulthood, and the best combination chemotherapy is not defined for this subtype.[3]

Radiotherapy

In most patients (85%), RT is required to obtain local control at the primary site, and is always required for pathologically involved lymph nodes.[25] There are only a few selected groups of patients with low-risk disease where RT can be safely avoided without potentially compromising cure, such as completely resected paratesticular RMS or vaginal RMS with a complete chemotherapy response. Intensity-modulated RT (IMRT), brachytherapy, and proton beam RT may achieve adequate tumor control with reduced radiation to normal surrounding tissues.[26]

SURGICAL TREATMENT
Primary Resection

Primary resection is indicated if the tumor can be excised with R0 margins (resection should be attempted only if it is anticipated that all gross tumor can be excised,

Table 4	
Intergroup Rhabdomyosarcoma Group surgical-pathologic (clinical) grouping classification	
IRS-I	Tumor completely removed
IRS-II	a. Microscopic residual tumor b. Involved regional nodes c. Both
IRS-III	Gross residual tumor after incomplete resection or biopsy only
IRS-IV	Distant metastatic disease

Table 5	
Favorable/unfavorable prognostic tumor sites	
Favorable Primary Tumor Sites	**Unfavorable Primary Tumor Sites**
Head and neck	Parameningeal
Orbital	Extremities
Genitourinary (now also includes bladder/prostate in EpSSG)	Bladder/prostate (remains unfavorable site in COG)
Biliary	Trunk
	Chest wall
	Other sites

Abbreviations: COG, Children's Oncology Group; EpSSG, European Pediatric Soft Tissue Sarcoma Study Group.

because leaving gross residual disease behind has a similar outcome to biopsy alone). Complete resection should include a rim of surrounding tissue with a margin of at least 0.5 cm without significant morbidity.[27,28]

Pretreatment Reexcision

Pretreatment reexcision (PRE) is a wide, nonmutilating reexcision to achieve a complete resection (R0 margin) in patients with microscopic residual disease after a primary procedure, which could have been a biopsy or incomplete tumor excision.[29] PRE needs to be done before other adjuvant therapies begin and as soon as possible after the primary resection. If R0 margins are obtained at the PRE operation, the patient should then be classified as IRS group I with its associated improved survival and potential for a decreased intensity of therapy.[30] PRE should only be offered if the resection of the entire tumor bed can occur with a margin without loss of function or form.

Delayed Primary Excision

Delayed primary excision (DPE) occurs after induction chemotherapy if the tumor can be macroscopically removed without danger or mutilation; this is most often combined with postoperative RT. Debulking operations are not recommended and there is no evidence that this improves oncological outcome compared with biopsy alone.[31] A complete R0 resection should be targeted; however, a microscopic residual R1 resection may decrease the amount of adjuvant RT needed.[32]

Fertility Preservation

Fertility-preserving procedures, such as gonadal transposition, should be considered before RT or ovarian/testicular cryopreservation.[33] In pubertal patients, sperm or egg

Table 6					
Pretreatment staging system					
Stage	**Site[b]**	**T Stage[a]**	**Size[a]**	**Node Stage[a]**	**Metastases[a]**
1	Favorable	T1 or T2	Any size	N0 or N1 or Nx	M0
2	Unfavorable	T1 or T2	a, ≤5 cm	N0 or Nx	M0
3	Unfavorable	T1 or T2	a, ≤5 cm	N1	M0
			b, >5 cm	N0 or N1 or Nx	
4	Any site	T1 or T2	Any size	N0 or N1 or Nx	M1

[a] Refer to TNM classification.
[b] Refer to **Table 5**.

Table 7
Children's Oncology Group risk-group assignment

Risk Group	Fusion Status	Stage	Group
Low risk	Fusion negative	1	I, II, III (orbit only)
	Fusion negative	2	I, II
Intermediate risk	Fusion negative	1	III (nonorbit)
		2, 3	III
		3	I, II
		4	IV (age<10 y)
	Fusion positive	1, 2, 3	I, II, III
High risk	Fusion positive	4	IV
	Fusion negative	4	IV(age $\geq$ 10 y)

storage should be offered if it can be performed without undue treatment delay, otherwise gonadal cryopreservation should be considered.

In prepubertal patients, gonadal cryopreservation should be discussed with the parents.[34,35]

Site-Specific Surgical Treatment

Bladder/prostate rhabdomyosarcoma
The aim of local treatment of bladder/prostate RMS is oncologic control in conjunction with preservation of bladder and sexual function.[36]

To achieve optimal outcomes an experienced multispeciality team needs to offer the spectrum of local treatment modalities, including surgery and reconstruction, as well as RT, including brachytherapy and proton beam RT.[36–39]

Vaginal rhabdomyosarcoma
Tumors at this site are generally very chemosensitive. Patients with favorable histology and biopsy-proven complete response to chemotherapy do not require any local therapy.[40] For those with residual disease after chemotherapy, local control is necessary. Patients with unfavorable histology must receive RT. Intracavitary brachytherapy has generally replaced surgery for local control, combined with temporary ovarian transposition away from the radiation field.[33]

Resection should only be considered if an R0 resection can be achieved with preservation of function and fertility.

Table 8
European Pediatric Soft Tissue Sarcoma Study Group risk-group assignment

Risk Group	Subgroup	Fusion Status	IRS Group	Site	Node Stage	Size or Age
Low risk	A	Negative	I	Any	N0	Both Favorable
Standard risk	B	Negative	I	Any	N0	One or both Unfavorable
	C	Negative	II, III	Favorable	N0	Any
High risk	D	Negative	II, III	Unfavorable	N0	Any
	E	Negative	II, III	Any	N1	Any
	F	Positive	I, II, III	Any	N0	Any
Very high risk	G	Positive	II, III	Any	N1	Any
	H	Any	IV	Any	Any	Any

Paratesticular rhabdomyosarcoma

Paratesticular RMS (PT-RMS) should be removed by radical orchidectomy through an inguinal approach.[41,42] The cord should be clamped at the internal ring before mobilization of the tumor. Care is taken not to breach the tunica vaginalis when the tumor, testis, and entire cord up to the internal ring are removed as a single specimen. When scrotal skin is fixed or invaded by tumor, it should be resected en bloc with the specimen, otherwise there is no indication for hemiscrotectomy.

PRE without formal hemiscrotectomy is required after incomplete resection to remove tumor-contaminated scrotal and/or cord tissue.[43]

Retroperitoneal lymph node assessment

Accurate staging of nodal metastases in PT-RMS is important because lymph node involvement is frequent (26% in IRS-I and IRS-II trials) and patients with positive nodes require intensified chemotherapy and RT.[44] All patients should have MRI/CT imaging of the retroperitoneal nodes, and those 10 years of age or older should also undergo surgical staging of the lymph nodes. A pooled analysis from North America and Europe of 319 patients 10 years of age or older with PT-RMS found that nodal involvement was present in approximately 30% and disease failures were most likely to occur in the nodes. Surgical evaluation of retroperitoneal lymph nodes was the only treatment variable that was associated with EFS.[45] There was a 30% lymph node relapse in patients 10 years of age or older who had nodal staging with imaging alone.[46–49]

Template retroperitoneal lymph node dissection (RPLND) has frequently been avoided because of concern about potential complications. Routh and colleagues[49] report that sampling between 7 and 12 lymph nodes taken from multiple areas in the ipsilateral retroperitoneum up to the renal vessels may be similarly efficacious to identify nodal involvement while minimizing the complications of template RPLND.

Extremity rhabdomyosarcoma

Several adverse prognostic factors are frequently associated with extremity RMS, including older age at presentation, PAX fusion–positive tumors, tumors that invade surrounding tissues, incomplete initial surgical resection, metastatic disease, and lymph node involvement.[18]

Aggressive surgical procedures resulting in loss of function are generally not indicated because the efficacy of chemotherapy and RT usually allows sparing of vital structures.[50] The primary goal of local tumor resection, which is usually a DPE, is limb-sparing complete (R0) resection. An incision is made along the major axis of the anatomic compartment containing the tumor and must include en bloc resection of previous biopsy and drain sites. An R1 (microscopically involved margins) resection with RT usually achieves oncological control while maintaining optimal functional outcome. Ablative procedures should only be performed after a second opinion from a specialized center.

Bile ducts and liver rhabdomyosarcoma

Patients with bile ducts and liver RMS usually present with jaundice, pruritus, and dilatation of the biliary tract. Ultrasonography and MRI with magnetic resonance cholangiopancreatography show the extent of the primary lesion and lymph node involvement, as well as ruling out other causes of biliary obstruction. Biopsy rather than primary excisional surgery is recommended because these tumors usually have a favorable subtype (fusion-negative/botryoid histopathology) that respond well to chemotherapy.[51]

Definitive local control is planned after induction chemotherapy.[51] Complete tumor resection can be considered, which may require partial hepatectomy; however, RT has similar outcomes to DPE, but the long-term effects of RT to the hepatic pedicle are unknown in young patients.[52]

Treatment of metastases
Current standard of care recommends systematic RT of all metastatic sites that can feasibly be treated without disruption of bone marrow function; however, it is not clear whether this strategy improves outcome. Surgical resection of end-of-therapy residual masses does not show any survival advantage.[53]

Follow-up
Following completion of treatment, the frequency of follow-up assessments is conventionally every 3 to 4 months for the first 2 years. There is a need for risk-adapted follow-up strategies to improve the efficiency of follow-up after RMS treatment.[54] RMS rarely relapses later than 3 years from diagnosis. At 5 years from end of treatment, patients can be referred to the long-term follow-up clinic.

Relapse
The commonest pattern of relapse in localized RMS is relapse at the primary site (75%) with or without nodal and distant metastases. Relapsed RMS carries a poor prognosis, although 35% of those who relapse following treatment of localized disease remain curable. Relapse of primary metastatic disease is usually fatal.

Local relapse patients should only be treated in tertiary cancer centers. When treatment with curative intent is deemed feasible after interdisciplinary consultation, the general principle of complete resection should be pursued, and in rare situations may include radical ablative procedures.[55,56]

Biopsies should be taken at relapse, because genomic profiling should be performed, so patients can be considered for targeted therapies or early-phase trials.[5,57]

New developments
SLNB using indocyanine green has been reported to stage lymph nodes in paratesticular and extremity RMS, and is likely to become more widely adopted, as has happened with cervical cancers in adult patients, because it offers a less invasive operative approach (**Fig. 2**).[58–61] With advances in understanding the biology of RMS, ways need to be found to optimize translation of preclinical findings into clinical trials, using rational combinations of targeted agents, conventional chemotherapeutics, and/or immunotherapeutics. International, multidisciplinary research teams are increasingly being established to facilitate discovery, share learning, and pool data[5] (https://cri-app02.bsd.uchicago.edu/instruct).

There are now more than 2 dozen preclinical biological targets with promising corresponding novel therapies in development; some of these are highlighted. WEE1 is a tyrosine kinase that is activated in response to DNA damage and halts progression of cells through the mitotic cycle, allowing DNA repair before cell division. A WEE1 inhibitor (AZD1775) administered in the setting of chemotherapy-induced DNA damage could lead to death of mitotic RMS cells.[62]

Aberrant activation of the receptor tyrosine kinase–mediated RAS signaling cascade is the primary driver of PAX fusion–negative RMS. Oncolytic virus-mediated RAS targeting in RMS can significantly reduce tumor growth and suggests that targeted gene-editing cancer therapies have promising translational applications.[63,64]

However, single-agent therapies do not seem to achieve durable responses because of the acquisition of resistance to treatment. Monoclonal antibodies can directly target cancer cells through several mechanisms, including inhibition of

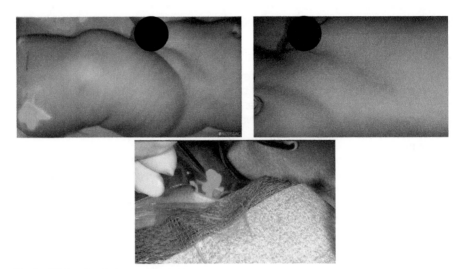

Fig. 2. SLNB using indocyanine green.

oncogenic signaling pathways, delivery of cytotoxic moieties to malignant cells, or induction of antibody-dependent cellular toxicity.[65] However, their role in treating RMS is not well established.

The clinical efficacy of CAR (chimeric antigen receptor) T-cell therapy to pediatric solid tumors has so far been limited, because of heterogeneous antigen expression; limited migration of T cells to tumor sites; and an immunosuppressive, hostile microenvironment.[66] RMS is a rare disease, so the incentives for pharmaceutical companies to develop specific therapeutic agents to directly target PAX-FOXO1 are neither strong nor imminent.

SUMMARY

Treatment of RMS involves a multimodality approach including chemotherapy, surgery, and RT while minimizing the long-term treatment-related morbidities. This article outlines the key points related to the diagnosis and management of RMS with a focus on current surgical management of RMS at specific tumor sites. There is a need for improved RT and surgical techniques as well as systemic therapy in RMS to reduce locoregional and metastatic relapse, reduce late sequelae of treatment, and improve functional outcomes. Better understanding of the biology of the RMS subtypes found in adult patients, with increased enrollment into cooperative group studies, is required.

CLINICS CARE POINTS

- The myriad clinical presentations of rhabdomyosarcoma are dependent on patient age, site of origin of the tumor and the pattern of tumor spread.
- Biopsy and appropriate staging should typically be completed before definitive local therapy, with paratesticular tumors being the only usual exception.
- Surgical lymph node assessment should be performed for certain named primary tumor sites where the risk for lymph node metastases and relapse are significant.
- Definitive locoregional treatment with multimodality approaches is integral, combined with chemotherapy, to control disease and minimize morbidity.

DISCLOSURE

The authors have nothing to disclose.

REFERENCES

1. Arndt CA. Common musculoskeletal tumors of childhood and adolescence. N Engl J Med 1999;342–52. https://doi.org/10.1056/NEJM199907293410507.
2. Ognjanovic S, Linabery AM, Charbonneau B, et al. Trends in childhood rhabdomyosarcoma incidence and survival in the United States, 1975-2005. Cancer 2009;115(18):4218–26.
3. Bompas E, Campion L, Italiano A, et al. Outcome of 449 adult patients with rhabdomyosarcoma: an observational ambispective nationwide study. Cancer Med 2018;7(8):4023–35.
4. Rossi S, Nascimento AG, Canal F, et al. Small round-cell neoplasms of soft tissues: An integrated diagnostic approach. Curr Diagn Pathol 2007;13(2):150–63.
5. Yohe ME, Heske CM, Stewart E, et al. Insights into pediatric rhabdomyosarcoma research: Challenges and goals. Pediatr Blood Cancer 2019;1–10. https://doi.org/10.1002/pbc.27869.
6. Skapek SX. PAX-FOXO1 Fusion Status Drives Unfavorable Outcome for Children With Rhabdomyosarcoma: A Children's Oncology Group Report. Pediatr Blood Cancer 2013;60(9):1411–7.
7. El Demellawy D, McGowan-Jordan J, de Nanassy J, et al. Update on molecular findings in rhabdomyosarcoma. Pathology 2017;49(3):238–46.
8. Selfe J, Olmos D, Al-Saadi R, et al. Impact of fusion gene status versus histology on risk-stratification for rhabdomyosarcoma: Retrospective analyses of patients on UK trials. Pediatr Blood Cancer 2017;64(7). https://doi.org/10.1002/pbc.26386.
9. Rudzinski ER, Anderson JR, Chi YY, et al. Histology, fusion status, and outcome in metastatic rhabdomyosarcoma: A report from the Children's Oncology Group. Pediatr Blood Cancer 2017;64(12):1–7.
10. Oberlin O, Rey A, Sanchez De Toledo J, et al. Randomized comparison of intensified six-drug versus standard three-drug chemotherapy for high-risk nonmetastatic rhabdomyosarcoma and other chemotherapy-sensitive childhood soft tissue sarcomas: Long-term results from the International Society of Pediatr. J Clin Oncol 2012;30(20):2457–65.
11. Oberlin O, Rey A, Lyden E, et al. Prognostic factors in metastatic rhabdomyosarcomas: Results of a pooled analysis from United States and European Cooperative Groups. J Clin Oncol 2008;26(14):2384–9.
12. Ferrari A, Bisogno G, Macaluso A, et al. Soft-tissue sarcomas in children and adolescents with neurofibromatosis type 1. Cancer 2007;109(7):1406–12.
13. Doros L. DICER1 Mutations in Embryonal Rhabdomyosarcomas From Children With and Without Familial PPB-Tumor Predisposition Syndrome. Pediatr Blood Cancer 2012;59(3):558–60.
14. Saletta F, Dalla Pozza L, Byrne JA. Genetic causes of cancer predisposition in children and adolescents. Transl Pediatr 2015;4(2):67–75.
15. Mallinson PI, Chou H, Forster BB, et al. Radiology of Soft Tissue Tumors. Surg Oncol Clin N Am 2014;23(4):911–36.
16. Wagner LM, Kremer N, Gelfand MJ, et al. Detection of lymph node metastases in pediatric and adolescent/young adult sarcoma: Sentinel lymph node biopsy versus fludeoxyglucose positron emission tomography imaging—A prospective trial. Cancer 2017;123(1):155–60.

17. Federico SM, Spunt SL, Krasin MJ, et al. Comparison of PET-CT and conventional imaging in staging pediatric rhabdomyosarcoma. Pediatr Blood Cancer 2013; 60(7):1128–34.

18. Oberlin O, Rey A, Brown KLB, et al. Prognostic Factors for Outcome in Localized Extremity Rhabdomyosarcoma. Pooled Analysis from Four International Cooperative Groups. Pediatr Blood Cancer 2015;62(12):2125–31.

19. Mitton B, Seeger LL, Eckardt MA, et al. Image-guided percutaneous core needle biopsy of musculoskeletal tumors in children. J Pediatr Hematol Oncol 2014; 36(5):337–41.

20. Weiss AR, Lyden ER, Anderson JR, et al. Histologic and clinical characteristics can guide staging evaluations for children and adolescents with rhabdomyosarcoma: A report from the children's oncology group soft tissue sarcoma committee. J Clin Oncol 2013;31(26):3226–32.

21. Meza JL, Anderson J, Pappo AS, et al. Analysis of prognostic factors in patients with nonmetastatic rhabdomyosarcoma treated on intergroup rhabdomyosarcoma studies III and IV: The children's oncology group. J Clin Oncol 2006; 24(24):3844–51.

22. Lawrence W, Anderson JR, Gehan EA, et al. Pretreatment TNM staging of childhood rhabdomyosarcoma: A report of the Intergroup Rhabdomyosarcoma Study Group. Cancer 1997;80(6):1165–70.

23. Dixon SB, Bjornard KL, Alberts NM, et al. Factors influencing risk-based care of the childhood cancer survivor in the 21st century. CA Cancer J Clin 2018;68(2): 133–52.

24. van der Graaf WTA, Orbach D, Judson IR, et al. Soft tissue sarcomas in adolescents and young adults: a comparison with their paediatric and adult counterparts. Lancet Oncol 2017;18(3):e166–75.

25. Mandeville HC. Radiotherapy in the Management of Childhood Rhabdomyosarcoma. Clin Oncol 2019;31(7):462–70.

26. Wolden SL, Wexler LH, Kraus DH, et al. Intensity-modulated radiotherapy for head-and-neck rhabdomyosarcoma. Int J Radiat Oncol Biol Phys 2005;61(5): 1432–8.

27. Lawrence W, Hays DM, Heyn R, et al. Surgical lessons from the Intergroup Rhabdomyosarcoma Study (IRS) pertaining to extremity tumors. World J Surg 1988; 12(5):676–84.

28. Dasgupta R, Rodeberg DA. Update on rhabdomyosarcoma. Semin Pediatr Surg 2012;21(1):68–78.

29. Cecchetto G. Primary re-excision : the Italian experience in patients with localized soft-tissue sarcomas 2001. p. 532–4. https://link-springer-com.bris.idm.oclc.org/content/pdf/10.1007%2Fs003830100580.pdf.

30. Hays DM, Lawrence W, Wharam M, et al. Primary reexcision for patients with 'microscopic residual' tumor following initial excision of sarcomas of trunk and extremity sites. J Pediatr Surg 1989;24(1):5–10.

31. Cecchetto G, Bisogno G, De Corti F, et al. Biopsy or debulking surgery as initial surgery for locally advanced rhabdomyosarcomas in children? The experience of the Italian Cooperative Group studies. Cancer 2007;110(11):2561–7.

32. Rodeberg DA, Wharam MD, Lyden ER, et al. Delayed primary excision with subsequent modification of radiotherapy dose for intermediate-risk rhabdomyosarcoma: A report from the Children's Oncology Group Soft Tissue Sarcoma Committee. Int J Cancer 2015;137(1):204–11.

33. De Lambert G, Haie-Meder C, Guérin F, et al. A new surgical approach of temporary ovarian transposition for children undergoing brachytherapy: Technical assessment and dose evaluation. J Pediatr Surg 2014;49(7):1177–80.

34. Lautz TB, Harris CJ, Laronda MM, et al. A fertility preservation toolkit for pediatric surgeons caring for children with cancer. Semin Pediatr Surg 2019;28(6):150861.

35. Burns KC, Hoefgen H, Strine A, et al. Fertility preservation options in pediatric and adolescent patients with cancer. Cancer 2018;124(9):1867–76.

36. Rodeberg DA, Anderson JR, Arndt CA, et al. Comparison of outcomes based on treatment algorithms for rhabdomyosarcoma of the bladder/prostate: Combined results from the Children's Oncology Group, German Cooperative Soft Tissue Sarcoma Study, Italian Cooperative Group, and International Society of P. Int J Cancer 2011;128(5):1232–9.

37. Arndt C, Rodeberg D, Breitfeld PP, et al. Does bladder preservation (as a surgical principle) lead to retaining bladder function in bladder/prostate rhabdomyosarcoma? Results from Intergroup Rhabdomyosarcoma Study IV. J Urol 2004; 171(6 I):2396–403.

38. Martelli H, Haie-Meder C, Branchereau S, et al. Conservative surgery plus brachytherapy treatment for boys with prostate and/or bladder neck rhabdomyosarcoma: a single team experience. J Pediatr Surg 2009;44(1):190–6.

39. Martelli H, Borrego P, Guérin F, et al. Quality of life and functional outcome of male patients with bladder-prostate rhabdomyosarcoma treated with conservative surgery and brachytherapy during childhood. Brachytherapy 2016;15(3):306–11.

40. Martelli H, Oberlin O, Rey A, et al. Conservative Treatment for Girls With Nonmetastatic Rhabdomyosarcoma of the Genital Tract: A Report From the Study Committee of the International Society of Pediatric Oncology. J Clin Oncol 1999;17(7): 2117.

41. Stewart RJ, Martelli H. Treatment of children with nonmetastatic paratesticular rhabdomyosarcoma: Results of the Malignant Mesenchymal Tumors studies (MMT 84 and MMT 89) of the International Society of Pediatric Oncology. J Clin Oncol 2003;21(5):793–8.

42. Rogers TN, De Corti F, Burrieza GG, et al. Paratesticular rhabdomyosarcoma—Impact of locoregional approach on patient outcome: A report from the European paediatric Soft tissue sarcoma Study Group (EpSSG). Pediatr Blood Cancer 2020. https://doi.org/10.1002/pbc.28479.

43. Seitz G, Dantonello TM, Kosztyla D, et al. Impact of hemiscrotectomy on outcome of patients with embryonal paratesticular rhabdomyosarcoma: Results from the Cooperative Soft Tissue Sarcoma Group Studies CWS-86, 91, 96 and 2002P. J Urol 2014;192(3):902–7.

44. Lawrence W, Hays D, Heyn R. Lymphatic Metastases with Childhood Rhabdomyosarcoma. Cancer 1987;60:910–5.

45. Walterhouse DO, Barkauskas DA, Hall D, et al. Demographic and Treatment Variables Influencing Outcome for Localized Paratesticular Rhabdomyosarcoma: Results From a Pooled Analysis of North American and European Cooperative Groups. J Clin Oncol 2018;36(35). JCO.2018.78.938.

46. Wiener ES, Anderson JR, Ojimba JI, et al. Controversies in the management of paratesticular rhabdomyosarcoma: Is staging retroperitoneal lymph node dissection necessary for adolescents with resected paratesticular rhabdomyosarcoma? Semin Pediatr Surg 2001;10(3):146–52.

47. Tomaszewski JJ, Sweeney DD, Kavoussi LR, et al. Laparoscopic retroperitoneal lymph node dissection for high-risk pediatric patients with paratesticular rhabdomyosarcoma. J Endourol 2010;24(1):31–4.

48. Rogers T, Minard-Colin V, Cozic N, et al. Paratesticular rhabdomyosarcoma in children and adolescents—Outcome and patterns of relapse when utilizing a nonsurgical strategy for lymph node staging: Report from the International Society of Paediatric Oncology (SIOP) Malignant Mesenchymal Tumour 89 a. Pediatr Blood Cancer 2017;64(9):1–8.

49. Routh JC, Dasgupta R, Chi Y, et al. Impact of Local Control and Surgical Lymph Node Evaluation in Localized Paratesticular Rhabdomyosarcoma: A Report from the Children's Oncology Group Soft Tissue Sarcoma Committee. Int J Cancer 2020;1–9. https://doi.org/10.1002/ijc.33143.

50. Donaldson SS, Meza J, Breneman JC, et al. Results from the irs-iv randomized trial of hyperfractionated radiotherapy in children with rhabdomyosarcoma-a report from the IRSG. Int J Radiat Oncol Biol Phys 2001;51:718–28.

51. Guérin F, Rogers T, Minard-Colin V, et al. Outcome of localized liver-bile duct rhabdomyosarcoma according to local therapy: A report from the European Paediatric Soft-Tissue Sarcoma Study Group (EpSSG)-RMS 2005 study. Pediatr Blood Cancer 2019;e27725. https://doi.org/10.1002/pbc.27725.

52. Spunt SL, Lobe TE, Pappo AS, et al. Aggressive surgery is unwarranted for biliary tract rhabdomyosarcoma. J Pediatr Surg 2000;35(2):309–16.

53. Lautz TB, Chi YY, Tian J, et al. Relationship between tumor response at therapy completion and prognosis in patients with Group III rhabdomyosarcoma: A report from the Children's Oncology Group. Int J Cancer 2020. https://doi.org/10.1002/ijc.32896.

54. Vaarwerk B, Mallebranche C, Affinita MC, et al. Is surveillance imaging in pediatric patients treated for localized rhabdomyosarcoma useful? The European experience. Cancer 2020;126(4):823–31.

55. Hayes-Jordan A, Doherty DK, West SD, et al. Outcome after surgical resection of recurrent rhabdomyosarcoma. J Pediatr Surg 2006;41(4):633–8.

56. Dantonello TM. Int-Veen C, Schuck A, et al. Survival following disease recurrence of primary localized alveolar rhabdomyosarcoma. Pediatr Blood Cancer 2013; 60(8):1267–73.

57. Chen C, Dorado Garcia H, Scheer M, et al. Current and Future Treatment Strategies for Rhabdomyosarcoma. Front Oncol 2019;9:1–18.

58. Mansfield SA, Murphy AJ, Talbot L, et al. Alternative approaches to retroperitoneal lymph node dissection for paratesticular rhabdomyosarcoma. J Pediatr Surg 2020;5–9. https://doi.org/10.1016/j.jpedsurg.2020.03.022.

59. Bedyńska M, Szewczyk G, Klepacka T, et al. Sentinel lymph node mapping using indocyanine green in patients with uterine and cervical neoplasms: restrictions of the method. Arch Gynecol Obstet 2019;299(5):1373–84.

60. Turpin B, Pressey JG, Nagarajan R, et al. Sentinel lymph node biopsy in head and neck rhabdomyosarcoma. Pediatr Blood Cancer 2019;66(3):1–4.

61. Lautz TB, Hayes-Jordan A. Recent progress in pediatric soft tissue sarcoma therapy. Semin Pediatr Surg 2019;28(6):150862.

62. Kahen E, Yu D, Harrison DJ, et al. Identification of clinically achievable combination therapies in childhood rhabdomyosarcoma. Cancer Chemother Pharmacol 2016;78(2):313–23.

63. Phelps MP, Yang H, Patel S, et al. Oncolytic Virus-Mediated RAS targeting in rhabdomyosarcoma. Mol Ther Oncolytics 2018;11:52–61.

64. Currier MA, Adams LC, Mahller YY, et al. Widespread intratumoral virus distribution with fractionated injection enables local control of large human rhabdomyosarcoma xenografts by oncolytic herpes simplex viruses. Cancer Gene Ther 2005;12(4):407–16.

65. Weiner GJ. Building better monoclonal antibody-based therapeutics. Nat Rev Cancer 2015;15(6):361–70.

66. Christopher DeRenzo, MD, MBA, Giedre Krenciute, PhD, and Stephen Go? Schalk M. The Landscape of CAR T Cells Beyond Acute Lymphoblas c. Christopher DeRenzo, MD, MBA, Gied Krenciute, PhD, Stephen Go? Schalk, MD. 2018:830-837. asco.org/edbook.

Treatment Concepts and Challenges in Nonrhabdomyosarcoma Soft Tissue Sarcomas

Joerg Fuchs, MD[a],*, Andreas Schmidt, MD[a],
Steven W. Warmann, MD[a], David A. Rodeberg, MD[b]

KEYWORDS

- Pediatric nonrhabdomyosarcoma • Myofibroblastic tumor
- Congenital infantile fibrosarcoma • Synovial sarcoma • Desmoid tumor
- Peripheral nerve sheath tumor • Desmoplastic small round cell tumor

KEY POINTS

- Nonrhabdomyosarcoma soft tissue sarcomas comprise a heterogeneous group of many different tumor entities.
- The therapeutic approach is similar despite the different tumor entities.
- Using a risk-adapted approach, low-grade tumors are mostly treated by surgery alone, whereas high-grade tumors require multimodal therapy.
- Surgery plays a crucial role for the oncological and functional outcome.
- New therapeutic concepts are necessary for the treatment of high-grade tumors in difficult localizations, unresectable tumors, tumor relapses, and stage IV disease.

INTRODUCTION

Nonrhabdomyosarcoma soft tissue sarcomas (NRSTSs) represent a heterogeneous group of soft tissue sarcomas with more than 50 histologies. NRSTSs show a variable clinical behavior with differing sensitivity to chemotherapy or radiotherapy, and variable prognosis. NRSTS account for approximately 4% of all childhood cancers. NRSTSs have an incidence of 550 to 600 cases per year in the United States with a bimodal age distribution.[1] The first peak occurs before than the age of 4 years, and

Conflict of interest: The authors have no conflict to disclose.
Funding: None.
[a] Department of Pediatric Surgery and Pediatric Urology, University Children's Hospital Tuebingen, Hoppe-Seyler-Str. 3, Tuebingen 72076, Germany; [b] Department of Surgery, Brody School of Medicine, East Carolina University, 600 Moye Boulevard, Greenville, NC 27834, USA
* Corresponding author.
E-mail address: joerg.fuchs@med.uni-tuebingen.de

surgonc.theclinics.com

comprises mostly infantile fibrosarcoma. The second peak is more commonly seen in the middle to late teenage years, and the histologic subtypes comprise predominantly synovial cell sarcoma, malignant peripheral nerve sheath tumor, or high-grade pleomorphic sarcoma. Male and female patients are equally affected, with the exception of desmoplastic small round blue cell tumors, which are predominantly male. Most NRSTS are sporadic, but survivors of childhood malignancies, with a history of radiation exposure, have an increased risk of sarcoma. Most patients with NRSTS have an extremity primary tumor (55%), localized disease (85%), high grade (72%), tumors less than 10 cm (69%), and deep tumors (83%).[2]

Genomic instability and specific chromosomal abnormalities have been implicated in the pathogenesis of NRSTS (**Table 1**). Children with certain cancer predisposition syndromes have an increased risk for developing NRSTS (Li-Fraumeni syndrome, neurofibromatosis [NF] type 1, Werner syndrome). Another predisposing factor is the development of secondary NRSTS within a radiation field after treatment of other malignancies.

In general, metastases, tumor grade, size, extent of resection, and margin status are strongly associated with event-free survival and overall survival.[3] Overall survival progressively declined with increasing age. Gender, race, ethnicity, primary site, and tumor histology were not significant predictors of outcomes. In comparing prognostic factors, tumor size and depth were stronger predictors of outcome in the pediatric population compared with an adult population.[4]

Most tumors are not responsive to chemotherapy. However, the more common pediatric NRSTSs, such as synovial sarcoma, unclassified sarcoma, and embryonal sarcoma of the liver, are chemosensitive. In these chemosensitive tumors, outcomes are superior to those in adults for the same tumor.[5,6]

This article gives a comprehensive overview of the impact of treatment modalities in NRSTS based on the experiences of the different international NRSTS trials.

GENERAL CONSIDERATIONS
Presentation and Diagnostic Evaluation

Most NRSTSs present as painless swellings with a wide range of specific clinical symptoms depending on the anatomic location of the tumor. Symptoms include neurologic abnormalities, lung or bowel dysfunction, and vascular compression. Systemic symptoms, such as loss of body weight, anemia, or fever, are rare. Regional lymph node involvement is unusual except in epithelioid (20%–30%) and clear cell (20%–30%) disease. The most common site of distant metastasis is in the lung, but it can also be seen in bone, liver, subcutaneous tissue, and the brain.[7]

The diagnostic work-up includes plain radiography, which might be useful for detecting the primary mass as well as a local or distant spread; for example, into the lungs or bones. It may also help to identify calcification, a classic sign for extraskeletal osteosarcoma or synovial sarcoma. Further imaging modalities are ultrasonography (including Doppler and contrast-enhanced sonography), contrast computed tomography (CT) scan, and MRI. These imaging techniques determine the presence of metastatic disease, tumor size/volume, extension, or infiltration into adjacent structures. They are essential for planning of surgical procedures and radiotherapy. It has not been well established whether a significant change in the size of the tumor mass, as determined by RECIST (Response Evaluation Criteria in Solid Tumours), is a meaningful surrogate of patient outcome in NRSTS. More than 15% of patients present with metastatic disease, which most commonly occurs in the lungs. A staging CT scan of the chest is therefore crucial in these patients. 2-[^{18}F]-fluoro-2-deoxy-D-glucose (FDG)

Table 1
Genetic alteration of selected nonrhabdomyosarcoma soft tissue sarcoma

Tumor Entity	Genetic Disorder	Genes Involved
Synovial sarcoma	t(X;18) (p11;q11)	SSX-SYT
MPNST	17Q11.2 loss rearrangement 10p, 11q, 17q, 22q	NF1
Infantile fibrosarcoma	t(12;15) (p13,q26)	ETV6-NTRK3
Inflammatory myofibroblastic tumor	2p23 rearrangement	ALK-TPM3, ALK-TPM4, ALK-clathrin and other
Ewing sarcoma	t(11;22) (q42;q12) t(21;22) (q22;q12)	EWSR1-FL11, EWSR1-ERG, EWSR1-ETS; FUS-ETS
Desmoplastic small round cell tumor	t(11;22) (p13;q12)	EWS-WT1
Undifferentiated pleomorphic sarcoma	t(2:22) (q33:q12) t(12:22) (q13:q12) t(12:16) (q13:p11)	EWSR1-CREB1 EWSR1-ATF1 FUS-ATF1
Desmoid tumor	Trisomy 8 or 20, loss of 5q21	CTNNB1 or APC

Abbreviation: MPNST, malignant peripheral nerve sheath tumor.

PET, used as PET/CT or PET/MRI, has increasingly been used in staging and surveillance (**Fig. 1**).[8,9] The prognostic implications of PET response in overall survival are still unclear.

Other modalities that may also be needed for adequate tumor staging depend on the tumor histology and potentially include radionuclide bone scan, bone marrow aspiration, sentinel lymph node biopsy, and cerebrospinal fluid examination.[10]

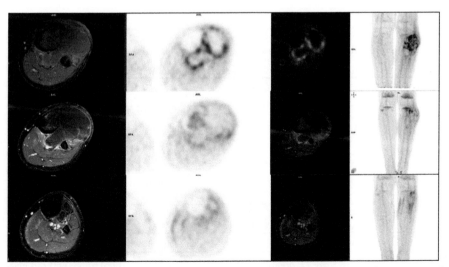

Fig. 1. FDG-PET/MRI of a 15-year-old boy with a low differentiated pleomorphic sarcoma of left lower leg. (*Upper row*) Baseline. (*Middle row*) Early response assessment (ERA). (*Lower row*) Late response assessment (LRA). In contrast with MRI, FDG uptake is decreasing from baseline to LRA. The MRI revealed a pseudoprogress at ERA (*arrow*).

Tumor biopsy plays an important role in the identification of the different tumor histologies comprising NRSTS. Therefore, an adequate amount of tissue should be obtained to allow microscopic, immunohistochemical, and other studies, such as molecular pathology and cytogenetics. Under these circumstances, fine-needle aspiration does not provide sufficient material. Core or open biopsies are recommended. However, planning of the biopsy approach should reflect that the biopsy tract has to be resected at the time of the definitive surgery. In selected cases with the possibility of a complete upfront primary tumor resection (superficial lesion with a diameter <3–5 cm with a safety margin of 1 cm) the tumor should just undergo a complete excision.[11]

Risk Stratification and Staging of Nonrhabdomyosarcoma Soft Tissue Sarcoma

Parameters for risk stratification of NRSTS can include presence of metastatic disease, primary tumor size, lymph node involvement, completeness of resection, histology, and tumor grading. However, a uniform method for staging and tumor grading has not been used by the different international study trials.

Staging of pediatric NRSTS can be performed according to the following methods: the American Joint Committee of Cancer (AJCC) staging (**Table 2**) used by the Children's Oncology Group (COG). The AJCC staging is a presurgical system and includes tumor size (T1, 5 cm; T2, 5 cm) and depth (a, superficial; b ,deep), nodal involvement, distant metastasis, and histologic grade. The AJCC staging system is in widespread use in adult soft tissue sarcoma clinical trials, and its ability to discriminate the overall survival of patients with soft tissue sarcomas has been validated. European groups developed a staging method, which includes aspects from presurgical and postsurgical systems (**Table 3**).

The grading of NRSTS represents one of the most debated and complex subjects. It describes the aggressiveness of the tumor based on degree of cellularity, mitotic activity, degree of necrosis, and anaplasia. However, a generally accepted grading system does not exist. Low-grade tumors are mostly localized, with a low tendency for

Table 2
The American Joint Committee on Cancer staging for soft tissue sarcoma

Stage	Tumor Size	LN Status	Metastases	Grading
IA	T1a	N0	M0	G1
	T1b	N0	M0	G1
IB	T2a	N0	M0	G1
	T2b	N0	M0	G1
IIA	T1a	N0	M0	G2
	T1b	N0	M0	G2, 3
IIB	T2a	N0	M0	G2
	T2b	N0	M0	G2
	T2b	N0	M0	G2
III	T2a, T2b	N0	M0	G3
	Any T	N1	M0	Any G
IV	Any T	Any N	M1	Any G

T1, less than or equal to 5 cm; T2, greater than or equal to 5 cm; a, superficial tumor without invasion of the fascia; b, deep tumor located either exclusively beneath the superficial fascia, superficial to the fascia with invasion of or through the fascia. N/M positive finding for nodal involvement or presence of metastases.
Abbreviations: G, grading; LN, lymph node.

Table 3
Risk stratification for nonrhabdomyosarcoma soft tissue sarcoma (Cooperative Weichteilsarkom Studiengruppe -2002-P protocol)

Risk Group	Histology	LN Status	IRS Group	Initial Tumor Size (cm)
Low	Any (except MRT, DSRCT)	N0	I	≤ 5
Standard	Any (except MRT, DSRCT)	N0	I	$\geq 5^a$
		N0	II	Any
		N0	III	$\leq 5^b$
High	MRT/DSRCT	N0/N1	I, II, III	Any
	Any	N0	III	≥ 5
	Any	N1	II, III	Any
Stage IV	Any	N0/N1	IV	Any

Abbreviations: DSRCT, desmoplastic small round cell tumor; MRT, malignant rhabdoid tumor.
  [a] Exception: typical low-grade tumor (grade1), greater than 5 cm, IRS group I might be treated in the low-risk group.
  [b] Exception: high-grade tumor (grade 2 and 3), less than 5 cm, IRS group III, might be treated in the high-risk group.

development of metastases. In contrast, high-grade tumors show an invasive behavior with a higher risk for metastatic spread. Two grading systems are commonly used: the Pediatric Oncology Group system for pediatric sarcoma (**Table 4**) and the system of the FNCLCC (Fédération National des Centres de Lutte Contre le Cancer; **Table 5**).

Recently, the COG published results from a prospective trial with the aim of a risk-based treatment strategy for NRSTS (ARST0332), which included 529 patients less than 30 years of age. The extent of tumor resection was defined as R0 (no malignant cells microscopically evident at the resection margin), R1 (malignant cells evident microscopically at the resection margin), or R2 (malignant cells grossly evident at the resection margin). The patients were allocated to 3 risk groups (**Box 1**).

The different treatment groups (surgery alone, radiotherapy, and multimodal treatment [both local treatment plus chemotherapy]) were also analyzed with regard to the outcome. The investigators observed that pretreatment clinical features could

Table 4
Pediatric Oncology Group grading system for pediatric nonrhabdomyosarcoma soft tissue sarcoma

Grade	Tumor Entities
1	Liposarcoma: myxoid and well differentiated
	Deep-seated dermatofibrosarcoma protuberans
	Fibrosarcoma: well differentiated or infantile (<5 y)
	Hemangiopericytoma well differentiated or infantile (<5 y)
	Well-differentiated MPNST
	Angiomatoid malignant fibrous histiocytoma
2	All NRSTSs not in grade 1 or 3; $\leq$15% of tumors show geographic necrosis or mitotic index is <5 mitoses/10 HPF
3	Fibrosarcoma with >15% of tumor with geographic necrosis or mitotic index $\geq$5 mitoses/10 HPF
	Liposarcoma pleomorphic, round cell; mesenchymal chondrosarcoma
	Extraskeletal osteosarcoma, malignant triton tumor, alveolar soft part sarcoma

Abbreviation: HPF, high-power field.

Table 5
Fédération National des Centres de Lutte Contre le Cancer system of grading soft tissue sarcoma

Parameter	Criterion
Tumor Differentiation	
Score = 1	Sarcoma histologically very similar to normal adult mesenchymal tissue
Score = 2	Sarcoma for defined histologic subtype (eg, myxoid MFH)
Score = 3	Sarcoma of uncertain type, embryonal and undifferentiated sarcomas
Mitosis Count	
Score = 1	0–9/10 HPF
Score = 2	10–19/10 HPF
Score = 3	≥20/10 HPF
Microscopic Tumor Necrosis	
Score = 0	No necrosis
Score = 1	≤50% tumor necrosis
Score = 2	≥50% tumor necrosis
Histologic Grade	
Grade 1	Total score 2 or 3
Grade 2	Total score 4 or 5
Grade 3	Total score 6, 7, or 8

Abbreviation: MFH, malignant histiocytoma.

be used for the stratification of the risk-adapted therapy. Most of the low-risk patients were cured without adjuvant therapy, thereby avoiding known long-term treatment complications.[3,8] Approximately a third of patients were treated with surgery alone, a third required adjuvant therapy, and a third required neoadjuvant therapy. Local control was almost 100%.

General Treatment Strategies

Cases discussion should occur within a multidisciplinary tumor board before initiation of treatment, to optimize treatment and outcomes.

Surgery is the mainstay of treatment of local tumor control. The completeness of resection has a prognostic impact for the outcome of the patients in nearly all tumor histologies. The ultimate goal of resection is complete surgical excision with negative margins. This goal can be achieved in approximately 48% of patients (39% at initial presentation) and with microscopic margins in 63% of patients. Primary reexcision may be necessary in tumors if residual disease (R1 or R2) is present after initial resection in order to avoid radiation. The optimal or appropriate size of the margins is unclear at this time; however, a margin of 0.5 cm or a fascial plane that is closer may

Box 1
Risk startification of NRSTS according to the COG Trial ARST0332

Low risk	Nonmetastatic tumors, resection status R0 or R1, low-grade tumors or high-grade tumors <5 cm
Intermediate risk	Nonmetastatic tumors, resection status R0 or R1 in tumors >5 cm, or unresected tumor of any size or grade
High risk	Metastatic tumor

be sufficient. Although an R0 complete resection is optimal, an R1 positive micro-scopic margin is also sufficient in low-grade tumors in low-risk patients.[3] For intermediate-risk patients, outcomes for R0 or R1 resection done before study entry were similar to delayed R0 or R1 resections. In addition, the proportion who had an R0 resection was higher when surgery was delayed (82%) compared with those done before study entry (57%). After neoadjuvant therapy, 92% of patients had either an R0 or R1 resection. However, outcome did not significantly differ between patients who had an R0 resection and patients who had an R1 resection. Intermediate-risk tu-mors should be treated with surgery and radiotherapy, depending on the histologic subtype.[12] The time interval between neoadjuvant radiotherapy and surgical resection does not seem to affect rates of wound complications in these patients. In addition, the wound complication rates are low (10%) in patients with prior neoadjuvant therapy. In high-risk patients, it is uncommon for patients to undergo complete resection of all disease. For unresectable tumors that are unresponsive to chemotherapy, a radical surgical approach may be necessary.[13] There is debate about the benefit of surgical resection of metastases.[14,15]

NRSTS tumors are much less sensitive to chemotherapy compared with rhabdo-myosarcoma (RMS). The most common cytotoxic drugs for the treatment of NRSTS are ifosfamide and doxorubicin. This chemotherapy regimen is used by the COG. Other drugs, such as vincristine, topotecan, etoposide, cyclophosphamide, and meth-otrexate have also been used.[12] New drugs such as kinase inhibitors (eg, sorafenib, temozolide, pazopanib) have shown promising treatment results in pilot studies on re-fractory sarcomas, although they are only considered investigational at this point.[15]

Radiation therapy may be used for local control in unresectable tumors. It can also be given preoperatively to facilitate negative margins at time of resection, or postop-eratively for tumors with positive margins. The radiation field margins are generally be-tween 2 and 4 cm encompassing the fascial planes axially. Although smaller margins of 1.5 to 2 cm may be equally efficacious for synovial sarcomas that are less than 5 cm in size.[16] Radiation doses range between 45 and 50 Gy in the preoperative period with an option to boost postoperatively to 10 to 20 Gy. In the postoperative setting, the ra-diation dose in NRSTS is generally between 55 and 60 Gy.

Management of Selected Nonrhabdomyosarcoma Soft Tissue Sarcoma Entities

Congenital infantile fibrosarcoma

Congenital infantile fibrosarcomas occur during the first months of life and are often misdiagnosed as hemangioma or vascular malformation. The tumors arise in the su-perficial and deep soft tissue layers of the extremities predominately, although trunk or head and neck region also occur. Sometimes the locally aggressive tumor mass can become very large compared with the size of the child and can lead to severe ul-ceration. Metastatic spread has rarely been reported (1%–13%). Spontaneous regres-sion in patients less than 3 months of age has been infrequently described.[17] A chromosomal translocation, t(12;15) (p13;q26), which leads to a fusion ETV6-NTRK3, has been reported.

Tumor biopsy confirms the diagnosis. On histology the tumors present with densely packed spindle cells arranged in bundles and fascicles with an infiltrative growth pattern. Variable myxoid and cystic degeneration, hemorrhage, and necrosis can be identified. The tumor cells are positive for vimentin and negative for desmin and S100 protein.

Complete surgical resection is the key for the best outcome. Primary reexcision af-ter initial R1 or R2 resection can improve the prognosis. In selected cases, a radical surgery is the only way for achieving survival (**Fig. 2**).

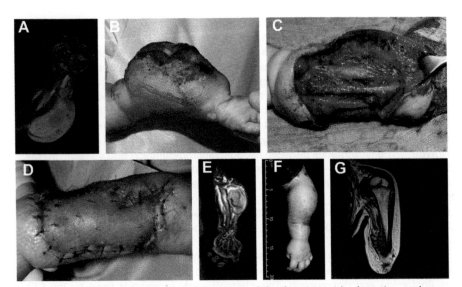

Fig. 2. Newborn with an infantile fibrosarcoma of the forearm with ulceration and recurrent local bleeding. (*A*) Initial MRI. (*B*) Clinical aspect. (*C, D*) Intraoperative view with R1 resection and decompression of the ulnar nerve. (*E*) Tumor progress despite adjuvant chemotherapy. (*F*) Forearm amputation (resected specimen). (*G*) MRI 5 years later with no evidence of disease (NED).

These tumors are chemosensitive, with a therapeutic pathologic response seen in up to 90% of patients. Neoadjuvant chemotherapy can downsize an unresectable tumor (extremely large mass and involvement of vital structures), allowing function-preserving delayed primary excision. The most common chemotherapy regimens are VA, VAC, or IVA.[17] Considering the typical age group, radiotherapy is not recommended because of the severe long-term side effects.

The 5-year overall survival rate lies between 80% and 100%.

Malignant peripheral nerve sheath tumor

Malignant peripheral nerve sheath tumor (MPNST) is a rare and aggressive soft tissue sarcoma, most often arising from previously benign peripheral neurofibromas or schwannomas (NF1, NF2, schwannomatosis). It accounts for approximately 2% of all NRSTS. Half of the children have an underlying NF1 mutation. A child with NF1 mutation has a cumulative lifetime risk of up to 13% for developing MPNST.[18] By comparison, the incidence of MPNST in the general population is only 0.01%.

On histology, there exists both a mesenchymal and an epithelioid variant. The most common mesenchymal element is RMS, but chondrosarcomatous and osteosarcomatous elements also occur. With immunostaining, neural antigens for S-100, CD 55, and Neuron-specific enolase can be observed.

Complete surgical en bloc removal plays the key role for survival and is the mainstay of treatment (**Fig. 3**). In initially unresectable tumors, neoadjuvant chemotherapy (ifosfamide and doxorubicin) may induce a partial tumor response in nearly half of the patients irrespective of NF1 mutations, although chemotherapy responsiveness is variable but largely has been reported as resistant.[19] The role of conventional radiotherapy in pediatric MPNST is not yet clear.[18] Van Noesel and colleagues[20] from the European Pediatric Soft Tissue Sarcoma Group (EpSSG) prospectively determined

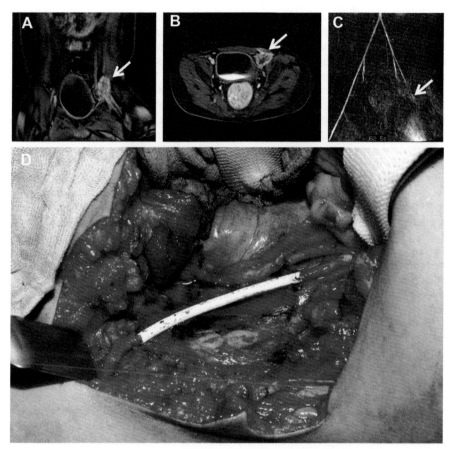

Fig. 3. An 11-year-old boy with an osteosarcoma and a secondary MPNST of the left stump. (*A*, *B*) MRI with tumor extension before surgery. (*C*) Angio-MRI with infiltration of the femoral artery. (*D*) Operative situs after en bloc tumor resection with vascular replacement of the femoral artery using Gore-Tex. Follow-up at 1.5 years, NED. Arrows in 3A, 3B, 3C indicate the tumor on imaging.

prognostic factors for MPNST. Negative prognostic factors for outcome were an R2 resection with gross residual disease and the presence of NF1 mutation. Surprisingly, the prognosis was not associated with age at diagnosis, tumor size, or tumor grade. However, other studies support the presence of NF1, invasive tumors, tumor size (>5 cm), R2 resection, and nonextremity primary site as poor prognostic factors.[21]

The 5-year overall survival rate is predominately affected by the completeness of surgical resection. Survival rates are 60% to 65% in R0 and R1 resections and 27% to 33% in R2 gross residual disease resections.

Rhabdomyosarcomalike tumors

Synovial sarcoma, soft tissue Ewing tumors (subgroup I, extraosseous Ewing sarcoma; subgroup II, peripheral primitive neuroectodermal tumor), and undifferentiated sarcoma can be summarized as RMS-like tumors. The 3 different subtypes of RMS-like tumors show a specific cytogenetic signature (see **Table 1**). Synovial sarcoma is the most common. Although it can affect all ages and locations, it is most commonly seen after 10 years of age and has a propensity for the lower extremities (usually around the knee). Most synovial sarcomas are considered intermediate-grade to high-grade tumors. Patients are treated according to the same guidelines in nearly all protocols. The rate of primary metastatic spread lies between 8% and 10% and most commonly is to the lungs.[10,22]

The tumor site is important for the surgical strategy. Most of the tumors are located in the limbs. Primary tumors located in the thigh are more frequent in older patients.[10,23] The axial site tumors (head and neck, trunk, lungs and pleura) are more difficult to excise, with a higher risk of incomplete tumor resection. Larger, invasive tumors and the presence of metastases are significantly associated with older patients in synovial sarcoma.

In low-risk tumors (initial tumor size <5 cm), primary surgery is recommended with the preoperative intent to perform a nonradical complete tumor resection. Both EpSSG and COG have published excellent treatment results of low-risk synovial sarcoma treated with surgery alone (100% 3 -year overall survival).[24]

In high-risk tumors, the optimal approach is tumor biopsy followed by neoadjuvant therapy. After neoadjuvant therapy, a complete clinical and radiological assessment of the tumor response is indicated.[25] Synovial sarcomas do not often respond with a significant reduction of tumor volume; however, the development of cysts and hemorrhage or necrosis within tumors may occur. Approximately 40% to 65% of synovial sarcomas are chemotherapy sensitive. In contrast, soft tissue Ewing tumors and undifferentiated sarcoma respond with significant tumor shrinkage after chemotherapy.[26–28] Radiotherapy may be administered before delayed primary tumor excision. Occasionally, despite adjuvant therapies, radical resections or the acceptance of functional impairments are unavoidable.[29]

The optimal local control modality should be discussed in a multidisciplinary tumor board. Radiotherapy can be avoided after primary complete R0 tumor resections. In all other patients, radiotherapy is indicated either preoperatively or postoperatively. The dosages range from 50.4 to 54 Gy (conventional fraction). A boost of 5.4 Gy makes sense in cases of progressive disease or poor response. An alternative approach is the hyperfractionated, accelerated irradiation with 44.8 Gy.[23] The advantage of preoperative radiotherapy is a smaller irradiation field, better oxygenation of the tumor, and a lower risk of tumor spillage during tumor removal. Preoperative radiotherapy is indicated in cases where the en bloc tumor resection is planned together with reconstructive surgical procedures (nerve interposition, vascular replacement, muscular flaps). The best time interval for surgery after radiotherapy is 6 weeks, because of the reduced risk of wound healing issues.

Because of the different histologic diagnoses and the locations, the 5-year overall survival for these entities ranges from 60% to 85%.[27,28,30–32] Improved survival is associated with smaller size, lower stage, and the use of radiotherapy. Poor prognostic factors include nonextremity tumors, proximal tumor location, greater tissue depth, and younger patients. Long-term follow-up is of utmost importance, because synovial sarcoma tends to recur locally and can present with metastatic disease well beyond 5 years.

Inflammatory myofibroblastic tumor

Inflammatory myofibroblastic tumor (IMT; synonyms include plasma cell granuloma, plasma cell pseudotumor, fibrous histiocytoma) is a rare tumor in the first decade of life with a median age of 9 years and a female predominance.

The clinical presentation depends on the localization and the tumor size. The lung is the most common site of occurrence, followed by the abdominal cavity. More than one-third of the patients present with systemic symptoms such as fever, weight loss, malaise, and anemia. Metastatic disease can occur in some cases.

On histology, the tumor is represented by myofibroblastic spindle cells and inflammatory infiltrates of plasma cells together with lymphocytes and eosinophils. The proliferation rate is sometimes very high. Cytogenetically there exist rearrangements of gene tmp-3(1q21), tpm-4(19p13), dtc(17q11), cars(11p15), or ranbp2(2q12) with ALK(2p23). Translocations involving ALK receptor tyrosine kinase have been described in nearly the half of IMTs and allows targeted therapy.[33–35]

The treatment of choice is complete surgical resection. In large tumors or tumors that are difficult to resect, a biopsy is indicated. For ALK-positive tumors, a primary treatment with crizotinib can reduce the tumor size significantly.[36] Mossé and colleagues[37] reported on a robust and sustained clinical response rate of 86% in primary unresectable IMTs. Under these circumstances, the reduction of tumor size can improve complete resection rates, which is associated with a lower rate of local relapse (**Fig. 4**).[37] Clinical symptoms and sometimes the tumor extension can be treated using steroids or nonsteroidal antiinflammatory drugs (cyclooxygenase-2 inhibitors). The role of chemotherapy is controversial. The Cooperative Weichteilsarkom Studiengruppe (CWS) showed a partial response after administration of dactinomycin, ifosfamide, and vincristine in 5 out of 18 patients. In addition, radiation has no role in the treatment of IMT.[33]

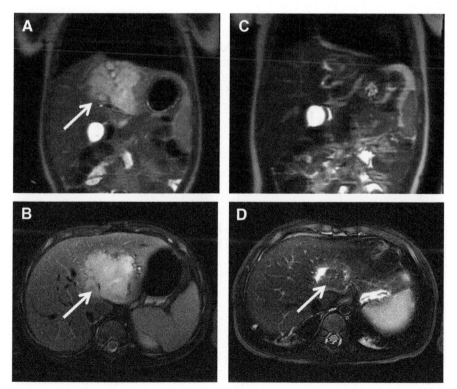

Fig. 4. IMT (*arrows*) in a 2-year-old girl. (*A, B*) Initial tumor extension with a tumor volume of 83 mL. (*C, D*) Response (tumor volume 5 mL) after tumor biopsy and treatment with larotrectinib for 4 months.

The prognosis of patients with IMT is good, with a 5-year overall survival of 85% to 90%, and depends on completeness of tumor resection and site.

Desmoplastic small round cell tumor

Desmoplastic small round cell tumor (DSRCT) is an extremely aggressive rare sarcoma typically affecting adolescent boys. The tumors occur primarily in the peritoneum or pleura. The liver, ovaries, lung, and retroperitoneal organs can also be involved.

On histology, tumors consist of small round cells embedded in desmoplastic stroma. There exists a coexpression of epithelial and mesenchymal antigens. A translocation t(11;22p12;13q), merging the EWS and the WT1 gene are present.

These tumors are highly chemosensitive. After several months of chemotherapy, complete resection is feasible even for patients with significant disease burden. The treatment options include chemotherapy after tumor biopsy, cytoreductive surgery, hyperthermic intraperitoneal chemotherapy (HIPEC), postoperative whole-abdominal irradiation (WART), and maintenance chemotherapy.[38,39] Cytoreductive surgery is challenging because all intra-abdominal or intrapleural implants have to be resected in an aggressive fashion, which may also include at least partial resection of organs (ovary, partial bowel resection, distal pancreatectomy, splenectomy, partial resection of the diaphragm, or partial liver resection) (**Fig. 5**). However, new agents, such as the tyrosine kinase inhibitor pazopanib, have not shown any improvement in the outcome of patients with DSRCT.[40,41]

Determination of prognostic factors such as response to chemotherapy, completeness of resection, liver involvement, ascites, and vascular thrombosis is impossible because of low case numbers and the worldwide differing treatment modalities.[42,43]

Despite all the intensive multimodal treatment options, DSRCT is associated with dismal outcomes (5-year overall survival 10%–25%). Treatment of DSRCT should be centralized, and prospective randomized international trials are necessary together with an international registry for judging treatment effects of HIPEC, the role of WART, or for testing new drug regimens.[44]

Desmoid tumors

Desmoid tumors arise from the fibrous tissue that forms tendons and ligaments. The cause of desmoid tumors remains unclear.

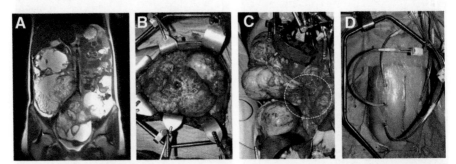

Fig. 5. A 16-year-old girl with a DSRCT and peritoneal carcinomatosis (T2bNxM0, IRS IIIA) after chemotherapy according to the CWS protocol. (A) MRI with tumor extension. (B, C) Intraoperative situs with peritoneal implants (dashed circle). (D) HIPEC with cisplatin and doxorubicin after cytoreductive surgery with complete macroscopic tumor resection.

These tumors are mostly located in the arms, legs, and abdomen (they can also occur in the head and neck region). When these tumors occur outside of the abdomen, they are referred to as aggressive fibromatosis. These benign tumors do not develop metastases. Nevertheless, they can adhere to and intertwine with surrounding structures and organs, making them difficult to control. The most common symptom of desmoid tumors is pain. Other signs and symptoms, which are often caused by the infiltration of the tumor into surrounding tissue, vary based on the size and location of the tumor (**Fig. 6**). Microscopically, they are well-differentiated, mature fibrous lesions composed of mature fibrocytes within an extensive collagen matrix.

Localized tumors should be observed unless they are causing symptoms, in which case they should be resected. Nevertheless, radical resections should not be performed because the frequency of local recurrence after excision is high. The current standard of care for pediatric unresectable or progressive desmoid-type fibromatosis is intravenous methotrexate/vinblastine.[45] Other medical treatment concepts include the kinase inhibitor sorafenib or pazopanib. The latter agents provide a promising,

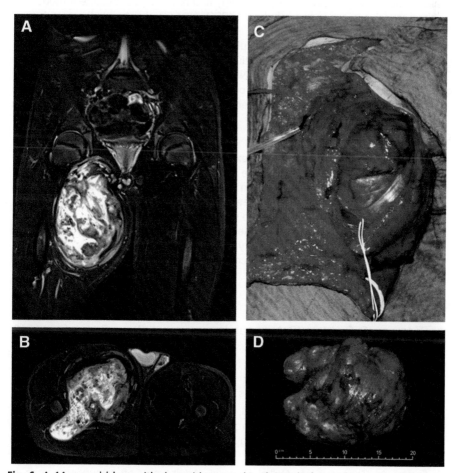

Fig. 6. A 14-year-old boy with desmoid tumor. (*A, B*) MRI before surgery showing tumor expansion through the obturator foramen into the lesser pelvis. (*C, D*) En bloc resection with preservation of the ischiadic nerve.

well-tolerated therapy for desmoid tumors and aggressive fibromatosis in the young and adolescent population and warrant further studies.[46] The role of radiotherapy is a controversial issue without relevant influence on the local recurrence rate, which is up to 30% even with negative margins.[47]

SUMMARY

Despite the progress in treatment regimens for NRSTS over the last 3 decades, the prognosis of children with metastatic disease, advanced tumors, or relapse disease is poor. New and innovative treatment concepts are necessary for improving the outcome of these challenging patient cohorts. In contrast, the close international collaboration between the different international trial groups is an important way for powerful data accrual and analysis in these rare tumor entities.

The international collaboration should establish common treatment guidelines for children with NRSTS and focus on research projects to investigate new drugs such as multikinase or gamma-secretase inhibitors and gene therapies. It is necessary to evaluate the efficacy of proton beam therapy and new surgical treatment modalities (minimal invasive surgery and robotics, HIPEC, surgery plus brachytherapy, hyperthermic isolated limb perfusion).[48]

One essential step for realizing these projects was the foundation of the INSTRuCT group (International Soft Tissue Consortium) group in 2017 with representatives from COG, EpSSG, and CWS. The aim of INSTRuCT is to establish common treatment guidelines and to build an international consensus for risk stratification similar to the risk stratification for neuroblastoma (International Neuroblastoma Risk Group).[49]

CLINICS CARE POINTS

- Metastases, tumor grade, size, extent of resection, and margin status are strongly associated with event-free survival and overall survival in NRSTS.
- A CT scan of the chest is crucial in affected patients because lung metastases occur in a relevant number of cases.
- Most NRSTS are not responsive to chemotherapy.
- Tumor biopsy plays a key role in the diagnostic workup. The biopsy tract should be excised during definitive surgery.
- Complete tumor resection with negative margins is the main goal of surgical treatment.

REFERENCES

1. Dasguptas R, Rodeberg D. Non-rhabdomyosarcoma. Semin Pediatr Surg 2016; 25(5):284–9.
2. Ferrari A, Miceli R, Rey A, et al. Non-metastatic unresected paediatric non-rhabdomyosarcoma soft tissue sarcomas: results of a pooled analysis from United States and European groups. Eur J Cancer 2011;47(5):724–31.
3. Spunt SL, Million L, Chi YY, et al. A risk-based treatment strategy for non-rhabdomyosarcoma soft-tissue sarcomas in patients younger than 30 years (ARST0332): a Children's Oncology Group prospective study. Lancet Oncol 2020;21(1):145–61.
4. Ferrari A, Casanova M, Collini P, et al. Adult-type soft tissue sarcomas in pediatric-age patients: experience at the Istituto Nazionale Tumori in Milan. J Clin Oncol 2005;23(18):4021–30.

5. Smolle MA, Parry M, Jeys L, et al. Synovial sarcoma: Do children do better? Eur J Surg Oncol 2019;45(2):254–60.

6. Murawski M, Scheer M, Leuschner I, et al. Undifferentiated sarcoma of the liver: Multicenter international experience of the Cooperative Soft-Tissue Sarcoma Group and Polish Paediatric Solid Tumor Group. Pediatr Blood Cancer 2020;e28598. https://doi.org/10.1002/pbc.28598.

7. Pappo AS, Rao BN, Jenkins JJ, et al. Metastatic nonrhabdomyosarcomatous soft-tissue sarcomas in children and adolescents: the St. Jude Children's Research Hospital experience. Med Pediatr Oncol 1999;33(2):76–82.

8. Kao SC. Overview of the clinical and imaging features of the most common non-rhabdomyosarcoma soft-tissue sarcomas. Pediatr Radiol 2019;49(11):1524–33.

9. Evilevitch V, Weber WA, Tap WD, et al. Reduction of glucose metabolic activity is more accurate than change in size at predicting histopathologic response to neo-adjuvant therapy in high-grade soft-tissue sarcomas. Clin Cancer Res 2008; 14(3):715–20.

10. Scheer M, Dantonello T, Hallmen E, et al. Primary metastatic synovial sarcoma: experience of the CWS Study Group. Pediatr Blood Cancer 2016;63(7): 1198–206.

11. Fujiwara T, Stevenson J, Parry M, et al. What is an adequate margin for infiltrative soft-tissue sarcomas? Eur J Surg Oncol 2020;46(2):277–81.

12. Dantonello TM, Int-Veen C, Harms D, et al. Cooperative trial CWS-91 for localized soft tissue sarcoma in children, adolescents, and young adults. J Clin Oncol 2009;27(9):1446–55.

13. Ferrari A, De Salvo GL, Brennan B, et al. Synovial sarcoma in children and ado-lescents: the European Pediatric Soft Tissue Sarcoma Study Group prospective trial (EpSSG NRSTS 2005). Ann Oncol 2015;26(3):567–72.

14. Scheer M, Dantonello T, Hallmen E, et al. Synovial sarcoma recurrence in children and young adults. Ann Surg Oncol 2016;23(Suppl 5):618–26.

15. Lautz TB, Hayes-Jordan A. Recent progress in pediatric soft tissue sarcoma ther-apy. Semin Pediatr Surg 2019;28(6):150862.

16. Tinkle CL, Fernandez-Pineda I, Sykes A, et al. Nonrhabdomyosarcoma soft tissue sarcoma (NRSTS) in pediatric and young adult patients: Results from a prospec-tive study using limited-margin radiotherapy. Cancer 2017;123(22):4419–29.

17. Orbach D, Brennan B, De Paoli A, et al. Conservative strategy in infantile fibrosar-coma is possible: The European paediatric Soft tissue sarcoma Study Group experience. Eur J Cancer 2016;57:1–9.

18. Martin E, Coert JH, Flucke UE, et al. Neurofibromatosis-associated malignant pe-ripheral nerve sheath tumors in children have a worse prognosis: A nationwide cohort study. Pediatr Blood Cancer 2020;67(4):e28138.

19. Ferrari A, Bisogno G, Carli M. Management of childhood malignant peripheral nerve sheath tumor. Paediatr Drugs 2007;9(4):239–48.

20. van Noesel MM, Orbach D, Brennan B, et al. Outcome and prognostic factors in pediatric malignant peripheral nerve sheath tumors: An analysis of the European Pediatric Soft Tissue Sarcoma Group (EpSSG) NRSTS-2005 prospective study. Pediatr Blood Cancer 2019;66(10):e27833.

21. Carli M, Ferrari A, Mattke A, et al. Pediatric malignant peripheral nerve sheath tu-mor: the Italian and German soft tissue sarcoma cooperative group. J Clin Oncol 2005;23(33):8422–30.

22. Martin E, Radomski S, Harley EH. Pediatric Ewing sarcoma of the head and neck: A retrospective survival analysis. Int J Pediatr Otorhinolaryngol 2019;117:138–42.

23. Scheer M, Blank B, Bauer S, et al. Synovial sarcoma disease characteristics and primary tumor sites differ between patient age groups: a report of the Cooperative Weichteilsarkom Studiengruppe (CWS). J Cancer Res Clin Oncol 2020; 146(4):953–60.

24. Ferrari A, Chi YY, De Salvo GL, et al. Surgery alone is sufficient therapy for children and adolescents with low-risk synovial sarcoma: A joint analysis from the European paediatric soft tissue sarcoma Study Group and the Children's Oncology Group. Eur J Cancer 2017;78:1–6.

25. Vlenterie M, Litiere S, Rizzo E, et al. Outcome of chemotherapy in advanced synovial sarcoma patients: Review of 15 clinical trials from the European Organisation for Research and Treatment of Cancer Soft Tissue and Bone Sarcoma Group; setting a new landmark for studies in this entity. Eur J Cancer 2016;58:62–72.

26. Smolle C, Holzer LA, Smolle MA, et al. Differences in intraosseous and extraosseous post-chemotherapy regression of Ewing sarcomas and their influence on prognosis. Pathol Res Pract 2019;215(10):152613.

27. Bouaoud J, Temam S, Cozic N, et al. Ewing's Sarcoma of the Head and Neck: Margins are not just for surgeons. Cancer Med 2018;7(12):5879–88.

28. Seitz G, Urla C, Sparber-Sauer M, et al. Treatment and outcome of patients with thoracic tumors of the Ewing sarcoma family: A report from the Cooperative Weichteilsarkom Studiengruppe CWS-81, -86, -91, -96, and -2002P trials. Pediatr Blood Cancer 2019;66(3):e27537.

29. Khan M, Rankin KS, Todd R, et al. Surgical excision and not chemotherapy is the most powerful modality in treating synovial sarcoma: the UK's North East experience. Arch Orthop Trauma Surg 2019;139(4):443–9.

30. Gurria JP, Dasgupta R. Rhabdomyosarcoma and extraosseous ewing sarcoma. Children (Basel) 2018;5(12):165.

31. Scheer M, Greulich M, Loff S, et al. Localized synovial sarcoma of the foot or ankle: A series of 32 Cooperative Weichteilsarkom Study Group patients. J Surg Oncol 2019;119(1):109–19.

32. Spunt SL, Francotte N, De Salvo GL, et al. Clinical features and outcomes of young patients with epithelioid sarcoma: an analysis from the Children's Oncology Group and the European paediatric soft tissue Sarcoma Study Group prospective clinical trials. Eur J Cancer 2019;112:98–106.

33. Kube S, Vokuhl C, Dantonello T, et al. Inflammatory myofibroblastic tumors-A retrospective analysis of the Cooperative Weichteilsarkom Studiengruppe. Pediatr Blood Cancer 2018;65(6):e27012.

34. Lee JC, Wu JM, Liau JY, et al. Cytopathologic features of epithelioid inflammatory myofibroblastic sarcoma with correlation of histopathology, immunohistochemistry, and molecular cytogenetic analysis. Cancer Cytopathol 2015;123(8): 495–504.

35. Mansfield AS, Murphy SJ, Harris FR, et al. Chromoplectic TPM3-ALK rearrangement in a patient with inflammatory myofibroblastic tumor who responded to ceritinib after progression on crizotinib. Ann Oncol 2016;27(11):2111–7.

36. Theilen TM, Soerensen J, Bochennek K, et al. Crizotinib in ALK(+) inflammatory myofibroblastic tumors-Current experience and future perspectives. Pediatr Blood Cancer 2018;65(4). https://doi.org/10.1002/pbc.26920.

37. Mossé YP, Voss SD, Lim MS, et al. Targeting ALK with crizotinib in pediatric anaplastic large cell lymphoma and inflammatory myofibroblastic tumor: a children's oncology group study. J Clin Oncol 2017;35(28):3215–21.

38. Hayes-Jordan A, Green HL, Lin H, et al. Complete cytoreduction and HIPEC improves survival in desmoplastic small round cell tumor. Ann Surg Oncol 2014; 21(1):220–4.
39. Hayes-Jordan AA, Coakley BA, Green HL, et al. Desmoplastic small round cell tumor treated with cytoreductive surgery and hyperthermic intraperitoneal chemotherapy: results of a phase 2 trial. Ann Surg Oncol 2018;25(4):872–7.
40. Honore C, Delhorme JB, Nassif E, et al. Can we cure patients with abdominal Desmoplastic Small Round Cell Tumor? Results of a retrospective multicentric study on 100 patients. Surg Oncol 2019;29:107–12.
41. Menegaz BA, Cuglievan B, Benson J, et al. Clinical activity of pazopanib in patients with advanced desmoplastic small round cell tumor. Oncologist 2018; 23(3):360–6.
42. Saltsman JA 3rd, Price AP, Goldman DA, et al. A novel image-based system for risk stratification in patients with desmoplastic small round cell tumor. J Pediatr Surg 2020;55(3):376–80.
43. Scheer M, Vokuhl C, Blank B, et al. Desmoplastic small round cell tumors: Multimodality treatment and new risk factors. Cancer Med 2019;8(2):527–42.
44. Honore C, Atallah V, Mir O, et al. Abdominal desmoplastic small round cell tumor without extraperitoneal metastases: Is there a benefit for HIPEC after macroscopically complete cytoreductive surgery? PLoS One 2017;12(2):e0171639.
45. Sparber-Sauer M, Seitz G, von Kalle T, et al. Systemic therapy of aggressive fibromatosis in children and adolescents: Report of the Cooperative Weichteilsarkom Studiengruppe (CWS). Pediatr Blood Cancer 2018;65(5):e26943.
46. Nishida Y, Sakai T, Koike H, et al. Pazopanib for progressive desmoid tumours: children, persistant effects, and cost. Lancet Oncol 2019;20(10):e555.
47. Bishop AJ, Zarzour MA, Ratan R, et al. Long-term outcomes for patients with desmoid fibromatosis treated with radiation therapy: a 10-year update and re-evaluation of the role of radiation therapy for younger patients. Int J Radiat Oncol Biol Phys 2019;103(5):1167–74.
48. Neuwirth MG, Song Y, Sinnamon AJ, et al. Isolated limb perfusion and infusion for extremity soft tissue sarcoma: a contemporary systematic review and meta-analysis. Ann Surg Oncol 2017;24(13):3803–10.
49. Cohn SL, Pearson AD, London WB, et al. The International Neuroblastoma Risk Group (INRG) classification system: an INRG Task Force report. J Clin Oncol 2009;27(2):289–97.

Pediatric Melanoma— Diagnosis, Management, and Anticipated Outcomes

Jennifer H. Aldrink, MD[a],*, Stephanie F. Polites, MD[b],
Mary Austin, MD[c]

KEYWORDS

• Melanoma • Sentinel lymph node • Pediatric • Skin lesion

KEY POINTS

- Pediatric melanoma is the most common skin cancer in children and often presents with atypical findings including Amelanosis, Bleeding or Bump, Color uniformity, De novo or any Diameter, and Evolution.
- Few pediatric-specific studies exist, and children have been excluded from most melanoma clinical trials; therefore, management is based on adult National Comprehensive Cancer Network guidelines.
- Survival for children with melanoma generally is favorable; however, disease stage strongly correlates with survival, with distant metastases portending a poor prognosis.

INTRODUCTION

Melanoma is one of the most common adult malignancies. In 2020, approximately 100,350 new cases of melanoma will be diagnosed in the United States, representing 5.6% of all adult cancer incidence, with an estimated 6850 melanoma-related deaths.[1] Of the adolescent and young adult age group (15–29 years), melanoma represents 8% of, or 7160, cases of new cancer diagnoses. Although only 0.4% of melanoma diagnoses and 0.1% of deaths from melanoma occur in patients under age 20 years, approximately 500 new diagnoses of melanoma are made in this youngest age group in the United States annually.[1] The incidence varies by race and ethnicity, with the highest incidence in the white population, at 6.68 per million in persons less than

[a] Division of Pediatric Surgery, Department of Surgery, Nationwide Children's Hospital, The Ohio State University College of Medicine, 700 Children's Drive, Faculty Office Building Suite 6B.1, Columbus, OH 43205, USA; [b] Division of Pediatric Surgery, Department of Surgery, Mayo Clinic, 200 1st Street Southwest, Rochester, MN 55905, USA; [c] Department of Surgical Oncology, Division of Surgery, The University of Texas MD Anderson Cancer Center, 1515 Holcombe Boulevard, Houston, TX 77030, USA
* Corresponding author.
E-mail address: Jennifer.Aldrink@nationwidechildrens.org

Surg Oncol Clin N Am 30 (2021) 373–388
https://doi.org/10.1016/j.soc.2020.11.005
1055-3207/21/© 2020 Elsevier Inc. All rights reserved.

surgonc.theclinics.com

19 years old.[2] The incidence of melanoma increases with age and is exceedingly rare in children less than 5 years old (0.87 per million children).[3] Although reports prior to 2008 suggested that the incidence of melanoma in children was increasing,[4] more recent studies show a declining incidence in both children and young adults.[2,3,5] This decline may be due in part to the increased use of sun protective clothing and sunscreen as well as the adoption of more strict indoor tanning regulations.[6]

The majority of childhood and adolescent melanoma occurs sporadically, with most attributed to UV pathophysiology exposure, especially in adolescents. Familial cases account for only 1% of melanoma in children,[7,8] but approximately 25% of pediatric patients have a preexisting condition known to be associated with melanoma.[9,10] The strongest risk factor for melanoma in adolescents is the presence of more than 100 nevi with a diameter greater than 2 mm.[11] Other less common predisposing conditions include dysplastic nevus syndrome, congenital melanocytic nevi, xeroderma pigmentosa, immunodeficiency, prior malignancy, and radiation therapy (**Box 1**).

DIAGNOSIS

In children and adolescents, a diagnosis of melanoma often is not considered due to its rarity and atypical presentation. Concerning features in a skin lesion include rapid growth, bleeding, and itching.[12] It has been shown that up to 60% of melanoma diagnoses in children under age 10 years and 40% of diagnoses in children ages 11 years to 19 years do not meet traditional asymmetry, border irregularity, color variegation, diameter greater than 6 mm, and evolution (ABCDE) criteria.[13] Thus, modified ABCDE criteria have been proposed to be used in addition to the traditional criteria to help identify suspicious skin lesions in children and adolescents. These criteria include amelanotic, bleeding or bump, color uniformity, de novo and any diameter, and evolution.[13] It is common for pediatric melanoma to be amelanotic, and amelanotic lesions more often are misdiagnosed as warts, pyogenic granulomas, or other benign skin lesions (**Fig. 1**). A recent study from the University of Michigan found approximately 80% of melanomas in prepubertal children and 25% in adolescents were amelanotic and that the lack of pigmentation was associated with a median delay in diagnosis of 9 months.[12]

Presentation patterns can vary by age, gender, and ethnicity. Melanoma of infancy presents almost exclusively either as malignant transformation of a congenital melanocytic nevus or via placental transmission with multiple cutaneous or visceral metastatic deposits.[14,15] Younger children are more likely to be male with a higher incidence of nonwhite ethnicity than seen in the adult population.[13,16] Tumors in young

---

Box 1
Preexisting conditions associated with pediatric melanoma

Congenital melanocytic nevus

Transplacental transmission

Xeroderma pigmentosa and other genetic disorders that affect tumor suppressor genes

Dysplastic nevi and dysplastic nevus syndrome

Immunosuppression

Sun-sensitive phenotype (facial freckling, inability to tan)

Family history of melanoma

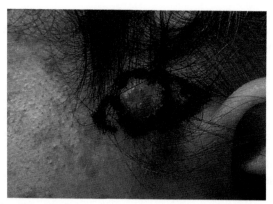

Fig. 1. Photograph of an amelanotic spitzoid melanoma in a 14-year-old girl.

children are thicker, and between 25% to 58% may present with regional nodal metastases.[17–19] In this younger age group, the role of UV exposure in children is uncertain because melanoma is more likely to arise from an existing congenital melanocytic nevus or dysplastic nevus. The clinical presentation of melanoma in adolescence mimics that of adults, with most tumors arising in previously healthy skin. Males tend to present with tumors of the face and trunk, whereas females more commonly present with extremity tumors.[4,18] According to the Surveillance, Epidemiology, and End Results (SEER) database, 85% of patients with melanoma under age 18 years are white, 5% Hispanic, and 2% Asian/Pacific Islander.[18]

There are 3 main categories of pediatric melanoma: conventional melanoma, melanoma arising in a congenital nevus, and spitzoid melanoma. Conventional melanoma genetically is similar to adult melanoma and demonstrates genomic characteristics secondary to UV damage, including an increased rate of single nucleotide variations.[20] In contrast, melanoma arising in congenital nevi demonstrates a much lower frequency of UV-related mutations.[9] There remains some debate among dermatopathologists regarding the distinction between atypical Spitz nevus, melanocytic tumors of uncertain malignant potential, and spitzoid melanoma.[21–23] In 1 study, 35% of spitzoid tumors initially were misdiagnosed as Spitz nevus and, on later review, were determined to be melanoma with epithelioid or spindle cells.[22] There is no single method to differentiate an atypical Spitz nevus from a melanoma; however, comparative genomic hybridization identifying chromosome copy number loss or gain often is helpful in that melanoma often has a variety of chromosomal aberrations compared with most Spitz nevi, which demonstrate a normal karyotype.[24] For this reason, it is essential that lesions concerning for melanoma be reviewed by a dermatopathologist with experience in diagnosing pediatric melanoma. If a lesion is determined to be a benign Spitz nevus or atypical Spitz nevus, excision with negative margins is indicated; however, spitzoid melanoma should be managed as melanoma per National Comprehensive Cancer Network (NCCN) guidelines.[25]

SURGICAL MANAGEMENT

The mainstay of treatment of pediatric cutaneous melanoma is cure by surgical resection. This process includes full-thickness biopsy for diagnosis, wide local excision (WLE) with margins based on lesion depth, and selective use of sentinel lymph node biopsy (SLNB) and completion lymph node dissection (CLND). Given the lack of pediatric-specific clinical trials guiding surgical management, adult guidelines are applied to children with some modifications based on expected differences in cosmetic and functional outcomes in younger patients.

Biopsy and Wide Local Excision

Suspicious lesions should undergo diagnostic evaluation either by punch biopsy or surgical biopsy. Surgical biopsy may be incisional or excisional but if the latter approach is used, margins should be less than 3 mm to maintain lymphatics for potential SLNB. The need for WLE should be considered when choosing the incision for initial surgical biopsy. After confirmation of diagnosis by a dermatopathologist experienced in pediatric melanoma, WLE is performed to the depth of the muscular fascia. Deeper resections involving fascia or muscle are not performed because these have not been shown to be beneficial in adult patients.[26]

Surgical margins for WLE of melanoma in pediatric patients utilize NCCN guidelines based on Breslow thickness of the lesion (**Table 1**).[25] Specifically, a 1.0-cm margin is recommended for lesions less than or equal to 1.0 mm in depth and a 2.0-cm margin for lesions greater than or equal to 2.0-mm deep. Although patients with lesions greater than or equal to 2.0 mm who underwent excision with 1.0-cm margins experienced worse disease-free survival (DFS) and melanoma-specific survival (MSS), no survival advantage has been shown for margins greater than 2.0 cm in several multi-center prospective randomized controlled trials.[27–29]

The clinical trials that informed the NCCN guidelines excluded pediatric patients. Retrospective cohort studies suggest children have lower risk of local recurrence compared with adults and have identified trends toward decreased recurrence in young children compared with adolescents.[30,31] With this in mind, smaller margins should be considered when form or function would be substantially compromised using standard NCCN recommendations. When smaller margins are used, it is important to obtain final pathology results prior to performing any major reconstruction.

Regional Lymph Nodes

Regional lymph nodes are the first site of metastases for melanoma, and lymph node metastases occur more frequently in pediatric patients than adults.[30,32] Because clinical examination and imaging studies do not detect microscopic metastases, SLNB is utilized in select patients for staging and prognostic purposes. Selection of pediatric patients with melanoma to undergo SLNB is based on adult guidelines. SLNB is not indicated in patients with lesions less than 0.8-mm thick without concerning features, such as ulceration, lymphovascular invasion, or greater than or equal to 2 mitoses per

Table 1	
Recommended surgical margins for wide local excision of melanoma based on Breslow thickness	
Melanoma Thickness	**Wide Local Excision Margin**
Melanoma in situ	0.5–1.0 cm
≤1.0 mm	1.0 cm
>1.0 mm–2.0 mm	1.0–2.0 cm
>2 mm	2.0 cm

Data from Fleming MD, Galan A, Gastman B, et al. *NCCN Guidelines Version 3.2020 Cutaneous Melanoma NCCN Evidence Blocks TM Continue NCCN Guidelines Panel Disclosures.*; 2020. www.nccn.org/patients. Accessed August 20, 2020.

millimeter.[2] It is utilized selectively after a discussion of risks and benefits with the patient and family for those with lesions between 0.8-mm and 1.0-mm deep.[33] For those with lesions greater than or equal to 1.0 mm in depth, it always should be performed, because more than 1 in 3 patients have a positive sentinel lymph node.[34]

The risk of complications after SLNB is less than 5% and the most frequent complication is seroma. CLND carries greater morbidity, with 1 in 4 adult patients developing lymphedema.[35] Approximately half of pediatric patients who undergo WLE with CLND experienced complications as opposed to 11% of those who underwent WLE with SLNB.[36] The highest postoperative morbidity is associated with inguinal node dissection followed by axillary location.[37] Current NCCN guidelines acknowledge that lymph node dissections should be anatomically complete; however, there is not consensus on the definition of a complete dissection or the number of nodes that should be excised.[25]

CLND should be used judiciously in pediatric patients, balancing the risk of morbidity with the risk of recurrence over their longer life expectancies compared with adults. This procedure is performed routinely for clinically or radiographically positive nodes and selectively utilized for occult metastases identified by SLNB.[33] This paradigm shift is based on the findings of 2 adult clinical trials in which patients with a positive sentinel node who were observed with routine clinical examinations and ultrasounds had a higher rate of regional nodal recurrence but without decreased survival compared with those who underwent immediate CLND.[35,38]

These data must be interpreted with caution in pediatric melanoma, because enrolled adults had significantly shorter life expectancies than children and access to frequent, high-quality surveillance at experienced centers. A discussion of risks and benefits of CLND and access to follow-up is recommended for pediatric patients with a positive SLNB. CLND also should be considered strongly for patients who cannot return regularly for follow-up evaluations and ultrasound surveillance of the affected nodal basin. Additionally, patients with high-risk features, including extracapsular extension, primary tumor microsatellitosis, greater than 3 involved sentinel nodes, greater than 2 involved nodal basis, or immunosuppression, should be offered CLND, because these patients were excluded in the adult trials.[39–49]

In a recent study, Parikh and colleagues[50] used propensity score matched analyses of SEER data and showed no difference in MSS between children and adolescents who underwent SLNB and/or lymphadenectomy versus those who did not undergo lymph node sampling. They noted worse overall survival (OS) in patients with positive lymph nodes, however, compared with those with either no lymph nodes sampled or negative lymph nodes. The prognostic impact of lymph node status on survival may be age related. Lorimer and colleagues[51] found that in children ages 1 year to 10 years, there was no difference in OS based on lymph node positivity; however, adolescents with node-positive disease were at higher risk of death compared with adolescents with node-negative disease (hazard ratio [HR] 4.82; 95% CI, 3.38–6.87). Most studies to date have shown that regional disease is associated with worse survival compared with localized disease[17,18,51–56]

MEDICAL MANAGEMENT

Pediatric patients with stages III and IV melanoma are considered for additional therapy (**Table 2**). Immune and targeted therapies comprise contemporary adjuvant and systemic treatment (**Table 3**). The safety and efficacy of these therapies largely are extrapolated from clinical trials that excluded pediatric patients. For completely resected stage III melanoma, the 2020 NCCN guidelines recommend considering

Table 2
American Joint Committee on Cancer clinical staging for melanoma

Stage	T	N	M
0	Tis	N0	M0
IA	T1a	N0	M0
IB	T1b	N0	M0
	T2a	N0	M0
IIA	T2b	N0	M0
	T3a	N0	M0
IIB	T3b	N0	M0
	T4a	N0	M0
IIC	T4b	N0	M0
III[a]	Any T/Tis	≥N1	M0
IV	Any T	Any N	M1

T Category	Thickness	Ulceration
TX[b]	N/A	N/A
T0	N/A	N/A
Tis	N/A	N/A
T1a	<0.8 mm	Not present
T1b	<0.8 mm	Present
	0.8–1.0 mm	Present or not present
T2a	>1.0–2.0 mm	Not present
T2b	>1.0–2.0 mm	Present
T3a	>2.0–4.0 mm	Not present
T3b	>2.0–4.0 mm	Present
T4a	>4.0 mm	Not present
T4b	>4.0 mm	Present

Abbreviations: N/A, not applicable; Tis, melanoma in situ.
[a] There is 1 clinical stage group for stage III melanoma. Stages IIIA, IIIB, IIIC, and IIID are pathologic stages based on the extent of lymph node involvement and clinical versus occult presentation.
[b] Thickness cannot be assessed due to inadequate tissue.

systemic adjuvant therapy given the reported benefits in DFS with contemporary agents.[25] It is not yet known if this will translate to improved OS; it should be noted that these trials included patients who underwent CLND after a positive SLNB, and those who received adjuvant therapy for occult nodal disease had at least 1 lymph node metastasis greater than 1 mm.

Interferon Alfa-2b

Adjuvant therapy with high-dose interferon alfa-2b utilized for node positivity or a deep lesion greater than 4.0 mm. Three adult clinical trials demonstrated improved DFS with inconclusive results on OS.[57–60] The approved regimen includes 1 month of intravenous induction therapy followed by 11 months of subcutaneous maintenance therapy, although with significant toxicities the 12-month course commonly is abandoned prior to completion. The addition of polyethylene glycol (PEG) formulation of interferon has improved efficacy whereas low-dose or intermediate-dose therapy is not efficacious and no longer recommended.[57,61,62] Several retrospective pediatric studies support the results of adult studies and showed improved tolerance compared with adults,

Table 3
Systemic therapies for advanced melanoma

Drug Name	Mechanism of Action/Target	Application in Melanoma
Interferon alfa-2b	Multifunctional immunoregulatory cytokine, stimulates B cells, activates NK cells	Stage III
Talimogene laherparepvec	Modified virus induces tumor cell lysis, granulocyte-monocyte colony stimulating factor expression	Unresectable subcutaneous or nodal disease
Melphalan	Alkylating agent inhibits DNA and RNA synthesis	Regionally advanced melanoma used in isolated limb perfusion/infusion
Dacarbazine	Methylation of guanine in DNA strands, preventing cell division	Metastatic
Ipilimumab	Monoclonal antibody against CTLA-4	Nodal recurrence or metastatic with prior anti–PD-1 exposure
Nivolumab	Monoclonal antibody against PD-1	Stage III, unresectable or metastatic
Pembrolizumab	Monoclonal antibody against PD-1	Stage III, unresectable or metastatic
Vemurafenib	BRAF inhibitor	BRAF V600E mutation–positive, unresectable or metastatic
Dabrafenib	BRAF inhibitor	BRAF V600E mutation–positive, unresectable or metastatic
Selumetinib	Selective MEK1 and MEK2 inhibitor (downstream of BRAF/MAPK/ERK pathway)	BRAF-activating mutation–positive
Trametinib	Selective MEK1 and MEK2 inhibitor (downstream of BRAF/MAPK/ERK pathway)	BRAF V600E–mutated, metastatic
Dabrafenib/trametinib	Combination therapy	BRAF V600E/K–mutated Stage III, unresectable or metastatic
Imatinib	Targeted c-kit inhibitor	c-kit mutated or amplified

with the exception of a higher rate of neutropenia in children.[63–66] A phase II clinical trial of PEG–interferon alfa-2b in pediatric patients is ongoing (NCT005539591).[67]

Immune Checkpoint Inhibitors

Immune checkpoint inhibitors reduce the immune response to cancer cells including ipilimumab, a monoclonal antibody that binds the T-cell receptor antigen CTLA-4. It has been shown to improve survival in adult patients with resected stage III and unresectable melanoma.[68,69] Side effects are dose dependent and occur in up to 60% of patients. NCCN does not recommend ipilimumab for adjuvant therapy of resected stage III melanoma at this time due to better tolerated and more efficacious alternatives.[25] Following a phase I study that found ipilimumab to be safe in adolescents with unresectable disease, a phase II study evaluating it as a single agent or in combination with nivolumab in pediatric patients with recurrent or refractory solid tumors, including melanoma is in process (NCT02304458).[70]

Other immune checkpoint inhibitors target the programmed death (PD)-1 protein expressed by T cells to prevent binding of tumor PD ligand protein. Nivolumab and pembrolizumab are 2 such therapies that are effective for both resected stage III and metastatic disease and now are the preferred immune checkpoint inhibitors for melanoma.[25] The former was better tolerated than ipilimumab when compared directly.[71] Although PD-1 expression in tumor cells was assessed in the clinical trials, patients with minimal expression responded as well and this should not be considered a contraindication. Pembrolizumab is being evaluated in children with melanoma and other malignancies in a phase 1 to phase 2 trial, with results expected in 2022.[72] A report of compassionate use in a pediatric patient with recurrent metastatic disease demonstrated remission at 1 year although the medication was discontinued due to adverse events.[73]

BRAF-Targeted Therapy

The signaling kinase BRAF is a target of therapy for melanoma with an activating mutation (BRAF V600).[74] Approximately half of patients with metastatic disease harbor this mutation and inhibitors of BRAF and downstream MEK have been developed. Tumors without BRAF mutations do not respond. BRAF inhibitors vemurafenib and dabrafenib have shorter response time and improved survival compared with chemotherapy; however, BRAF inhibitors have a high rate of relapse within 6 months , and vemurafenib has an approximately 20% risk of hyperproliferative cutaneous adverse events, including squamous cell carcinoma and, therefore, is not recommended as adjuvant monotherapy.[75–78] Although MEK inhibitor (trametinib, cobimetinib, and binimetinib) monotherapy also is more effective than chemotherapy for those with BRAF mutations, response rates are lower than BRAF inhibitors.[79]

For resected stage III disease, combination dabrafenib/trametinib therapy was Food and Drug Administration approved after it was shown to have improved DFS and decreased risk of developing metastatic disease.[80] The combination is better tolerated than BRAF inhibitor monotherapy. Clinical trials of BRAF and MEK inhibitors in pediatric patients are challenged by low enrollment, highlighting the importance of including this population in larger adult studies. A phase I study of vemurafenib in adolescents could not identify a safe and effective dose. Phase I studies of trametinib alone and in combination with dabrafenib for other pediatric malignancies, including gliomas, have shown it to be safe in children.[81–84]

Second-Line Systemic Therapies

Pediatric case series with dacarbazine, paclitaxel and temozolomide suggested improved response in children compared with adults, although exclusion of children from larger clinical trials has limited further investigation of chemotherapy in this population.[85–88] At least 2 children have been treated with systemic interleukin 2 for melanoma but literature is insufficient to conclude pediatric efficacy.[89–91]

OUTCOMES

Although studies evaluating long-term survival of children and adolescents with melanoma are limited, several reports have demonstrated improved survival over the past 40 years.[18,50,51] Five-year and 10-year OS rates for all stages range from 88.9% to 94.7% and 80.9% to 88%, respectively.[17,51,92–94] Studies lack consistency in reporting, but most report favorable outcomes with disease-specific survival rates greater than 80% at 5 years.[18,92,95] Similar to adults, the strongest predictor of survival for children and adolescents with melanoma is stage of disease at presentation. In 2007, Lange and colleagues[17] reported the following 5-year OS by stage using data from the SEER program: 97.8% for in situ, 93.6% for localized melanoma, 68% for melanoma with regional metastases, and 11.8% for distant metastatic disease. More recent studies have confirmed the importance of stage as a strong predictor of survival in children and adolescents with melanoma.[50,51,92,93] Fortunately, most patients present with either localized (77%) or regional disease (15%), with only 1% presenting with distant metastases.[50] A significant limitation to both SEER and the National Cancer Database (NCDB) is a failure to collect all of the variables included in the American Joint Committee on Cancer (AJCC) staging for melanoma.[96]

It is not surprising that health disparities play a role in both disease presentation and outcomes for children and adolescents with melanoma. Using Texas Cancer Registry data, Hamilton and colleagues[97] demonstrated that Hispanic race/ethnicity was independently associated with increased odds of presenting with advanced disease (HR 3.5; 95% CI, 1.4–8.8) and Hispanics were 3 times more likely to die from melanoma than non-Hispanic whites. In a SEER study of pediatric and adult melanoma patients, black race was independently associated with increased risk of death (HR 1.84; 95% CI, 1.64–2.04) after controlling for age, sex, primary site, stage, type of therapy, and year of diagnosis.[51]

The data are conflicting regarding the prognostic importance of age, gender, primary site, histology, tumor thickness, mitoses per square millimeter, and lymph node status. Several studies have shown that younger children ($\leq$10 years age) are more likely to present with thicker lesions[17,18,51,92] and nodal disease compared with adolescents and adults.[17,18,50,52,98] Survival results vary, however, with Lange and colleagues[17] reporting a poorer 5-year OS rate for children ages 1 year to 9 years (77.0% $\pm$ 4.5%) compared with older age groups, whereas other studies either show no significant difference in survival by age[52,92] or improved survival for children less than or equal to 10 years of age at diagnosis.[18,51] Using the NCDB, Lorimer and colleagues[51] found that both children ages 1 year to 10 years and adolescents ages 11 years to 20 years had improved OS compared with adults greater than 20 years old (HR 0.11; 95% CI, 0.06–0.21, and HR 0.22; 95% CI, 0.19–0.26, respectively).

Several studies report favorable outcomes for females compared with males[18,50,51]; however, other studies found no significant differences in survival between genders.[92,93] Head and neck primary sites have been associated with worse prognosis compared with other sites.[18,51,94] In a recent study using SEER program data, Shi and colleagues[94] showed that pediatric and adolescent patients with head and neck melanoma had an increased risk of mortality (HR 1.6; 95% CI, 1.3–2.1) compared with those with non–head and neck melanoma after adjusting for gender, age, and race/ethnicity. In addition, nodular histology may portend a worse prognosis.[18,50,93]

There is debate about the role of tumor thickness and mitoses per square millimeter in prognosis of pediatric and adolescent melanoma. Lange and colleagues[17] reported that tumor thickness was not associated with OS, using a cutoff of greater than or equal to 1.5 mm to define thick melanoma. Several other studies have demonstrated the importance of Breslow thickness as a prognostic factor in pediatric and adolescent melanoma, including Averbook and colleagues,[92] who found that both OS and DFS were independently associated with tumor thickness greater than 1.0 mm in patients less than or equal to 20 years of age at diagnosis.[93] In the most recent version of the AJCC melanoma staging, mitotic rate greater than or equal to $1/mm^2$ replaces level of invasion as the primary criterion for defining T1b melanomas[96]; however, the significance of mitotic rate for pediatric and adolescent melanoma remains unknown. In a recent study from the Melanoma Institute Australia, mitotic rate greater than or equal to $1/mm^2$ was found to be the only factor independently associated with worse relapse-free survival and MSS for children less than or equal to 19 years old after adjusting for gender, age, Breslow thickness, primary tumor site, histology, and lymph node status.[95]

Data also are limited on time to recurrence for pediatric patients and adolescents with melanoma. In a report from the Melanoma Institute Australia, the time between diagnosis of the primary melanoma and first recurrence ranged from 3 months to 13 years, with 5 patients (31%) experiencing a recurrence more than 5 years after diagnosis.[95] This emphasizes the importance of long-term follow-up, including regular comprehensive skin examinations by a physician with expertise in pediatric melanoma.

SUMMARY

Although rare, melanoma is the most common skin cancer in children and adolescents, with approximately 500 new diagnoses per year in the United States in persons less than 20 years of age. It often presents in an atypical fashion with modified ABCDE criteria. The mainstay of treatment is surgical resection. All suspicious skin lesions should undergo punch biopsy, incisional biopsy, or excisional biopsy. SLNB is indicated for all T1b and above lesions as well as those 0.8-mm to 1-mm thickness with concerning features (mitoses $>2/mm^2$, ulceration, or lymphovascular invasion). There has been a paradigm shift in the management of positive SLNB based on 2 large multi-institutional clinical trials in adults that demonstrated increased regional recurrence but no difference in OS for SLNB-positive patients who were managed with nodal observation versus those who underwent immediate CLND. The results of these trials have been applied to pediatric and adolescent patients; however, it is critical that patients undergoing observation be followed with regular ultrasounds performed in a center with experience in nodal surveillance by ultrasound. Targeted therapies and immunotherapy have changed the landscape for melanoma patients with advanced disease; and, although most clinical trials to date have excluded children, several have demonstrated safety and efficacy of these newer treatment modalities in adolescent patients. Survival generally is favorable in pediatric melanoma, with the exception of those with distant metastases, but even this is rapidly evolving field of immunotherapy.

DISCLOSURE

The authors have nothing to disclose.

REFERENCES

1. National Cancer Institute. Melanoma of the Skin — Cancer Stat Facts. Available at: https://seer.cancer.gov/statfacts/html/melan.html. Accessed August 26, 2020.

2. Siegel DA, King J, Tai E, et al. Cancer incidence rates and trends among children and adolescents in the United States, 2001-2009. Pediatrics 2014;134(4): e945–55.

3. Campbell LB, Kreicher KL, Gittleman HR, et al. Melanoma incidence in children and adolescents: Decreasing trends in the United States. J Pediatr 2015;166(6): 1505–13.

4. Austin MT, Xing Y, Hayes-Jordan AA, et al. Melanoma incidence rises for children and adolescents: An epidemiologic review of pediatric melanoma in the United States. J Pediatr Surg 2013;48(11):2207–13.

5. Barr RD, Ries LAG, Lewis DR, et al. Incidence and incidence trends of the most frequent cancers in adolescent and young adult Americans, including "nonmalignant/noninvasive" tumors. Cancer 2016;122(7):1000–8.

6. Ghiasvand R, Weiderpass E, Green AC, et al. Sunscreen use and subsequent melanoma risk: A population-based cohort study. J Clin Oncol 2016;34(33): 3976–83.

7. Aoude LG, Wadt KAW, Pritchard AL, et al. Genetics of familial melanoma: 20 years after CDKN2A. Pigment Cell Melanoma Res 2015;28(2):148–60.

8. Kefford RF, Newton Bishop JA, Bergman W, et al. Counseling and DNA testing for individuals perceived to be genetically predisposed to melanoma: A consensus statement of the melanoma genetics consortium. J Clin Oncol 1999;17(10): 3245–51.

9. Pappo AS. Melanoma in children and adolescents. Eur J Cancer 2003;39(18): 2651–61.

10. Wong JR, Harris JK, Rodriguez-Galindo C, et al. Incidence of childhood and adolescent melanoma in the United States: 1973-2009. Pediatrics 2013;131(5): 846–54.

11. Youl P, Aitken J, Hayward N, et al. Melanoma in adolescents: A case-control study of risk factors in Queensland, Australia. Int J Cancer 2002;98(1):92–8.

12. Bailey KM, Durham AB, Zhao L, et al. Pediatric melanoma and aggressive Spitz tumors: a retrospective diagnostic, exposure and outcome analysis. Transl Pediatr 2018;7(3):203–10.

13. Cordoro KM, Gupta D, Frieden IJ, et al. Pediatric melanoma: Results of a large cohort study and proposal for modified ABCD detection criteria for children. J Am Acad Dermatol 2013;68(6):913–25.

14. Trumble ER, Smith RM, Pearl G, et al. Transplacental transmission of metastatic melanoma to the posterior fossa: Case report. J Neurosurg 2005;103(SUPPL. 2):191–3.

15. Alomari AK, Glusac EJ, Choi J, et al. Congenital nevi versus metastatic melanoma in a newborn to a mother with malignant melanoma - Diagnosis supported by sex chromosome analysis and Imaging Mass Spectrometry. J Cutan Pathol 2015; 42(10):757–64.

16. Braam KI, Overbeek A, Kaspers GJL, et al. Malignant melanoma as second malignant neoplasm in long-term childhood cancer survivors: A systematic review. Pediatr Blood Cancer 2012;58(5):665–74.

17. Lange JR, Palis BE, Chang DC, et al. Melanoma in children and teenagers: An analysis of patients from the National Cancer Data Base. J Clin Oncol 2007; 25(11):1363–8.

18. Strouse JJ, Fears TR, Tucker MA, et al. Pediatric melanoma: Risk factor and survival analysis of the Surveillance, Epidemiology and End Results database. J Clin Oncol 2005;23(21):4735–41.

19. Han D, Zager JS, Han G, et al. The unique clinical characteristics of melanoma diagnosed in children. Ann Surg Oncol 2012;19(12):3888–95.

20. Tracy ET, Aldrink JH. Pediatric melanoma. Semin Pediatr Surg 2016;25(5):290–8.

21. Berk DR, Labuz E, Dadras SS, et al. Melanoma and melanocytic tumors of uncertain malignant potential in children, adolescents and young adults - The stanford experience 1995-2008. Pediatr Dermatol 2010;27(3):244–54.

22. Massi D, Tomasini C, Senetta R, et al. Atypical Spitz tumors in patients younger than 18 years. J Am Acad Dermatol 2015;72(1):37–46.
23. Zhao G, Lee KC, Peacock S, et al. The utilization of spitz-related nomenclature in the histological interpretation of cutaneous melanocytic lesions by practicing pathologists: results from the M-Path study. J Cutan Pathol 2017;44(1):5–14.
24. Bauer J, Bastian BC. Distinguishing melanocytic nevi from melanoma by DNA copy number changes: Comparative genomic hybridization as a research and diagnostic tool. Dermatol Ther 2006;19(1):40–9.
25. Fleming MD, Galan A, Gastman B, et al. NCCN guidelines version 3.2020 cutaneous melanoma NCCN evidence Blocks TM Continue NCCN guidelines Panel Disclosures 2020. Available at: www.nccn.org/patients. Accessed August 20, 2020.
26. Kenady DE, Brown BW, McBride CM. Excision of underlying fascia with a primary malignant melanoma: effect on recurrence and survival rates. Surgery 1982; 92(4):615–8. Available at: http://www.ncbi.nlm.nih.gov/pubmed/7123480. Accessed January 5, 2019.
27. Ethun CG, Delman KA. The importance of surgical margins in melanoma. J Surg Oncol 2016;113(3):339–45.
28. Thomas JM, Newton-Bishop J, A'Hern R, et al. Excision margins in high-risk malignant melanoma. N Engl J Med 2004;350(8):757–66.
29. Hayes AJ, Maynard L, Coombes G, et al. Wide versus narrow excision margins for high-risk, primary cutaneous melanomas: long-term follow-up of survival in a randomised trial. Lancet Oncol 2016;17(2):184–92.
30. Livestro DP, Kaine EM, Michaelson JS, et al. Melanoma in the young: differences and similarities with adult melanoma: a case-matched controlled analysis. Cancer 2007;110(3):614–24.
31. Aldrink JH, Selim MA, Diesen DL, et al. Pediatric melanoma: a single-institution experience of 150 patients. J Pediatr Surg 2009;44(8):1514–21.
32. Howman-Giles R, Uren RF, Thompson J. Sentinel lymph node biopsy in pediatric and adolescent patients. Ann Surg 2014;259(6):e86.
33. Wong SL, Faries MB, Kennedy EB, et al. Sentinel lymph node biopsy and management of regional lymph nodes in melanoma: American Society of Clinical Oncology and Society of Surgical Oncology Clinical Practice Guideline Update. J Clin Oncol 2018;36(4):399–413.
34. Sreeraman Kumar R, Messina JL, Reed D, et al. Pediatric melanoma and atypical melanocytic neoplasms. Cancer Treat Res 2016;167:331–69.
35. Faries MB, Thompson JF, Cochran AJ, et al. Completion Dissection or Observation for Sentinel-Node Metastasis in Melanoma. N Engl J Med 2017;376(23): 2211–22.
36. Palmer PE, Warneke CL, Hayes-Jordan AA, et al. Complications in the surgical treatment of pediatric melanoma. J Pediatr Surg 2013;48(6):1249–53.
37. Moody JA, Botham SJ, Dahill KE, et al. Complications following completion lymphadenectomy versus therapeutic lymphadenectomy for melanoma – A systematic review of the literature. Eur J Surg Oncol 2017;43(9):1760–7.
38. Leiter U, Stadler R, Mauch C, et al. Complete lymph node dissection versus no dissection in patients with sentinel lymph node biopsy positive melanoma (DeCOG-SLT): a multicentre, randomised, phase 3 trial. Lancet Oncol 2016;17(6): 757–67.
39. Fayne RA, MacEdo FI, Rodgers SE, et al. Evolving management of positive regional lymph nodes in melanoma: Past, present and future directions. Oncol Rev 2019;13(2):175–82.

40. Louie RJ, Perez MC, Jajja MR, et al. Real-world outcomes of talimogene laherparepvec therapy: a multi-institutional experience. J Am Coll Surg 2019;228(4): 644–9.
41. Lens MB, Dawes M. Isolated limb perfusion with melphalan in the treatment of malignant melanoma of the extremities: A systemic review of randomised controlled trials. Lancet Oncol 2003;4(6):359–64.
42. Beasley GM, Caudle A, Petersen RP, et al. A multi-institutional experience of isolated limb infusion: defining response and toxicity in the US. J Am Coll Surg 2009; 208(5):706–15.
43. Perone JA, Farrow N, Tyler DS, et al. Contemporary approaches to in-transit melanoma. J Oncol Pract 2018;14(5):292–300.
44. Kroon HM, Lin DY, Kam PCA, et al. Efficacy of repeat Isolated limb infusion with melphalan and actinomycin D for Recurrent melanoma. Cancer 2009;115(9): 1932–40.
45. Cornett WR, McCall LM, Petersen RP, et al. Randomized multicenter trial of hyperthermic isolated limb perfusion with melphalan alone compared with melphalan plus tumor necrosis factor: American College of Surgeons Oncology Group trial Z0020. J Clin Oncol 2006;24(25):4196–201.
46. Boesch CE, Meyer T, Waschke L, et al. Long-term outcome of hyperthermic isolated limb perfusion (HILP) in the treatment of locoregionally metastasised malignant melanoma of the extremities. Int J Hyperthermia 2010;26(1):16–20.
47. Baas PC, Hoekstra HJ, Koops HS, et al. Hyperthermic isolated regional perfusion in the treatment of extremity melanoma in children and adolescents. Cancer 1989;63(1):199–203.
48. Hohenberger P, Tunn PU. Isolated limb perfusion with rhTNF-α and melphalan for locally recurrent childhood synovial sarcoma of the limb. J Pediatr Hematol Oncol 2003;25(11):905–9.
49. Gutman M, Inbar M, Lev-Shlush D, et al. High dose tumor necrosis factor-α and melphalan administered via isolated limb perfusion for advanced limb soft tissue sarcoma results in a >90% response rate and limb preservation. Cancer 1997; 79(6):1129–37.
50. Parikh PP, Tashiro J, Rubio GA, et al. Incidence and outcomes of pediatric extremity melanoma: A propensity score matched SEER study. J Pediatr Surg 2018;53(9):1753–60.
51. Lorimer PD, White RL, Walsh K, et al. Pediatric and Adolescent Melanoma: A National Cancer Data Base Update. Ann Surg Oncol 2016;23(12):4058–66.
52. Moore-Olufemi S, Herzog C, Warneke C, et al. Outcomes in pediatric melanoma: comparing prepubertal to adolescent pediatric patients. Ann Surg 2011;253(6): 1211–5.
53. Offenmueller S, Leiter U, Bernbeck B, et al. Clinical characteristics and outcome of 60 pediatric patients with malignant melanoma registered with the German Pediatric Rare Tumor Registry (STEP). Klin Pädiatr 2017;229(06):322–8.
54. Lisy K, Lai-Kwon J, Ward A, et al. Patient-reported outcomes in melanoma survivors at 1, 3 and 5 years post-diagnosis: a population-based cross-sectional study. Qual Life Res 2020;29(8):2021–7.
55. Stump TK, Aspinwall LG, Kohlmann W, et al. Genetic test reporting and counseling for melanoma risk in minors may improve sun protection without inducing distress. J Genet Couns 2018;27(4):955–67.
56. Wu YP, Aspinwall LG, Parsons B, et al. Parent and child perspectives on family interactions related to melanoma risk and prevention after CDKN2A/p16 testing of minor children. J Community Genet 2020;11(3):321–9.

57. Kirkwood JM, Ibrahim JG, Sondak VK, et al. High- and low-dose interferon alfa-2b in high-risk melanoma: First analysis of intergroup trial E1690/S9111/C9190. J Clin Oncol 2000;18(12):2444–58.

58. Kirkwood JM, Strawderman MH, Ernstoff MS, et al. Interferon alfa-2b adjuvant therapy of high-risk resected cutaneous melanoma: The Eastern Cooperative Oncology Group trial EST 1684. J Clin Oncol 1996;14(1):7–17.

59. Kirkwood JM, Manola J, Ibrahim J, et al. A Pooled Analysis of Eastern Cooperative Oncology Group and Intergroup Trials of Adjuvant High-Dose Interferon for Melanoma. Clin Cancer Res 2004;10(5):1670–7.

60. Kirkwood JM, Ibrahim JG, Sosman JA, et al. High-dose interferon alfa-2b significantly prolongs relapse-free and overall survival compared with the GM2-KLH/QS-21 vaccine in patients with resected stage IIB-III melanoma: Results of intergroup trial E1694/S9512/C509801. J Clin Oncol 2001;19(9):2370–80.

61. Raef HS, Friedmann AM, Hawryluk EB. Medical options for the adjuvant treatment and management of pediatric melanoma. Pediatr Drugs 2019;21(2):71–9.

62. Moschos SJ, Kirkwood JM, Konstantinopoulos PA. Present status and future prospects for adjuvant therapy of melanoma: Time to build upon the foundation of high-dose interferon alfa-2b. J Clin Oncol 2004;22(1):11–4.

63. Navid F, Furman WL, Fleming M, et al. The feasibility of adjuvant interferon α-2b in children with high-risk melanoma. Cancer 2005;103(4):780–7.

64. Shah NC, Ted Gerstle J, Stuart M, et al. Use of sentinel lymph node biopsy and high-dose interferon in pediatric patients with high-risk melanoma: The Hospital for Sick Children experience. J Pediatr Hematol Oncol 2006;28(8):496–500.

65. Navid F, Herzog CE, Sandoval J, et al. Feasibility of pegylated interferon in children and young adults with resected high-risk melanoma. Pediatr Blood Cancer 2016;63(7):1207–13.

66. Chao MM, Schwartz JL, Wechsler DS, et al. High-risk surgically resected pediatric melanoma and adjuvant interferon therapy. Pediatr Blood Cancer 2005;44(5):441–8.

67. Phase II Study Incorporating Pegylated Interferon In the Treatment For Children With High-Risk Melanoma - Full Text View - ClinicalTrials.gov. Available at: https://clinicaltrials.gov/ct2/show/NCT00539591. Accessed August 24, 2020.

68. Hodi FS, O'Day SJ, McDermott DF, et al. Improved survival with ipilimumab in patients with metastatic melanoma. N Engl J Med 2010;363(8):711–23.

69. Robert C, Thomas L, Bondarenko I, et al. Ipilimumab plus dacarbazine for previously untreated metastatic melanoma. N Engl J Med 2011;364(26):2517–26.

70. Geoerger B, Bergeron C, Gore L, et al. Phase II study of ipilimumab in adolescents with unresectable stage III or IV malignant melanoma. Eur J Cancer 2017;86:358–63.

71. Weber J, Mandala M, Del Vecchio M, et al. Adjuvant nivolumab versus ipilimumab in resected stage III or IV melanoma. N Engl J Med 2017;377(19):1824–35.

72. Geoerger B, Kang HJ, Yalon-Oren M, et al. Pembrolizumab in paediatric patients with advanced melanoma or a PD-L1-positive, advanced, relapsed, or refractory solid tumour or lymphoma (KEYNOTE-051): interim analysis of an open-label, single-arm, phase 1–2 trial. Lancet Oncol 2020;21(1):121–33.

73. Marjanska A, Galazka P, Marjanski M, et al. Efficacy and toxicity of pembrolizumab in pediatric metastatic recurrent melanoma. Anticancer Res 2019;39(7):3945–7.

74. Flaherty KT, Puzanov I, Kim KB, et al. Inhibition of mutated, activated BRAF in metastatic melanoma. N Engl J Med 2010;363(9):809–19.

75. Chapman PB, Hauschild A, Robert C, et al. Improved survival with vemurafenib in melanoma with BRAF V600E mutation. N Engl J Med 2011;364(26):2507–16.
76. McArthur GA, Chapman PB, Robert C, et al. Safety and efficacy of vemurafenib in BRAFV600E and BRAFV600K mutation-positive melanoma (BRIM-3): Extended follow-up of a phase 3, randomised, open-label study. Lancet Oncol 2014; 15(3):323–32.
77. Hauschild A, Grob JJ, Demidov LV, et al. Dabrafenib in BRAF-mutated metastatic melanoma: A multicentre, open-label, phase 3 randomised controlled trial. Lancet 2012;380(9839):358–65.
78. Sosman JA, Kim KB, Schuchter L, et al. Survival in BRAF V600-mutant advanced melanoma treated with vemurafenib. N Engl J Med 2012;366(8):707–14.
79. Dummer R, Schadendorf D, Ascierto PA, et al. Binimetinib versus dacarbazine in patients with advanced NRAS-mutant melanoma (NEMO): a multicentre, open-label, randomised, phase 3 trial. Lancet Oncol 2017;18(4):435–45.
80. Long GV, Hauschild A, Santinami M, et al. Adjuvant Dabrafenib plus Trametinib in Stage III BRAF-Mutated Melanoma. N Engl J Med 2017;377(19):1813–23.
81. Chisholm JC, Suvada J, Dunkel IJ, et al. BRIM-P: A phase I, open-label, multicenter, dose-escalation study of vemurafenib in pediatric patients with surgically incurable, BRAF mutation-positive melanoma. Pediatr Blood Cancer 2018;65(5). https://doi.org/10.1002/pbc.26947.
82. Kieran MW, Geoerger B, Dunkel IJ, et al. A phase I and pharmacokinetic study of oral dabrafenib in children and adolescent patients with recurrent or refractory BRAF V600 mutation–positive solid tumors. Clin Cancer Res 2019;25(24): 7294–302.
83. Eggermont AMM, Kirkwood JM. Re-evaluating the role of dacarbazine in metastatic melanoma: What have we learned in 30 years? Eur J Cancer 2004; 40(12):1825–36.
84. Middleton MR, Grob JJ, Aaronson N, et al. Randomized phase III study of temozolomide versus dacarbazine in the treatment of patients with advanced metastatic malignant melanoma. J Clin Oncol 2000;18(1):158–66.
85. Boddie AW, Cangir A. Adjuvant and neoadjuvant chemotherapy with dacarbazine in high-risk childhood melanoma. Cancer 1987;60(8):1720–3.
86. Hayes FA, Green AA. Malignant melanoma in childhood: Clinical course and response to chemotherapy. J Clin Oncol 1984;2(11):1229–34.
87. Atkins MB, Lotze MT, Dutcher JP, et al. High-dose recombinant interleukin 2 therapy for patients with metastatic melanoma: Analysis of 270 patients treated between 1985 and 1993. J Clin Oncol 1999;17(7):2105–16.
88. Davar D, Ding F, Saul M, et al. High-dose interleukin-2 (HD IL-2) for advanced melanoma: A single center experience from the University of Pittsburgh Cancer Institute. J Immunother Cancer 2017;5(1). https://doi.org/10.1186/s40425-017-0279-5.
89. Ribeiro RC, Rill D, Roberson PK, et al. Continuous infusion of interleukin-2 in children with refractory malignancies. Cancer 1993;72(2):623–8.
90. Bauer M, Reaman GH, Hank JA, et al. A phase II trial of human recombinant Interleukin-2 administered as a 4-day continuous infusion for children with refractory neuroblastoma, non-Hodgkin's lymphoma, sarcoma, renal cell carcinoma, and malignant melanoma. A childrens cancer group study. Cancer 1995;75(12): 2959–65.
91. Curtin JA, Busam K, Pinkel D, et al. Somatic activation of KIT in distinct subtypes of melanoma. J Clin Oncol 2006;24(26):4340–6.

92. Averbook BJ, Lee SJ, Delman KA, et al. Pediatric melanoma: Analysis of an international registry. Cancer 2013;119:4012–9.
93. Brecht IB, Garbe C, Gefeller O, et al. 443 paediatric cases of malignant melanoma registered with the German Central Malignant Melanoma Registry between 1983 and 2011. Eur J Cancer 2015;51(7):861–8.
94. Shi K, Camilon PR, Roberts JM, et al. Survival differences between pediatric head and neck versus body melanoma in the surveillance, epidemiology, and end results program. Laryngoscope 2020. https://doi.org/10.1002/lary.28711.
95. Ipenburg NA, Lo SN, Vilain RE, et al. The prognostic value of tumor mitotic rate in children and adolescents with cutaneous melanoma: A retrospective cohort study. J Am Acad Dermatol 2020;82(4):910–9.
96. Balch CM, Gershenwald JE, Soong SJ, et al. Final version of 2009 AJCC melanoma staging and classification. J Clin Oncol 2009;27(36):6199–206.
97. Hamilton EC, Nguyen HT, Chang YC, et al. Health Disparities Influence Childhood Melanoma Stage at Diagnosis and Outcome. J Pediatr 2016;175:182–7.
98. Richards MK, Czechowicz J, Goldin AB, et al. Survival and Surgical Outcomes for Pediatric Head and Neck Melanoma. JAMA Otolaryngol Neck Surg 2017; 143(1):34.

A Surgical Approach to Pulmonary Metastasis in Children

Jonathan Karpelowksy, MBBCh, PhD[a,b,c],*, Guido Seitz, MD[d]

KEYWORDS

- Pulmonary metastasis • Embryonal cancer • Surgery

KEY POINTS

- The aims of resection are localized resections with clear margins with the aim of preserving adequate lung volume.
- Unnecessary toxic therapy sometimes can be avoided with accurate diagnosis.
- Tumor type is of utmost importance.
- The number of metastases and the disease-free interval are not contraindications to metastasectomy.
- Staged or synchronous bilateral resections are well tolerated.

BACKGROUND

Approximately 10% to 40% of all children with solid tumors present with lung metastases at the time of diagnosis.[1] Although there have been significant improvements in the outcomes of children with embryonal malignancies, those with metastatic disease, however, have not mirrored the outcomes of those of nonmetastatic solid malignancies, with overall survival (OS) rates ranging from 20% to 70%, depending primarily on histology[1,2]

The decision regarding the role of surgery in pulmonary metastasis needs to take into account the histology and hence the biology of the cancer being treated. Response to chemotherapy and radiotherapy, balanced with the relative toxicities of these therapies, factors into the decision about metastasectomy. In general, the less sensitive the tumor is to adjuvant therapy, the more likely it is that metastasectomy may be beneficial.

[a] Pediatric Oncology and Thoracic Surgery, The Children's Hospital, Westmead, Sydney, Australia; [b] Children's Cancer Research Unit, Kids Research Institute, Sydney, Australia; [c] Faculty of Medicine and Health, The University of Sydney, Sydney, Australia; [d] Department of Pediatric Surgery, University Hospital Marburg, Baldingerstraße, Marburg 35043, Germany
* Corresponding author. Locked Bag 4001, Westmead, New South Wales 2145, Australia.
E-mail address: Jonathan.karpelowsky@health.nsw.gov.au
Twitter: @DrJonathanK (J.K.)

Surg Oncol Clin N Am 30 (2021) 389–399
https://doi.org/10.1016/j.soc.2020.11.007
1055-3207/21/© 2020 Elsevier Inc. All rights reserved.

Through numerous historical cases series, the following broad principles have been established:

1. The aims of resection are localized resections with clear margins, with the aim of preserving adequate lung volume.
2. Unnecessary toxic therapy sometimes can be avoided with accurate diagnosis.
3. Tumor type is of utmost importance.
4. The number of metastases and the disease-free interval are not contraindications to metastasectomy,
5. Staged or synchronous bilateral resections are well tolerated.[3]

TECHNICAL ASPECTS TO PULMONARY METASTASECTOMY

The goal of metastasectomy is localized resection with maximal preservation of normal lung tissue; lobectomies or segmentectomies are used only in specific circumstances with central lesion adjacent to hilar structures.

Computed tomography (CT) scan remains the current standard for identifying pulmonary lesions. Although the high sensitivity of CT can be beneficial, its lack of specificity with respect to differentiating malignant from benign nodules can lead to false-positive interpretations.[4] Conversely, for osteosarcoma, the number of lesions reported on CT scan often can underestimate the true burden of disease by at least 30% to 40%.[1,5–7]

Several techniques have been utilized to aid intraoperative lesion localization. This is particularly relevant in patients undergoing a thoracoscopic approach, where the lack of tactile feel makes localization even more challenging. Preoperative localization using CT-guided placement of localized dye (methylene blue ± and autologous blood patch),[8–11] hook wires, or coils[12] has been used in isolation or in combination.[13] Each technique has a failure rate of either coil/wire dislodgment or dye spill but rarely both[5–7]; as such, some investigators have advocated for the use of more than 1 technique to avoid technical failures.

Recently, newer techniques, using indocyanine green (ICG) and near-infrared fluorescence imaging, have gained in popularity. ICG may be used either as a localized dye injected under CT guidance or by systemic intravenous administration. When injected systemically, its use typically has been in hepatic neoplasms, including hepatoblastoma. Although both normal hepatocytes and tumor cells can take up ICG, the excretion by tumor cells is significantly slower, leading to relative retention. Its use in identifying hepatoblastoma metastasis is both sensitive and specific.[14–16] More recently, ICG use also has been studied in identifying sarcoma pulmonary metastasis, although at 10-fold the doses of ICG used in heptoblastoma.[14] The exact underlying physiologic basis for this is uncertain (**Fig. 1**).

When presented with bilateral pulmonary metastasis, several approaches are possible. Some surgeons prefer metachronous bilateral thoracotomy[17] with a 2-week to 6-week interval between exploration. Although this provides optimal exposure to the ipsilateral hemithorax, it has the disadvantages of requiring 2 surgeries and potential delays in chemotherapy. To ensure optimal exposure and to minimize delays in chemotherapy, 1 of the authors (JK) routinely undertakes bilateral synchronous muscle-sparing posterolateral thoracotomies together with epidural analgesia for postoperative recovery. Because the epidural provides bilateral pain relief, the stay does not exceed that for a unilateral thoracotomy, and patients are discharged on the fourth or fifth postoperative day. Two well-established alternative approaches are the median or the transverse sternotomy.[18] The latter improves the exposure (but still provides limited posterosuperior access) but is performed infrequently. The

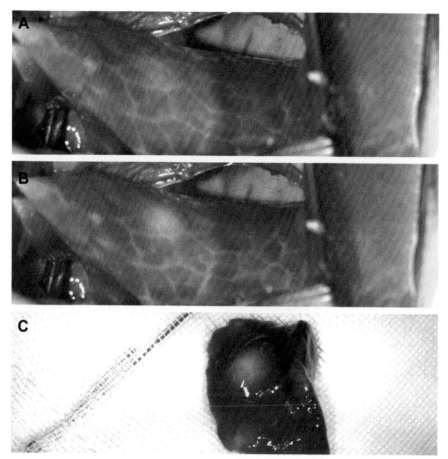

Fig. 1. ICG identification of a hepatoblastoma pulmonary metastasis, 8 mm in size and 9 mm below the pleural surface. (*A*) Without ICG near-infrared fluorescence. (*B*) With ICG near-infrared fluorescence to identify the lesion. (*C*) Confirmation of the excised pulmonary metastasis using ICG near-infrared fluorescence.

sternotomy is a well-tolerated approach in children. In cases of sternotomy, some investigators remark that exploration or exposure of the basal or posterior lung segments is difficult.[1] Access, especially to the posterior aspect of the left lower lobe, can be challenging due to cardiac compression but can be improved by the transection of the pulmonary ligament and anesthetic management.[19] Finally, a bilateral synchronous thoracoscopic approach has been reported but has the limitation of localizing deeper lesions.[20]

WILMS TUMOR

Approximately 10% of Wilms tumor patients present with pulmonary metastasis.[1,2,21] Traditionally, pulmonary metastases were treated with the addition of an anthracycline to chemotherapy and whole-lung radiotherapy.[22] The addition of these, however, increases long-term morbidity, including pulmonary disease, cardiac disease, and an increased risk of breast cancer, especially in females.[22,23] To avoid these, both the International Society of Paediatric Oncology (SIOP) protocol and the recently closed

Children's Oncology Group (COG) AREN0533 protocol now avoid whole-lung radiation in those patients who achieve a complete pulmonary response (CR) with 6 weeks of 3-drug chemotherapy. The current role of pulmonary metastasectomy to achieve CR was assessed in the SIOP protocol 93-01. Patients achieving CR either by chemotherapy alone or a combination of chemotherapy and surgery had a good OS rate, of 88%, without pulmonary radiotherapy.[24] This approach will be incorporated into the next COG study. Finally, there is a role for biopsy of small CT only lesions at presentation to confirm pulmonary disease.

HEPATOBLASTOMA

At the time of diagnosis, 20% of children with hepatoblastoma present with metastases to distant sites.[25] Metastatic hepatoblastoma has a much worse prognosis, with an OS rate of approximately 50% to 65%.[26–28] Although hepatoblastoma pulmonary metastases often resolve with chemotherapy alone, surgery of lung metastases is an important tool. In the European high-risk SIOPEL 4 study, among the patients with initial lung metastases, of the 39 patients with initial lung metastases, a CR of the lung lesions was achieved in 20 patients and partial response in 18 patients, with preoperative chemotherapy alone[28]

Radical surgery for pulmonary metastatic relapse is not futile in hepatoblastoma; it may provide a durable cure in approximately 30% of patients.[29–31] Indications for surgery of pulmonary metastases are persistent nodules after primary chemotherapy and pulmonary relapse off treatment.[27] Metastasectomy also should be performed in children with locally advanced liver disease that may require transplantation.[1,32] The timing of metastasectomy depends on degree residual disease after chemotherapy and whether a partial hepatectomy or transplantation is required. Usually, metastasectomy is delayed to after definitive local control for the former but undertaken to clear metastatic disease prior to undertaking transplantation.[27,33] There are groups that have demonstrated the feasibility of synchronous resection of both the local primary tumor and the metastatic disease.[34]

RHABDOMYOSARCOMA

Rhabdomyosarcoma (RMS) is the most common pediatric soft tissue sarcoma, accounting for two-thirds of all soft tissue sarcomas and 7% to 8% of all solid malignant tumors in children.[35] Multimodal therapy has led to an improved survival of patients in low-risk localized disease, and OS rates of more than 90% can be achieved.[36] In infants younger than 1 year, the OS rate is lower (69%) in comparison to older children.[37] In contrast, the survival rates of patients with metastatic disease still are sobering and have not improved: 15% of RMS patients present with metastatic disease.[38,39] Currently, the risk stratification for metastatic RMS is based on the Oberlin score, involving age, primary tumor site, number of metastases, histology, and bone marrow involvement.[36,39]

In the European intergroup studies (MMT4-89 and MMT4-91), the 5-year OS rates were 24% for patients with metastatic disease, with no difference between high-dose and standard-dose chemotherapy.[40] A large retrospective analysis of 101 children treated in France showed that metastatic patients undergoing aggressive local treatment had a better outcome (OS 44%) than patients treated with less aggressive surgery. The conclusion was that isolated debulking surgery is associated with a very poor outcome and should be avoided, whereas aggressive local treatment even in metastatic patients should be considered.[41–43] A large pooled international analysis of 787 metastatic RMS patients treated in 9 European and North American cooperative group trials revealed a 3-year OS of 34% and a 3-year event-free survival (EFS) of 27%.[39] The investigators carried out a univariate analysis and found that the 3-year EFS was influenced by age, alveolar histology, unfavorable primary tumor localization, and 3 or more sites of metastatic disease as well as bone or bone marrow involvement.[39] The multivariate analysis correlated all factors except the histology.[39] The EFS was 50% for patients without these factors, whereas it was 42% for 1 factor, 18% for 2 factors, 12% for 3 factors, and 5% for 4 factors with statistical significance.[39]

Local control of metastatic RMS depends on the site of metastatic disease. Mohan and colleagues[44] showed that the survival of patients with lung metastases can be improved by whole-lung irradiation. Additionally, they could show that local therapy at all distant metastatic sites led to a significant increase in the progression-free survival.[44] Dantonello and colleagues[45] reported on 29 patients with embryonal RMS and lung metastases. Lung metastases were in remission in 22 children after induction chemotherapy, 3 had pulmonary metastasectomy, and 9 underwent lung irradiation. Complete remission was achieved in 24 of 29 children, with a 5-year OS rate of 48.7%. Local treatment of metastases did not improve the outcome in this cohort.[45] Reports on pulmonary metastasectomy in RMS are rare.[46,47]

Taken together, aggressive local control seems justified in patients with metastatic RMS. Local control also should be applied to lung metastases, particularly if still present at end of therapy. Other novel treatment options clearly are required to improve the outcome of these patients.

NONRHABDOMYOSARCOMA

Pediatric non-RMS soft tissue sarcoma includes a heterogeneous group of more than 50 different tumor entities.[48] Relevant subtypes in children are, among others, synovial sarcoma, malignant peripheral nerve sheath tumor (MPNST), and alveolar soft part sarcoma. Metastases can occur at different sites, including lung, bone, bone marrow, lymph nodes, brain, and others.[49]

The COG recently published a risk-based treatment regimen for non-RMS soft tissue sarcoma based on the prospective trial (ARST0332).[50] They included, in a study period of 5 years, 80 patients with metastatic disease, and these patients were treated with surgery alone, chemotherapy alone, or neoadjuvant radiochemotherapy.[50] Cross-resection of all metastases was carried out in 20 patients, and 8 patients were treated with radiotherapy at 1 or more metastatic sites.[50] The 5-year OS rate for all metastatic patients was 35.5% with a 5-year EFS rate of 21.2%. Due to the low number of patients with gross resection of the primary tumor and metastases (n = 18), it was not possible for the investigators to draw conclusions if this approach would result in a better outcome.[50]

The Cooperative Weichteilsarkom Studiengruppe (CWS) group recently published their experience with primary metastatic synovial sarcoma. They found that the prognosis of patients was best if they had oligometastatic lung metastases (5-year OS 85%) and was worse for multiple bilateral lung metastases (5-year OS 13%). Whole-lung irradiation was not correlated with better outcomes.[51] Pulmonary metastasectomy also can be used for synovial sarcoma. Stanelle and colleagues[52] showed in 31 patients undergoing at least 1 pulmonary metastasectomy that 2-year and 5-year OS rates of 65% and 24%, respectively, could be achieved, whereas all other patients died within 2 years from diagnosis of pulmonary disease. The conclusion was that pulmonary metastasectomy may be associated with improved survival if a complete resection could be carried out.[52]

Alveolar soft part sarcoma is a rare tumor entity often arising at the extremities. Lung metastases may occur. An analysis from the CWS study group showed that patients with metastatic disease had a 5-year OS rate of 61% and that a complete resection seemed to be a prognostic factor for outcome. Pulmonary metastasectomy was carried out in some patients.[53] Patients suffering from metastatic MPNSTs also have been shown to have a poor prognosis. In a current COG analysis, the OS rate was 13%.[54] There are no clear data on the influence of the surgical management of metastases in the literature.

In conclusion, non-RMSs are a heterogeneous group of tumors, which might be accompanied by metastatic disease. The numbers in children are low, and, therefore, it is difficult to give general treatment advices for the management of metastatic disease.

EWING SARCOMA

Ewing sarcoma (ES) is the second most common bone tumor in children and adolescence. Besides the bone, it also can arise in the soft tissue. The survival rate for patients with metastatic disease is approximately 30%, and tumors can metastasize into the lungs, bone, and bone marrow.[55] Irradiation of the lungs has shown an improvement in survival in metastatic disease.[56] Therefore, radiation therapy has been included in several ES treatment protocols.[57] A smaller analysis from Houston, with 22 patients suffering from metastatic ES, has shown that patients undergoing pulmonary metastasectomy had a significantly better OS rate than patients with whole-lung irradiation or chemotherapy only. Patients with pulmonary metastasectomy also did better than patients who underwent radiation and PM. The conclusion of the trial was that ES patients possibly benefit from pulmonary metastasectomy.[57,58] Another study, which included, among other histologies, 28 pediatric ES patients, showed that 3 or more metastases, histology other than osteosarcoma, and incomplete resection were unfavorable prognostic factors for survival.[59] Morbidity and mortality were low.[59] It still is unclear if there is benefit to surgical metastasectomy in patients with ES.

OSTEOSARCOMA

Osteosarcoma is the most common malignant bone tumor in children and young adults.[60] High-grade osteosarcomas usually are treated by neoadjuvant and adjuvant chemotherapy and surgery, whereas low-grade osteosarcomas often are treated by surgery only.[61] Lungs are the most common metastatic site; however, they may occur in bone and other sites.[61] The overall outcome of patients with metastatic osteosarcoma is poor. In an international multivariate analysis of the EURAMOS-1 study, it was shown that the most adverse prognostic factors at diagnosis were pulmonary metastases, nonpulmonary metastases, and axial skeleton tumor site.[60]

Imaging of lung metastases is performed by CT scan of the thorax. It has been described that it is helpful for the treating surgeon and radiologist to achieve consensus when reviewing the CT scans prior to surgery to achieve the best surgical results.[19] There is a relevant difference in the number of preoperatively detected lung metastases on CT scan and the intraoperative findings.[19] Different investigators demonstrated that there is a 30% to 40% difference in numbers of metastases, and there is an underestimation of lung nodules on CT scans.[19,47] The risk of underestimation increases with the number of nodules, and there is a cutoff point for the exact correlation between 5 and 10 metastases.[1,19,47] On the other hand, there is a discrimination problem between small lung metastases and small benign lesions, which sometimes leads to an overestimation of small metastases on imaging compared with intraoperative findings.[61,62]

Curative treatment of primary metastatic osteosarcoma is identical to that of localized disease with the addition of removal of all metastatic lesions. More than 40% of metastatic patients achieving a complete surgical remission can become long-term survivors.[63–65] Survival is correlated significantly with age, site of the primary tumor, number and location of metastases, response to preoperative chemotherapy, and completeness and time point of surgical resection of all tumor sites. Kager and colleagues[64] stated that the number of metastases at diagnosis and the completeness of surgical resection of all clinically detected tumor sites are of independent prognostic value. Additionally, patients with unilateral lung metastases have a better outcome than patients with bilateral lung metastases.[66] Patients with solitary nodules have a better 5-year OS rate (75%) than those with 2 to 5 metastases (26%) and those with more than 5 metastases (23%).[66]

Stereotactic radiosurgery also has been described for the management of osteosarcoma metastases. Yu and colleagues[67] described a series of 73 osteosarcoma patients, of whom 33 were treated with stereotactic radiosurgery with a total dose of 70 Gy to the gross target volume compared with 40 patients who underwent pulmonary metastasectomy. The results of both groups were comparable in regard to 4-year progression-free survival and 4-year survival rates. The investigators stated the radiosurgery was tolerated well with fewer complications and advocated this technique especially for inoperable patients or patients refusing surgery.[67] Percutaneous CT-guided thermal ablation might be another minimally invasive treatment approach, which was used in patients after surgical metastasectomy. Thermal ablation may be useful in patients with oligometastatic pulmonary disease in whom a surgical approach is contraindicated.[68]

SUMMARY

Despite significant improvements in the survival of childhood cancer patients, those with metastatic disease have not shown the same equivalent outcomes. Although chemotherapy and radiotherapy remain the main modalities in the treatment of metastatic disease, surgery is playing an increasingly important role in the treatment of several pediatric metastatic solid tumors. In some cases, this is diagnostic to confirm metastatic disease or, alternatively, to obtain tissue at the time of diagnosis or relapse for further analysis to guide targeted therapy. There is, however, a subset of cancers where surgery to remove all remaining metastasis can provide a survival benefit.

DISCLOSURE

Nothing to disclose.

REFERENCES

1. Fuchs J, Seitz G, Handgretinger R, et al. Surgical treatment of lung metastases in patients with embryonal pediatric solid tumors: an update. Semin Pediatr Surg 2012;21:79–87.
2. Heij HA, Vos A, de Kraker J, et al. Prognostic factors in surgery for pulmonary metastases in children. Surgery 1994;115:687–93.
3. Heaton TE, Davidoff AM. Surgical treatment of pulmonary metastases in pediatric solid tumors. Semin Pediatr Surg 2016;25:311–7.
4. Rosenfield NS, Keller MS, Markowitz RI, et al. CT differentiation of benign and malignant lung nodules in children. J Pediatr Surg 1992;27:459–61.

5. Kayton ML, Huvos AG, Casher J, et al. Computed tomographic scan of the chest underestimates the number of metastatic lesions in osteosarcoma. J Pediatr Surg 2006;41:200–6 [discussion: 200–6].

6. McCarville MB, Lederman HM, Santana VM, et al. Distinguishing benign from malignant pulmonary nodules with helical chest CT in children with malignant solid tumors. Radiology 2006;239:514–20.

7. Parsons AM, Detterbeck FC, Parker LA. Accuracy of helical CT in the detection of pulmonary metastases: is intraoperative palpation still necessary? Ann Thorac Surg 2004;78:1910–6 [discussion: 1916–8].

8. Karpelowsky J. Paediatric thoracoscopic surgery. Paediatr Respir Rev 2012;13: 244–50 [quiz: 250–1].

9. Choi BG, Kim HH, Kim BS, et al. Pulmonary nodules: CT-guided contrast material localization for thoracoscopic resection. Radiology 1998;208:399–401.

10. Nomori H, Horio H. Colored collagen is a long-lasting point marker for small pulmonary nodules in thoracoscopic operations. Ann Thorac Surg 1996;61:1070–3.

11. Wicky S, Mayor B, Cuttat JF, et al. CT-guided localizations of pulmonary nodules with methylene blue injections for thoracoscopic resections. Chest 1994;106: 1326–8.

12. Gaffke G, Stroszczynski C, Rau B, et al. [CT-guided resection of pulmonary metastases]. RoFo 2005;177:877–83.

13. Martin AE, Chen JY, Muratore CS, et al. Dual localization technique for thoracoscopic resection of lung lesions in children. J Laparoendosc Adv Surg Tech A 2009;19(Suppl 1):S161–4.

14. Keating J, Newton A, Venegas O, et al. Near-infrared intraoperative molecular imaging can locate metastases to the lung. Ann Thorac Surg 2017;103:390–8.

15. Yamamichi T, Oue T, Yonekura T, et al. Clinical application of indocyanine green (ICG) fluorescent imaging of hepatoblastoma. J Pediatr Surg 2015;50:833–6.

16. Kitagawa N, Shinkai M, Mochizuki K, et al. Navigation using indocyanine green fluorescence imaging for hepatoblastoma pulmonary metastases surgery. Pediatr Surg Int 2015;31:407–11.

17. Hacker FM, von Schweinitz D, Gambazzi F. The relevance of surgical therapy for bilateral and/or multiple pulmonary metastases in children. Eur J Pediatr Surg 2007;17:84–9.

18. Abbo O, Guatta R, Pinnagoda K, et al. Bilateral anterior sternothoracotomy (clamshell incision): a suitable alternative for bilateral lung sarcoma metastasis in children. World J Surg Oncol 2014;12:233.

19. Fuchs J, Seitz G, Ellerkamp V, et al. Analysis of sternotomy as treatment option for the resection of bilateral pulmonary metastases in pediatric solid tumors. Surg Oncol 2008;17:323–30.

20. Han KN, Kang CH, Park IK, et al. Thoracoscopic approach to bilateral pulmonary metastasis: is it justified? Interactive Cardiovasc Thorac Surg 2014;18:615–20.

21. Green DM, Breslow NE, Ii Y, et al. The role of surgical excision in the management of relapsed Wilms' tumor patients with pulmonary metastases: a report from the National Wilms' Tumor Study. J Pediatr Surg 1991;26:728–33.

22. Green DM, Lange JM, Qu A, et al. Pulmonary disease after treatment for Wilms tumor: a report from the national wilms tumor long-term follow-up study. Pediatr Blood Cancer 2013;60:1721–6.

23. Lange JM, Takashima JR, Peterson SM, et al. Breast cancer in female survivors of Wilms tumor: a report from the national Wilms tumor late effects study. Cancer 2014;120:3722–30.

24. Verschuur A, Van Tinteren H, Graf N, et al. Treatment of pulmonary metastases in children with stage IV nephroblastoma with risk-based use of pulmonary radiotherapy. J Clin Oncol 2012;30:3533–9.

25. Emre S, Umman V, Rodriguez-Davalos M. Current concepts in pediatric liver tumors. Pediatr Transplant 2012;16:549–63.

26. Towbin AJ, Meyers RL, Woodley H, et al. 2017 PRETEXT: radiologic staging system for primary hepatic malignancies of childhood revised for the Paediatric Hepatic International Tumour Trial (PHITT). Pediatr Radiol 2018;48:536–54.

27. Wanaguru D, Shun A, Price N, et al. Outcomes of pulmonary metastases in hepatoblastoma–is the prognosis always poor? J Pediatr Surg 2013;48:2474–8.

28. Zsiros J, Brugieres L, Brock P, et al. Dose-dense cisplatin-based chemotherapy and surgery for children with high-risk hepatoblastoma (SIOPEL-4): a prospective, single-arm, feasibility study. Lancet Oncol 2013;14:834–42.

29. Meyers RL, Czauderna P, Otte JB. Surgical treatment of hepatoblastoma. Pediatr Blood Cancer 2012;59:800–8.

30. Meyers RL, Tiao GM, Dunn SP, et al. Liver transplantation in the management of unresectable hepatoblastoma in children. Front Biosci (Elite Ed) 2012;4:1293–302.

31. Angelico R, Grimaldi C, Gazia C, et al. How do synchronous lung metastases influence the surgical management of children with hepatoblastoma? an update and systematic review of the literature. Cancers 2019;11:1693.

32. Meyers RL, Katzenstein HM, Krailo M, et al. Surgical resection of pulmonary metastatic lesions in children with hepatoblastoma. J Pediatr Surg 2007;42:2050–6.

33. Seng MS, Berry B, Karpelowsky J, et al. Successful treatment of a metastatic hepatocellular malignant neoplasm, not otherwise specified with chemotherapy and liver transplantation. Pediatr Blood Cancer 2019;66:e27603.

34. Urla C, Seitz G, Tsiflikas I, et al. Simultaneous resection of high-risk liver tumors and pulmonary metastases in children. Ann Surg 2015;262:e1–3.

35. McDowell HP. Update on childhood rhabdomyosarcoma. Arch Dis Child 2003;88:354–7.

36. Chen C, Dorado Garcia H, Scheer M, et al. Current and future treatment strategies for rhabdomyosarcoma. Front Oncol 2019;9:1458.

37. Sparber-Sauer M, Stegmaier S, Vokuhl C, et al. Rhabdomyosarcoma diagnosed in the first year of life: Localized, metastatic, and relapsed disease. Outcome data from five trials and one registry of the Cooperative Weichteilsarkom Studiengruppe (CWS). Pediatr Blood Cancer 2019;66:e27652.

38. Breneman JC, Lyden E, Pappo AS, et al. Prognostic factors and clinical outcomes in children and adolescents with metastatic rhabdomyosarcoma–a report from the Intergroup Rhabdomyosarcoma Study IV. J Clin Oncol 2003;21:78–84.

39. Oberlin O, Rey A, Lyden E, et al. Prognostic factors in metastatic rhabdomyosarcomas: results of a pooled analysis from United States and European cooperative groups. J Clin Oncol 2008;26:2384–9.

40. Carli M, Colombatti R, Oberlin O, et al. European intergroup studies (MMT4-89 and MMT4-91) on childhood metastatic rhabdomyosarcoma: final results and analysis of prognostic factors. J Clin Oncol 2004;22:4787–94.

41. Ben Arush M, Minard-Colin V, Mosseri V, et al. Does aggressive local treatment have an impact on survival in children with metastatic rhabdomyosarcoma? Eur J Cancer 2015;51:193–201.

42. Gosiengfiao Y, Reichek J, Walterhouse D. What is new in rhabdomyosarcoma management in children? Paediatric Drugs 2012;14:389–400.

43. Yamazaki F, Osumi T, Shigematsu N, et al. Successful treatment of metastatic rhabdomyosarcoma with radiochemotherapy and allogeneic hematopoietic stem cell transplantation. Jpn J Clin Oncol 2015;45:225–8.

44. Mohan AC, Venkatramani R, Okcu MF, et al. Local therapy to distant metastatic sites in stage IV rhabdomyosarcoma. Pediatr Blood Cancer 2018;65. https://doi.org/10.1002/pbc.26859.

45. Dantonello TM, Winkler P, Boelling T, et al. Embryonal rhabdomyosarcoma with metastases confined to the lungs: report from the CWS Study Group. Pediatr Blood Cancer 2011;56:725–32.

46. Erginel B, Gun Soysal F, Keskin E, et al. Pulmonary metastasectomy in pediatric patients. World J Surg Oncol 2016;14:27.

47. Kayton ML. Pulmonary metastasectomy in pediatric patients. Thorac Surg Clin 2006;16:167–83, vi.

48. Dasgupta R, Rodeberg D. Non-rhabdomyosarcoma. Semin Pediatr Surg 2016; 25:284–9.

49. Pappo AS, Devidas M, Jenkins J, et al. Phase II trial of neoadjuvant vincristine, ifosfamide, and doxorubicin with granulocyte colony-stimulating factor support in children and adolescents with advanced-stage nonrhabdomyosarcomatous soft tissue sarcomas: a Pediatric Oncology Group Study. J Clin Oncol 2005;23: 4031–8.

50. Spunt SL, Million L, Chi YY, et al. A risk-based treatment strategy for non-rhabdomyosarcoma soft-tissue sarcomas in patients younger than 30 years (ARST0332): a Children's Oncology Group prospective study. Lancet Oncol 2020;21:145–61.

51. Scheer M, Dantonello T, Hallmen E, et al. Primary Metastatic Synovial Sarcoma: Experience of the CWS Study Group. Pediatr Blood Cancer 2016;63:1198–206.

52. Stanelle EJ, Christison-Lagay ER, Wolden SL, et al. Pulmonary metastasectomy in pediatric/adolescent patients with synovial sarcoma: an institutional review. J Pediatr Surg 2013;48:757–63.

53. Sparber-Sauer M, Seitz G, von Kalle T, et al. Alveolar soft-part sarcoma: Primary metastatic disease and metastatic relapse occurring during long-term follow-up: Treatment results of four Cooperative Weichteilsarkom Studiengruppe (CWS) trials and one registry. Pediatr Blood Cancer 2018;65:e27405.

54. Waxweiler TV, Rusthoven CG, Proper MS, et al. Non-rhabdomyosarcoma soft tissue sarcomas in children: a surveillance, epidemiology, and end results analysis validating COG risk stratifications. Int J Radiat Oncol Biol Phys 2015;92:339–48.

55. Grünewald TGP, Cidre-Aranaz F, Surdez D, et al. Ewing sarcoma. Nat Rev Dis Primers 2018;4:5.

56. Briccoli A, Rocca M, Ferrari S, et al. Surgery for lung metastases in Ewing's sarcoma of bone. Eur J Surg Oncol 2004;30:63–7.

57. Dirksen U, Brennan B, Le Deley MC, et al. High-dose chemotherapy compared with standard chemotherapy and lung radiation in ewing sarcoma with pulmonary metastases: results of the european ewing tumour working initiative of national groups, 99 trial and EWING 2008. J Clin Oncol 2019;37:3192–202.

58. Letourneau PA, Shackett B, Xiao L, et al. Resection of pulmonary metastases in pediatric patients with Ewing sarcoma improves survival. J Pediatr Surg 2011; 46:332–5.

59. Temeck BK, Wexler LH, Steinberg SM, et al. Metastasectomy for sarcomatous pediatric histologies: results and prognostic factors. Ann Thorac Surg 1995;59: 1385–9 [discussion: 1390].

60. Smeland S, Bielack SS, Whelan J, et al. Survival and prognosis with osteosarcoma: outcomes in more than 2000 patients in the EURAMOS-1 (European and American Osteosarcoma Study) cohort. Eur J Cancer 2019;109:36–50.
61. Bielack SS, Hecker-Nolting S, Blattmann C, et al. Advances in the management of osteosarcoma. F1000Research 2016;5:2767.
62. Dix DB, Seibel NL, Chi YY, et al. Treatment of stage IV favorable histology wilms tumor with lung metastases: a report from the Children's Oncology Group AREN0533 Study. J Clin Oncol 2018;36:1564–70.
63. Ciccarese F, Bazzocchi A, Ciminari R, et al. The many faces of pulmonary metastases of osteosarcoma: retrospective study on 283 lesions submitted to surgery. Eur J Radiol 2015;84:2679–85.
64. Kager L, Zoubek A, Pötschger U, et al. Primary metastatic osteosarcoma: presentation and outcome of patients treated on neoadjuvant Cooperative Osteosarcoma Study Group protocols. J Clin Oncol 2003;21:2011–8.
65. Ritter J, Bielack SS. Osteosarcoma. Ann Oncol 2010;21(Suppl 7):vii320–5.
66. Kager L, Kempf-Bielack B, Bielack S. Synchronous and metachronous lung metastases in high-grade osteosarcoma. Jpn J Clin Oncol 2010;40:94–5.
67. Yu W, Liu Z, Tang L, et al. Efficacy and safety of stereotactic radiosurgery for pulmonary metastases from osteosarcoma: Experience in 73 patients. Sci Rep 2017; 7:17480.
68. Yevich S, Gaspar N, Tselikas L, et al. Percutaneous computed tomography-guided thermal ablation of pulmonary osteosarcoma metastases in children. Ann Surg Oncol 2016;23:1380–6.

Fertility Considerations in Pediatric and Adolescent Patients Undergoing Cancer Therapy

Timothy B. Lautz, MD[a],[*],[1], Karen Burns, MD[b],[1], Erin E. Rowell, MD[a]

KEYWORDS

- Pediatric • Cancer • Survivorship • Infertility • Fertility preservation

KEY POINTS

- Survivors of pediatric cancer are at increased risk for infertility and premature hormonal failure.
- Surgeons caring for children with cancer have an important role to play in understanding this risk, as well as advocating for and performing appropriate fertility preservation procedures.
- Fertility preservation options in males and females vary by pubertal status and include nonexperimental (oocyte harvest, ovarian tissue cryopreservation, sperm cryopreservation) and experimental (testicular tissue cryopreservation) options.

BACKGROUND

A baseline risk of infertility exists in the general population. Approximately 1% of women will experience premature menopause, leading to infertility, and 1% of males will have abnormal or absent sperm counts or function.[1] However, for survivors of pediatric and adolescent cancer, this risk can be much higher owing to the effects of therapy.[2–4] This circumstance may lead to the inability to conceive a biological child and to hormonal dysfunction.

As childhood and adolescent cancer survival rates continue to increase, the number of survivors is growing. With current 5-year survival rate of more than 85%, it is estimated that there are now 500,000 survivors living in the United States, a number that is

[a] Northwestern Feinberg School of Medicine, Ann & Robert H. Lurie Children's Hospital of Chicago, 225 East Chicago Avenue, Box 63, Chicago, IL 60611, USA; [b] University of Cincinnati College of Medicine, Cincinnati Children's Hospital Medical Center, 3333 Burnet Avenue, Cincinnati, OH 45229-3039, USA
[1] Both authors contributed equally to this work.
* Corresponding author.
E-mail address: tlautz@luriechildrens.org

Surg Oncol Clin N Am 30 (2021) 401–415
https://doi.org/10.1016/j.soc.2020.11.009
1055-3207/21/© 2020 Elsevier Inc. All rights reserved.

increasing each year.[5] This circumstance has led to an increased emphasis on managing the late effects related to the therapies used to cure these diseases. In particular, the gonadotoxic effect of radiation therapy (RT) and chemotherapy have been identified as one of the most important concerns of parents and young adult survivors of childhood cancer.[6,7]

It is therefore of critical importance to address the risk of gonadotoxicity and the potential impact of the treatment plan on future fertility with each patient and family as early as possible after diagnosis. This process enables the medical team to begin discussions with the patient and family regarding possible fertility preservation options. Surgeons caring for children with cancer have an important role to play in (1) understanding which patients are at increased risk of infertility, (2) advocating for appropriate fertility preservation services, and (3) performing fertility preservation procedures and working to coordinate these with other sedated procedures to minimize anesthesia exposures.

BASICS OF RISK ASSESSMENT

The risk of gonadotoxicity is not uniform across all patients and treatment plans; thus, patients and families must be counseled about their individual risk so they can make the most informed decision regarding their fertility preservation options. Their risk depends on their sex, age at the time of treatment exposure, and treatment specific to their cancer diagnosis.

Age and Sex

Male patients are at similar risk of gonadotoxicity regardless of age at time of therapy.[8] The risk is present beginning with the first doses of chemotherapy or RT. Sertoli cells (sperm-producing cells) in the testes are exquisitely sensitive to the gonadotoxic effects of therapy, even at a young age. Therapy-induced loss of Sertoli cells leads to temporary azoospermia, allowing for recovery over time, typically within the first 5 years after chemotherapy. However, if too many Sertoli cells are lost, as with more intense therapy, the azoospermia may be permanent.[9]

Leydig cells are responsible for testosterone production and necessary for progression through puberty. These cells are more resistant to the gonadotoxic effects of therapy.[10] Therefore, this article focuses on the effects of chemotherapy on gamete production and preservation. Because Leydig cells are much more resistant to therapy than the Sertoli cells, it is common to have a loss of sperm production (fertility) while still preserving normal testosterone levels and the ability to progress through puberty.[10]

Females are born with a defined number of primordial follicles (bank of potential eggs) and this number decreases over their lifetime. The primordial follicles have 3 potential fates:

1. Remain quiescent as the "ovarian reserve,"
2. Become activated to grow and ovulate at puberty and beyond, or
3. Become activated to grow and undergo atresia.

Over time, the ovarian reserve is gradually depleted, and at the point the primordial follicle reserve falls below a critical level (typically 1000 primordial follicles), menopause occurs.[11] Owing to the effects of chemotherapy and radiation on the ovary, the primordial follicle reserve can be depleted prematurely, resulting in premature ovarian insufficiency (POI), which is defined as women who experience menopause-like symptoms before the age of 40 years.[12] Because prepubertal patients have significantly more primordial follicles and their ovaries have not yet begun folliculogenesis, they have a higher threshold for POI from gonadotoxic chemotherapy.[13] Patients who do not resume ovarian function within 5 years after cancer therapy are said to have acute ovarian failure.[14]

It is important to note that, although menses and oocyte function are closely related, it is possible to have menstrual cycles without follicle development and release of an oocyte. This condition is known as an anovulatory cycle and is a result of disruption in the hypothalamus–pituitary–ovarian axis. Thus, resumption of menses after therapy is not always a reliable indicator of ovarian reserve. A female childhood cancer survivor could experience POI in her teenage years, in her 20s, or in her 30s, depending on her treatment regimen.[15] Current risk assessment aims to predict who will undergo POI at the youngest ages to provide tissue preservation opportunities.

Treatment-Related Factors

Surgery
Surgery is a mainstay of cancer therapy in pediatric and young adult patients for many diagnoses. Surgery involving removal of gonadal tissue or reproductive organs may impact future fertility and the ability to have one's own biological child. Certainly, males who require bilateral orchiectomy will no longer produce sperm and will not be able to sire a pregnancy. More common is the removal of 1 testis, in which case the remaining testis will continue sperm production. Although the rate of sperm production will now be roughly 50% of prior, it is unlikely to affect fertility.[16] Males are also at risk of nerve damage during abdominal surgery, most commonly with retroperitoneal lymph node dissection.[17] These patients have impaired ejaculation, but may continue to produce normal sperm that can be extracted by testicular sperm extraction (TESE) or aspiration.

As with male patients, it is rare for the treatment of childhood and adolescent cancer in females to require bilateral oophorectomy. Should this be the case, the ability to conceive a biological child would be lost. In cases of planned bilateral oophorectomy, patients may have the option to undergo ovarian stimulation and oocyte retrieval before surgery or to have a small portion of ovarian tissue cryopreserved based on an intraoperative assessment of the surgical specimen. The removal of 1 ovary does decrease the oocyte pool for that individual, theoretically increasing the risk of POI. Because of compensatory mechanisms in the remaining ovary, to date it is unclear if removing 1 ovary decreases the remaining oocyte pool to any clinically significant degree.[18]

Radiation therapy
Male gonadal tissue is exquisitely sensitive to damage from RT.[9] Doses of more than 4 Gy to the testes are likely to result in permanent azoospermia. Even as little as 2 Gy may cause abnormalities with low sperm counts or abnormal function that are unlikely to recover.[9,19]

Ovarian tissue is also quite sensitive to RT. Prepubertal females do show some relative resistance to the effects of radiation, but permanent dysfunction can be seen with as little as 15 Gy. Postpubertal females are likely to see ovarian insufficiency with greater than 10 Gy[2,19] (**Fig. 1**).

Owing to the low dose thresholds at which permanent damage is seen, direct radiation to gonadal tissue is not necessary to experience severe dysfunction. Rather, scatter radiation alone can cause significant damage.[4] The use of proton radiation may help to limit the field of scatter radiation, but photon radiation still offers superior disease control under some circumstances and thus is still commonly used.[20]

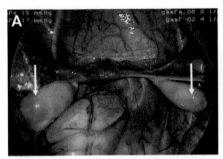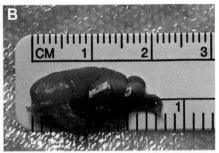

Fig. 1. (*A*) Ovarian tissue cryopreservation (OTC) in prepubertal girl. Note the follicles (*arrows*) on the ovarian cortical surface. (*B*) Size of unilateral oophorectomy specimen in 2.5-year-old girl.

Discussion with the treating radiation oncologist can help to predict the degree of scatter and potential exposure to gonadal tissues.

Chemotherapy

Multiagent chemotherapy remains the mainstay of cancer treatment for children and adolescents. Alkylating agents carry the greatest risk of gonadotoxicity and are the most widely studied.[21] The cyclophosphamide equivalent dose (CED) is discussed elsewhere in this article and was developed to help ascertain the risk of gonadotoxicity with cumulative doses of alkylating agents in pediatric and adolescent chemotherapy regimens. Guidelines recently published by the Pediatric Interest Network of the Oncofertility Consortium focus solely on this patient population. Males receiving a CED of more than 4 g/m^2 are at significant risk of permanent damage to Sertoli cells resulting in abnormal or absent sperm count. Doses of cisplatin of more than 500 mg/m^2 place males at risk of abnormal sperm motility or number.[8,19]

In postpubertal female patients, a cumulative CED of 4 g/m^2 increases the risk of POI significantly, and 8 g/m^2 will categorize a similar patient as at high risk of POI. As with RT, prepubertal females are relatively protected from gonadotoxic effects, with cumulative doses of 8 g/m^2 placing survivors at significant risk and more than 12 g/m^2 necessary to be categorized as being at high risk of POI.[12,19]

There is some preliminary evidence that anthracycline chemotherapy may increase the risk of gonadotoxicity, particularly in mouse models, but more investigation is needed before factoring this point into the patient risk assessment.[22] Likewise, newer classes of anticancer medications such as antibody therapy, immune-modulating agents, and targeted drug therapy are playing an increased role in the treatment of childhood and adolescent cancers, and their effects on fertility are not yet clear.

The effects of chemotherapy regimens (as in multiple treatment regimens with relapsed disease) and RT are additive when determining the risk of gonadotoxicity for any patient.[23,24] Patients undergoing stem cell transplantation are at high risk for gonadotoxicity and future infertility.[19] Many conditioning regimens contain high doses of alkylating agents with or without total body irradiation, particularly those for myeloablative conditioning. Patients receiving a reduced intensity conditioning regimen may have a less intense conditioning regimen and particular attention will need to be paid to the medications and dosages in use to assess the risk properly.

Risk Calculation Tools

Calculating the risk of gonadotoxicity and potential infertility from any cancer treatment is an evolving science. As the number of childhood and adolescent cancer survivors grows, so does the information regarding their outcomes and toxicities from prior therapy. In addition, as this population ages, the effect on biological reproduction becomes more apparent. There are several tools available to clinicians to aid in providing the most up-to-date information in counseling patients at the start of therapy and continuing into survivorship.

1. Cyclophosphamide equivalent dosing: The cumulative dosing of cyclophospha- mide and its relationship to gonadotoxicity has been well-established.[24] It is also established that alkylating agents, as a class of chemotherapy drugs, are gonado- toxic. However, dosing regimens for various alkylating agents are not interchange- able. Thus, Green and colleagues[24] developed the CED equation to standardize dosing regimens and allow universal risk stratification. Calculations can be done by hand using cumulative doses of various agents, or completed via an online calculator (https://fertilitypreservationpittsburgh.org/fertility-resources/fertility- risk-calculator/).
2. The Pediatric Interest Network of the Oncofertility Consortium recently published updated risk tables specific to the pediatric and adolescent population.[19] These ta- bles are specific to males and females and include radiation exposure.
3. There is an online calculator available to help determine the risk of acute ovarian failure published by Clark and colleagues.[14] This tool helps to predict which female patients will not recover ovarian function after therapy, as with high-dose alkylating agent chemotherapy or RT.
4. The International Guideline Harmonization Group has published evidence-based guidelines on who is at risk of gonadotoxicity, who should receive fertility preserva- tion counseling, and how to monitor survivors to aid practitioners and provide con- sistency in counseling this population.[21]

FERTILITY PRESERVATION OPTIONS STRATIFIED BY TREATMENT TIMING, PUBERTAL STATUS, AND SEX

The age and pubertal status of the pediatric patient are critical when considering fertility preservation options. The American Society for Reproductive Medicine (ASRM) released a committee statement in December 2019, which states that "ovarian tissue banking is an acceptable fertility-preservation technique and is no longer considered experimental."[25] This statement includes pediatric ovarian tissue cryopreservation (OTC), although leaders in pediatric fertility preservation continue to recommend treating prepubertal patients on investigational protocols.[26,27] Orga- nizing females and males based on age and pubertal status is a useful way to begin to examine the fertility preservation options (**Table 1**). Whenever possible, removal of ovarian tissue before the start of therapy ensures the healthiest and most numerous pool of primordial follicles.[15] For males undergoing testicular tissue cryo- preservation or postpubertal males, surgical tissue removal before the start of ther- apy results in the highest quality tissue for preservation, but tissue can have identifiable germ cells after chemotherapy, with a CED of more than 7 g/m^2 repre- senting the accepted cut-off point for sterility.[28] For both OTC and testicular tissue cryopreservation (TTC), chemotherapy may begin within 24 hours and RT in 5 to 7 days after surgery.

Prepubertal Males

Until the onset of puberty, males do not produce mature sperm. The only pretreatment option for males at significant risk of infertility is to undergo unilateral testicular biopsy for TTC. This option is experimental and has not produced any human live births to

Table 1
Gonadal tissue preservation options based on timing of treatment, sex, and pubertal status

		Before Treatment	During Treatment	After Treatment
Males[a]	Prepubertal	TTC	TTC	N/A
	Peripubertal	Sperm baking TESE TTC	TTC	N/A
	Postpubertal	Sperm banking TESE TTC[b]	TTC	TESE
Females[a]	Prepubertal	OTC	OTC	Oocyte harvest OTC
	Postpubertal	Oocyte harvest OTC	OTC	Oocyte harvest OTC

Abbreviations: N/A, not applicable; OTC, ovarian tissue cryopreservation; TTC, testicular tissue cryopreservation.
[a] Natal designation.
[b] If inadequate sperm specimen.

date. However, the recent report of a live birth from transplanted cryopreserved testicular tissue in a primate represents very promising scientific progress.[29] The testicle biopsy provides a source of spermatogonial stem cells for future maturation and reimplantation.[28,29] Typically, 0.5 cm³ of tissue is sufficient for cryopreservation and results in an acceptable cosmetic outcome, size, and growth of the remainder of the testicle (**Fig. 2**). The procedure has a very low complication risk and is most often combined with other necessary surgery or procedures requiring general anesthesia.[30]

Postpubertal Males

Sperm banking is always the first-choice option for fertility preservation in any male able to produce an adequate specimen. Compared with their female counterparts, males are much less likely to experience hormonal failure as a result of their therapy, so preserving sperm is satisfactory for future fertility. Unlike other fertility preservation options that can be performed in patients who have already received limited doses of chemotherapy, including alkylating agents, it is essential that sperm banking be performed before any therapy owing to the risk of DNA damage to any mature sperm that

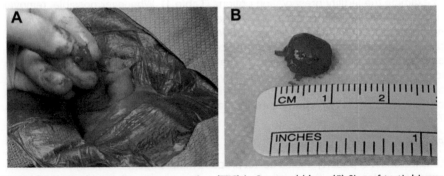

Fig. 2. (*A*) Testicular tissue cryopreservation (TTC) in 3-year-old boy. (*B*) Size of testis biopsy specimen in 3-year-old boy.

would be collected.[31] Predicting which patients will be able to produce an adequate specimen is challenging, but this option can be offered to any male who has reached Tanner 3 stage of development or has begun having nocturnal emissions. The next potential barrier is determining the child's familiarity with and comfort with masturbation. Streamlining this discussion through a dedicated fertility preservation clinician (nurse, advanced practice provider, or physician) with a fixed routine for this conversation can help to alleviate any patient discomfort about engaging in this discussion. For patients who are not able to produce a sperm sample, TTC for cryopreservation of testicular tissue and TESE for extraction and freezing of mature sperm are options.

Prepubertal Females

Until the onset of menarche, a female is considered prepubertal, and ovarian stimulation for oocyte cryopreservation (egg freezing) is not an option for fertility preservation. For these patients, the only pretreatment fertility preservation option is OTC, typically under a combined anesthesia for another needed medical procedure and involving unilateral oophorectomy by laparoscopic approach.[32] A patient can typically recover from the surgery and begin chemotherapy within 24 hours and begin RT within 5 to 7 days. If the therapy needs to begin imminently and time does not allow for surgery before beginning therapy, then the OTC may be scheduled after 1 or 2 rounds of therapy, possibly in combination with interim procedures that may require general anesthesia and before the patient approaches gonadotoxic doses of therapy.

For girls who are unable to harvest oocytes before chemotherapy initiation, including those who undergo OTC, there may be an option for harvesting oocytes in the late teen or early adult years when their remaining ovarian reserve is at its maximum. Although this post-therapy fertility preservation option should not preclude appropriate upfront fertility preservation counseling, it can be considered as an adult for survivors of pediatric cancer who want to maximize their options for future pregnancy.

Postpubertal Females

For a teenage or young adult patient who has achieved menarche, ovarian stimulation for mature oocyte cryopreservation (egg freezing) is recommended if possible, and the ASRM advocates this method as the most reliable way to preserve fertility.[25] However, many postpubertal females cannot delay the start of therapy for the approximately 2 weeks needed for hormone stimulation before egg retrieval. In addition, this fertility preservation option preserves fertility, but does not provide an option for the restoration of hormone function in the future. For some patients, both egg freezing and OTC are options and can be done in sequence, which provides the maximum range of fertility preservation options. Thorough fertility preservation counseling for postpubertal patients and families should include a discussion of these options and the opportunity to do both if time and patient circumstances allow, especially now that OTC is no longer considered experimental by ASRM. Counseling should include an explanation of the need for a transvaginal ultrasound examination and needle retrieval for egg freezing, because these procedures may be challenging for some teenagers. For patients who undergo OTC, the procedure can be combined with other necessary surgery or procedures under 1 anesthetic exposure. The Fertility and Hormone Preservation and Restoration team at Lurie Children's in Chicago advocates laparoscopic unilateral oophorectomy to provide high-quality ovarian tissue for long-term storage and for the most reliable hemostasis, with a minimal impact on the patient's own innate ovarian function as the remaining ovary compensates.[18,33,34]

UNIQUE CONSIDERATIONS IN PEDIATRIC FERTILITY PRESERVATION
Success of Sperm Banking in Adolescent Males

Sperm banking is the preferred approach for fertility preservation in any male patient who is able to provide an ejaculated semen specimen before the initiation of chemotherapy. This process must take into account both the physical and emotional maturity of the patient, as well as the religious and cultural views of the family. However, with the proper fertility counseling resources, the chances of successful sperm cryopreservation can be maximized. Providers often underestimate the chance of successful sperm cryopreservation, and these biases or preconceptions should not interfere with offering and encouraging this option.

Sperm banking continues to be underused in adolescent male patients. A Canadian study found that fewer than 25% of eligible male adolescents attempt to bank sperm.[35] In a survey of pediatric oncology providers, only 46% reported they refer male pubertal patients with cancer to a fertility specialist before cancer treatment more than 50% of the time.[36] More encouragingly, in a French multicenter study, it was noted that referrals for sperm banking increased 9.5% annually from 1973 to 2007.[37] Additionally, the percentage of younger patients with cancer who cryopreserved sperm increased, particularly in the 11- to 14-year-old age group, where it increased from 1% in 1986 to 9% in 2006. With a continued emphasis on the importance of fertility preservation counseling and services, this use will hopefully continue to increase.

Efforts to increase the use of sperm cryopreservation techniques require providers to better understand the factors predictive of successful banking attempts. The age range of pubertal development varies widely, and patients who have begun having nocturnal emissions or reached Tanner stage 3 should be offered this option, even if they are at a younger chronologic age. In a multi-institutional study of 146 male patients surveyed at the start of chemotherapy, meeting with a fertility specialist (odds ratio [OR], 3.44), parent (OR, 3.02) or provider (OR, 2.67) recommendation to bank, and greater adolescent self-efficacy to bank (OR, 1.16) were associated with successful sperm banking.[38] They also found that banking was successful in 23% of Tanner stage 3, 31% of Tanner stage 4, and 52% of Tanner stage 5 patients. It was also successful in 40% of patients who denied a history of nocturnal emission and 15% of patients who denied a history of masturbation. In another study of 80 males aged 13 to 19 years, 84% were able to produce semen by masturbation and 66% had adequate quality for cryopreservation.[39] A follow-up report of 114 males from the same institution reported a 93% rate of semen production by masturbation and 68% rate of successful sperm cryopreservation.[40] Among 11 patients with a median Tanner stage of 3 who were unable to produce an ejaculated specimen by masturbation, 100% had successful cryopreservation after electroejaculation in the this study.

The Role of Hybrid Testicular Tissue Cryopreservation and Testicular Sperm Extraction in Peripubertal Males Unable to Sperm Bank or Those Who Produce an Inadequate Specimen

A hybrid approach to fertility preservation is often beneficial for peripubertal males. It is not uncommon for these efforts to produce an oligospermatic specimen or even be unsuccessful in their attempt at banking. The sperm is stored in aliquot vials with each vial representing 1 opportunity for future insemination. We recommend consideration of additional fertility preservation interventions to males unable to store 5 to 10 good vials of sperm. For peripubertal males who are likely to have mature sperm in the testicle but are unable to produce a semen sample, TTC can be combined with TESE. These patients are typically Tanner stage 3 to 4, with testicular volumes large enough to allow taking a 1.0 × 0.5-cm wedge for TTC plus a similar size wedge for sperm extraction through the same incision. This hybrid approach ensures that all future restoration options using spermatogonial stem cells remain available to the patient, while also maximizing the opportunity to store mature sperm for in vitro fertilization.

The Role of Gonadotropin-Releasing Hormone Agonists in Female Fertility Preservation

The role of ovarian suppression with gonadotropin-releasing hormone agonists during chemotherapy to help preserve fertility and prevent ovarian failure remains controversial.[41] A meta-analysis of adults with early stage breast cancer demonstrated that patients who received gonadotropin-releasing hormone agonist therapy had their risk of POI decreased by one-half ($P<.001$).[42] However, in a randomized trial of young patients with lymphoma after 5 years of clinical follow-up, there was no difference in the rate of primary ovarian failure or pregnancy rate in the treatment and control groups.[43] The ASRM practice guidelines indicate that gonadotropin-releasing hormone analogs may be given to select patients with breast cancer, but should not be used in place of other fertility preservation measures.[25]

The Usefulness of Ovarian Transposition

Ovarian transposition is a consideration for girls receiving radiation to the pelvis. Transposition can be permanent or temporary. The standard approach for girls undergoing pelvic radiation involves transposition of the ovary to the paracolic gutters with the division of the ligamentous attachments.[44] The effect of dividing these attachments and relocating the tube and ovary out of the pelvis on future fertility is poorly understood. In some cases, relocation back to the pelvis after therapy completion is performed. Alternatively, temporary transposition for the short duration of treatment for girls receiving brachytherapy can be achieved without division of the ligamentous attachments using a laparoscopic approach.[45] A transcutaneous suture is used to fixate the ovary to the abdominal wall as far out of the pelvis as possible and the suture is cut after completion of therapy to allow the ovary to fall back into the pelvis.

Ovarian transposition has been reported in at least 37 patients from 6 studies in patients under the age of 20.[46] One study reported 4 associated complications, including small bowel obstruction, dyspareunia, and pelvic adhesions causing tubal obstruction.[47] Despite the sound logic behind moving the ovary out of the radiation field, the benefit of transposition for decreasing the risk of ovarian failure or infertility is unproven. In fact, in patients who received pelvic RT for Hodgkin's lymphoma, ovarian transposition did not seem to modify the risk of ovarian insufficiency.[48]

FUTURE DIRECTIONS IN PEDIATRIC OVARIAN TISSUE CRYOPRESERVATION
Optimal Surgical Approach for Pediatric Ovarian Tissue Cryopreservation

For female patients undergoing OTC, debate exists over the optimal extent of the ovarian harvest procedure. A recent systematic review found that 57% of patients underwent total oophorectomy and 43% had partial oophorectomy.[46] Advocates for unilateral oophorectomy cite (1) a potential improved safety profile, (2) the maximization of the amount of cortical tissue for cryopreservation and future reimplantation, and (3) evidence that unilateral oophorectomy is not associated with reduced fertility or premature menopause.[32] The cut surface on the ovary for partial oophorectomy is a potential source of hemorrhagic complications, which are avoided with unilateral oophorectomy. The few reported cases of postoperative bleeding requiring transfusion or re-exploration occurred in patients who had undergone partial oophorectomy.[46] Furthermore, when cortical strips are reimplanted, the duration of fertility restoration is limited. Preserving multiple cortical strips from the entire ovary allows for multiple attempts at reimplantation, as well as repeat reimplantation if the hormonal restoration effect abates. The rate of pregnancy after reimplantation is 29% and live birth rate is 23% based on the most reliable data from 5 major centers published in a 2017 review.[49] In a review of 210 women who underwent ovarian transplantation, 170 of which were from their own frozen ovarian tissue, more than 78% achieved restoration of ovarian function.[50] However, the duration of the restored ovarian function was quite variable, ranging from less than 1 year to more than 5 years. In a systematic review of worldwide data on transplantation of thawed ovarian tissue, 360 ovarian transplant procedures were performed in 318 women. In this review, endocrine function was restored in 95% of those for whom data were available, and 131 pregnancies were achieved in 95 patients, with a total of 93 children born to 69 women. This review also noted that the youngest reported patient to undergo OTC with tissue use was 9 years of age, and that younger patients (average, 26.4 years; range, 9–38 years) who underwent OTC were more likely to succeed in having a live birth than older patients.[51]

With regard to the effect of unilateral oophorectomy on ovarian reserve, a systematic review and meta-analysis compared the success of assisted reproduction in women who had undergone unilateral oophorectomy with those with 2 ovaries. It found a comparable overall weighted odds of clinical pregnancy, although those who had undergone oophorectomy demonstrated evidence of decreased ovarian reserve.[52] In a population-based study from Norway, women who had undergone unilateral oophorectomy progressed through menopause only 1 year earlier than those with both ovaries.[18]

Proponents of partial oophorectomy cite the principle of "first do no harm" and emphasize the importance of preserving a maximal amount of native ovarian reserve. There are no data to suggest that women with ovarian tissue exposed to gonadotoxic chemotherapy have a higher chance of spontaneous pregnancy after partial compared with total oophorectomy. Further work is required to determine the optimal surgical approach, which may vary based on the exact treatment regimen. For females whose treatment includes very high CEDs and significant pelvic radiation, which places them at extremely high risk of infertility and premature ovarian failure, unilateral oophorectomy maximizes the options for fertility and hormone restoration while minimizing surgical risks. However, for those females whose treatment places them at a more modest risk of infertility, there may be an advantage to preserving as much native ovarian function as possible. This goal must be balanced against increasing evidence of successful restoration of endocrine and fertility function from OTC. The long-term effects on fertility and hormone restoration are required to determine if the theoretic benefits of partial oophorectomy outweigh the potential increased surgical complication rate and decreased volume of stored tissue compared with unilateral oophorectomy.

Optimal Processing Technique for Prepubertal Ovarian Tissue Cryopreservation

The protocols for processing pediatric ovarian tissue for OTC use the same technique established for adult patients.[53] The process involves thinning the ovarian tissue while removing the medullary region, where growing follicles are located, while preserving the cortical region, where the primordial follicles exist in dense stroma. The thinning process allows cryoprotectant to penetrate the tissue, which is then cut into cortical strips that are stored in individual vials so that they may be thawed individually in the future. The prepubertal ovary is fundamentally different from the postpubertal ovary because it is much smaller, typically 1 to 2 cm^2, and lacks a clear cortical–medullary junction.[53] In postpubertal patients, the tissue processing involves thinning the cortex with a tissue slicer, and then cutting the tissue into cortical strips that are stored in individual vials so that they may be thawed individually in the future. Our experience with processing ovarian tissue from prepubertal patients has revealed that primordial follicles exist within the tissue fragments of OTC processing media, which does not occur in media processed from adult patients and is thought to only contain the medullary regions **(Fig. 3)**. More research is required to optimize the technique for processing in an effort to preserve the most primordial follicles that could restore both fertility and hormones in these pediatric patients once transplanted. Although the main objective in OTC is to preserve the ovarian cortex, which contains the majority of primordial follicles or ovarian reserve, during the tissue processing, small antral follicles in the medulla are disrupted and cumulus oocyte complexes are released into the media.[54,55] In a process referred to as ex vivo in vitro maturation, these cumulus oocyte complexes can be recovered and matured in vitro to obtain eggs arrested at metaphase of meiosis II, which may be possible to cryopreserve for future use.[27]

SUMMARY AND FUTURE DIRECTIONS

Advances in clinical pediatric oncology care leading to dramatically improved survival now present challenges of long-term quality-of-life issues in survivorship, including fertility and hormone function. Multicenter data will be essential to refine the risk assessment for future pediatric patients based on the outcomes of adult patients who had gonadal tissue preservation before gonadotoxic therapy compared with those who did not. Further research into fertility and hormone restoration options and outcomes is necessary for adult survivors of childhood cancer who underwent gonadal tissue preservation. Surgeons caring for pediatric patients with cancer can remain knowledgeable advocates in fertility preservation, incorporate fertility preservation options pretreatment or early in treatment, and perform procedures to preserve pediatric ovarian and testicular tissue when safe and necessary for those children at most significant risk of infertility.

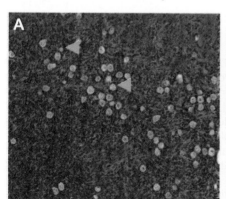 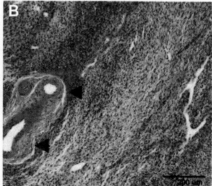

Fig. 3. Tissue fragments collected from OTC processing media. (*A*) A 7-year-old girl with no previous treatment, containing primordial follicles (*green arrow*) and (*B*) a 21-year-old woman with no previous treatment, containing stroma and vessels (*black arrow*) (indicating medullary tissue without ovarian reserve).

CLINICS CARE POINTS

- Fertility preservation options exist for both prepubertal and postpubertal males and females.
- A fertility consultation should be offered to the families of all children receiving therapies that place them at increased risk for infertility or premature hormonal failure, and standardized risk assessment tools exist to help quantify this risk.
- There are both nonexperimental (oocyte harvest, OTC, sperm cryopreservation) and experimental (testicular tissue cryopreservation) options for fertility preservation, depending on the patient's sex and pubertal status.

DISCLOSURE

The authors have no commercial or financial conflicts of interest to disclose. The authors have no sources of funding to report.

REFERENCES

1. Cocuzza M, Alvarenga C, Pagani R. The epidemiology and etiology of azoospermia. Clinics (Sao Paulo) 2013;68(Suppl 1):15–26.
2. Green DM, Kawashima T, Stovall M, et al. Fertility of female survivors of childhood cancer: a report from the childhood cancer survivor study. J Clin Oncol 2009; 27(16):2677–85.
3. Green DM, Kawashima T, Stovall M, et al. Fertility of male survivors of childhood cancer: a report from the Childhood Cancer Survivor Study. J Clin Oncol 2010;28(2):332–9.
4. van Dorp W, Haupt R, Anderson RA, et al. Reproductive function and outcomes in female survivors of childhood, adolescent, and young adult cancer: a review. J Clin Oncol 2018;36(21):2169–80.
5. Robison LL, Hudson MM. Survivors of childhood and adolescent cancer: life-long risks and responsibilities. Nat Rev Cancer 2014;14(1):61–70.
6. Ellis SJ, Wakefield CE, McLoone JK, et al. Fertility concerns among child and adolescent cancer survivors and their parents: a qualitative analysis. J Psychosoc Oncol 2016;34(5):347–62.
7. Klosky JL, Simmons JL, Russell KM, et al. Fertility as a priority among at-risk adolescent males newly diagnosed with cancer and their parents. Support Care Cancer 2015;23(2):333–41.
8. Green DM, Liu W, Kutteh WH, et al. Cumulative alkylating agent exposure and semen parameters in adult survivors of childhood cancer: a report from the St Jude Lifetime Cohort Study. Lancet Oncol 2014;15(11):1215–23.
9. Kenney LB, Antal Z, Ginsberg JP, et al. Improving male reproductive health after childhood, adolescent, and young adult cancer: progress and future directions for survivorship research. J Clin Oncol 2018;36(21):2160–8.
10. Chemaitilly W, Liu Q, van Iersel L, et al. Leydig cell function in male survivors of childhood cancer: a report from the St Jude Lifetime Cohort study. J Clin Oncol 2019;37(32):3018–31.
11. Wallace WH, Kelsey TW. Human ovarian reserve from conception to the menopause. PLoS One 2010;5(1):e8772.
12. Levine JM, Whitton JA, Ginsberg JP, et al. Nonsurgical premature menopause and reproductive implications in survivors of childhood cancer: a report from the Childhood Cancer Survivor Study. Cancer 2018;124(5):1044–52.

13. Johnston RJ, Wallace WH. Normal ovarian function and assessment of ovarian reserve in the survivor of childhood cancer. Pediatr Blood Cancer 2009;53(2): 296–302.

14. Clark RA, Mostoufi-Moab S, Yasui Y, et al. Predicting acute ovarian failure in female survivors of childhood cancer: a cohort study in the Childhood Cancer Survivor Study (CCSS) and the St Jude Lifetime Cohort (SJLIFE). Lancet Oncol 2020; 21(3):436–45.

15. Wallace WH, Smith AG, Kelsey TW, et al. Fertility preservation for girls and young women with cancer: population-based validation of criteria for ovarian tissue cryopreservation. Lancet Oncol 2014;15(10):1129–36.

16. Ferreira U, Netto Junior NR, Esteves SC, et al. Comparative study of the fertility potential of men with only one testis. Scand J Urol Nephrol 1991;25(4):255–9.

17. Hudson MM. Reproductive outcomes for survivors of childhood cancer. Obstet Gynecol 2010;116(5):1171–83.

18. Bjelland EK, Wilkosz P, Tanbo TG, et al. Is unilateral oophorectomy associated with age at menopause? A population study (the HUNT2 Survey). Hum Reprod 2014;29(4):835–41.

19. Meacham LR, Burns K, Orwig KE, et al. Standardizing risk assessment for treatment-related gonadal insufficiency and infertility in childhood adolescent and young adult cancer: the pediatric initiative network risk stratification system. J Adolesc Young Adult Oncol 2020. https://doi.org/10.1089/jayao.2020.0012.

20. Proton Beam Therapy versus Photon Radiotherapy for Adult and Pediatric Oncology Patients: A Review of the Clinical and Cost-Effectiveness [Internet]. Ottawa (ON): Canadian Agency for Drugs and Technologies in Health; 2016 May 20. SUMMARY OF EVIDENCE. Available at: https://www.ncbi.nlm.nih.gov/books/NBK368355/.

21. Skinner R, Mulder RL, Kremer LC, et al. Recommendations for gonadotoxicity surveillance in male childhood, adolescent, and young adult cancer survivors: a report from the International Late Effects of Childhood Cancer Guideline Harmonization Group in collaboration with the PanCareSurFup Consortium. Lancet Oncol 2017;18(2):e75–90.

22. Xiao S, Zhang J, Liu M, et al. Doxorubicin has dose-dependent toxicity on mouse ovarian follicle development, hormone secretion, and oocyte maturation. Toxicol Sci 2017;157(2):320–9.

23. Vakalopoulos I, Dimou P, Anagnostou I, et al. Impact of cancer and cancer treatment on male fertility. Hormones (Athens) 2015;14(4):579–89.

24. Green DM, Nolan VG, Goodman PJ, et al. The cyclophosphamide equivalent dose as an approach for quantifying alkylating agent exposure: a report from the Childhood Cancer Survivor Study. Pediatr Blood Cancer 2014;61(1):53–67.

25. Practice Committee of the American Society for Reproductive Medicine. Electronic address AAO. Fertility preservation in patients undergoing gonadotoxic therapy or gonadectomy: a committee opinion. Fertil Steril 2019;112(6):1022–33.

26. Nahata L, Woodruff TK, Quinn GP, et al. Ovarian tissue cryopreservation as standard of care: what does this mean for pediatric populations? J Assist Reprod Genet 2020;37(6):1323–6.

27. Rowell EEDF, Laronda MM. ASRM removes the experimental label from ovarian tissue cryopreservation (OTC): pediatric research must continue. Fertility and Sterility 2020. Available at: https://www.fertstertdialog.com/posts/asrm-removes-the-experimental-label-from-ovarian-tissue-cryopreservation-otc-pediatric-research-must-continue. Accessed July 20, 2020.

28. Valli-Pulaski H, Peters KA, Gassei K, et al. Testicular tissue cryopreservation: 8 years of experience from a coordinated network of academic centers. Hum Reprod 2019;34(6):966–77.

29. Fayomi AP, Peters K, Sukhwani M, et al. Autologous grafting of cryopreserved prepubertal rhesus testis produces sperm and offspring. Science 2019; 363(6433):1314–9.

30. Corkum KS, Lautz TB, Johnson EK, et al. Testicular wedge biopsy for fertility preservation in children at significant risk for azoospermia after gonadotoxic therapy. J Pediatr Surg 2019;54(9):1901–5.

31. Beaud H, Tremblay AR, Chan PTK, et al. Sperm DNA damage in cancer patients. Adv Exp Med Biol 2019;1166:189–203.

32. Rowell EE, Corkum KS, Lautz TB, et al. Laparoscopic unilateral oophorectomy for ovarian tissue cryopreservation in children. J Pediatr Surg 2019;54(3):543–9.

33. Corkum KS, Laronda MM, Rowell EE. A review of reported surgical techniques in fertility preservation for prepubertal and adolescent females facing a fertility threatening diagnosis or treatment. Am J Surg 2017;214(4):695–700.

34. Rowell EE, Corkum KS, Even KA, et al. Ovarian tissue health after laparoscopic unilateral oophorectomy: a porcine model for establishing optimized fertility preservation techniques in children. J Pediatr Surg 2020;55(8):1631–8.

35. Chong AL, Gupta A, Punnett A, et al. A cross Canada survey of sperm banking practices in pediatric oncology centers. Pediatr Blood Cancer 2010;55(7): 1356–61.

36. Kohler TS, Kondapalli LA, Shah A, et al. Results from the survey for preservation of adolescent reproduction (SPARE) study: gender disparity in delivery of fertility preservation message to adolescents with cancer. J Assist Reprod Genet 2011; 28(3):269–77.

37. Daudin M, Rives N, Walschaerts M, et al. Sperm cryopreservation in adolescents and young adults with cancer: results of the French national sperm banking network (CECOS). Fertil Steril 2015;103(2):478–486 e471.

38. Klosky JL, Lehmann V, Flynn JS, et al. Patient factors associated with sperm cryopreservation among at-risk adolescents newly diagnosed with cancer. Cancer 2018;124(17):3567–75.

39. van Casteren NJ, Dohle GR, Romijn JC, et al. Semen cryopreservation in pubertal boys before gonadotoxic treatment and the role of endocrinologic evaluation in predicting sperm yield. Fertil Steril 2008;90(4):1119–25.

40. Adank MC, van Dorp W, Smit M, et al. Electroejaculation as a method of fertility preservation in boys diagnosed with cancer: a single-center experience and review of the literature. Fertil Steril 2014;102(1):199–205 e1.

41. Blumenfeld Z. Fertility preservation using GnRH agonists: rationale, possible mechanisms, and explanation of controversy. Clin Med Insights Reprod Health 2019;13. 1179558119870163.

42. Lambertini M, Moore HCF, Leonard RCF, et al. Gonadotropin-releasing hormone agonists during chemotherapy for preservation of ovarian function and fertility in premenopausal patients with early breast cancer: a systematic review and meta-analysis of individual patient-level data. J Clin Oncol 2018;36(19):1981–90.

43. Demeestere I, Brice P, Peccatori FA, et al. No evidence for the benefit of gonadotropin-releasing hormone agonist in preserving ovarian function and fertility in lymphoma survivors treated with chemotherapy: final long-term report of a prospective randomized trial. J Clin Oncol 2016;34(22):2568–74.

44. Moawad NS, Santamaria E, Rhoton-Vlasak A, et al. Laparoscopic ovarian transposition before pelvic cancer treatment: ovarian function and fertility preservation. J Minim Invasive Gynecol 2017;24(1):28–35.

45. de Lambert G, Haie-Meder C, Guerin F, et al. A new surgical approach of temporary ovarian transposition for children undergoing brachytherapy: technical assessment and dose evaluation. J Pediatr Surg 2014;49(7):1177–80.

46. Corkum KS, Rhee DS, Wafford QE, et al. Fertility and hormone preservation and restoration for female children and adolescents receiving gonadotoxic cancer treatments: a systematic review. J Pediatr Surg 2019;54(11):2200–9.

47. Thibaud E, Ramirez M, Brauner R, et al. Preservation of ovarian function by ovarian transposition performed before pelvic irradiation during childhood. J Pediatr 1992;121(6):880–4.

48. Fernandez-Pineda I, Davidoff AM, Lu L, et al. Impact of ovarian transposition before pelvic irradiation on ovarian function among long-term survivors of childhood Hodgkin lymphoma: a report from the St. Jude Lifetime Cohort Study. Pediatr Blood Cancer 2018;65(9):e27232.

49. Donnez J, Dolmans MM. Fertility preservation in women. N Engl J Med 2017; 377(17):1657–65.

50. Sheshpari S, Shahnazi M, Mobarak H, et al. Ovarian function and reproductive outcome after ovarian tissue transplantation: a systematic review. J Transl Med 2019;17(1):396.

51. Gellert SE, Pors SE, Kristensen SG, et al. Transplantation of frozen-thawed ovarian tissue: an update on worldwide activity published in peer-reviewed papers and on the Danish cohort. J Assist Reprod Genet 2018;35(4):561–70.

52. Younis JS, Naoum I, Salem N, et al. The impact of unilateral oophorectomy on ovarian reserve in assisted reproduction: a systematic review and meta-analysis. BJOG 2018;125(1):26–35.

53. Rosendahl M, Schmidt KT, Ernst E, et al. Cryopreservation of ovarian tissue for a decade in Denmark: a view of the technique. Reprod Biomed Online 2011;22(2): 162–71.

54. Segers I, Mateizel I, Van Moer E, et al. In vitro maturation (IVM) of oocytes recovered from ovariectomy specimens in the laboratory: a promising "ex vivo" method of oocyte cryopreservation resulting in the first report of an ongoing pregnancy in Europe. J Assist Reprod Genet 2015;32(8):1221–31.

55. Yin H, Jiang H, Kristensen SG, et al. Vitrification of in vitro matured oocytes collected from surplus ovarian medulla tissue resulting from fertility preservation of ovarian cortex tissue. J Assist Reprod Genet 2016;33(6):741–6.

Minimally Invasive Techniques in Pediatric Surgical Oncology

Marc W.H. Wijnen, MD[a], Andrew M. Davidoff, MD[b],*

KEYWORDS

- Minimally invasive surgery • Laparoscopy • Thoracoscopy • Pediatric cancer
- Solid tumors

KEY POINTS

- Minimally invasive approaches to pediatric cancer surgery are increasingly used, not only for the benefits of smaller incisions, but also for better field visualization and precise dissection.
- Advances in technology and surgeon experience have facilitated this trend.
- However, the appropriate indications for its use remain to be determined, and oncologic principles should not be compromised.

INTRODUCTION

Classically, minimally invasive surgery (MIS) refers to surgical techniques that limit the size of incisions to access a body cavity or specific anatomic region. However, many other advantages of MIS are being appreciated. These advantages include better visualization of the surgical field, potentially more precise dissection, and less disruption of normal tissue.

MIS use has markedly increased over the last 2 decades and is now widely applied in adult and pediatric general surgery. More recently, MIS has been increasingly used in pediatric surgical oncology.[1,2] The traditionally espoused benefits of MIS include smaller incisions, resulting in a better cosmetic outcome; smaller wounds and therefore less postoperative pain, translating into shorter hospital stays; a more rapid return to regular activities; and, importantly for patients with cancer, the opportunity to begin adjuvant therapy more quickly. Another theoretic benefit of MIS is a decreased incidence of bowel adhesions, a surgical complication that can be quite problematic, particularly when surgery is combined with other treatment modalities such as

[a] Department of Surgery, Princess Maxima Center, Heidelberglaan 25, 3584 CS Utrecht, Netherlands; [b] Department of Surgery, St. Jude Children's Research Hospital, 262 Danny Thomas Place, Memphis, TN 38105, USA
* Corresponding author.
E-mail address: Andrew.Davidoff@STJUDE.ORG

Surg Oncol Clin N Am 30 (2021) 417–430
https://doi.org/10.1016/j.soc.2020.11.008
1055-3207/21/© 2020 Elsevier Inc. All rights reserved.

radiation therapy. MIS may also provide immunologic advantages because there is less tissue trauma. Finally, visualization of the operative field with a laparoscope or thoracoscope is often enhanced for some locations, particularly deep in the pelvis and apex of the chest cavity. However, the advantage of tactile sense for localization is lost. Importantly, the conduct and goals of operations that are consistent with an open approach should not be compromised when using a minimally invasive approach.

Early reports described the use of MIS in pediatric patients with cancer for performing biopsies, staging solid tumors, assessing tumor resectability, and evaluating and potentially resecting metastatic disease.[3,4] Shortly thereafter, a randomized clinical trial sponsored by the National Institutes of Health was conducted to assess the efficacy and safety of MIS as compared with standard open approaches for surgical procedures in children with cancer. However, the trial closed early, primarily because of a lack of patient accrual. The reasons for poor accrual included a lack of buy-in by pediatric oncologists, a lack of surgical expertise with MIS procedures, and a preconceived surgeon bias toward either endoscopic or traditional open approaches.[5] Additional theoretic concerns, which were largely unfounded, regarding tumor cell disbursement with insufflation and port site recurrence also contributed to the poor accrual. In addition to these issues, performing MIS in pediatric patients without appropriately sized instrumentation was technically challenging. Finally, anesthesia had and still does introduce challenges, including the requirement for lung collapse for most thoracoscopic procedures, abdominal insufflation pushing the diaphragm up, and CO_2 diffusion from insufflation resulting in hypercapnia. Finally, the need to remove tumors intact often necessitates a large incision, negating some of the benefits of MIS. The limited tactile feedback of MIS may also be important when trying to locate small lesions, particularly for metastatic lesions in the lungs.

More recently, Cecchetto and colleagues,[6] representing the Italian Group of Pediatric Surgical Oncology, made recommendations on the use of MIS for pediatric solid tumors. The basic operative principles of open pediatric cancer surgery should be followed during the conduct of the operation. Tumor spill and positive margins should be avoided, particularly in tumor types in which an R0 resection is critical for good oncologic outcomes. Lymph node dissection or sampling should still be performed when indicated. Additionally, the authors discussed a number of histology-specific considerations, such as removing intact Wilms tumors intact (in contrast with neuroblastoma tumors, which can be removed piecemeal), and purpose-specific considerations for biopsies, staging, or therapeutic solid tumor resections.

Spurbeck and colleagues[7] described the early pediatric oncology experience with MIS at St. Jude Children's Research Hospital. This experience was updated more recently by Abdelhafeez and colleagues[8] Over nearly 20 years, more than 350 minimally invasive procedures were performed. Thirty-eight percent were laparoscopic and 62% were thoracoscopic. Of all abdominal procedures, only 15% were performed with a minimally invasive approach, whereas more than one-half of chest procedures were performed with a minimally invasive approach. The majority of these procedures (60%) were performed for diagnostic purposes. Approximately 25% of these procedures were performed to resect primary solid tumors and 17% were performed for adjuvant or supportive indications for disease or treatment-related complications (ie, cholecystectomy, gastrostomy tube placement or fundoplication, splenectomy, or oophoropexy for female patients before receiving pelvic irradiation). Of the therapeutic resections in the abdominal cavity, approximately two-thirds were performed for neuroblastic tumors and one-third were performed for germ cell tumors. Of the therapeutic resections performed with a thoracoscopic approach, most were for metastatic nodules in the lung; a few were for neuroblastic tumors in the chest and germ cell tumors.

THE ROLE OF MINIMALLY INVASIVE SURGERY IN SPECIFIC PEDIATRIC SOLID TUMORS

The usefulness and appropriateness of MIS in the management of pediatric solid tumors is very much tumor histology dependent. The following is an overview of the role of MIS in the most common pediatric solid tumors and scenarios (**Table 1**).

Adrenal Tumors

Most adrenal tumors in children are neuroblastic tumors, although differential diagnoses may include adrenocortical tumors and pheochromocytomas. The goals of surgery differ depending on the suspected histology. For neuroblastic tumors, the goals can be variable, but margin-negative, R0 resections are never required (and often not feasible). In most circumstances, even gross tumor can be left behind without compromising oncologic outcomes. MIS is commonly used for resection of L1 tumors (ie, no encasement of major blood vessels or other image-defined risk factors) (**Fig. 1**). For neuroblastic tumors with 1 or more preoperative image-defined risk

Table 1 Appropriate use of MIS for pediatric solid tumors	
Tumor	**Appropriateness of MIS**
Adrenal	
Neuroblastic tumors	
Image-defined risk factors absent (L1)	Yes
Image-defined risk factor present (L2)	Depends on surgeon skill/experience
Adrenocortical tumors	
Likely malignant	Rarely
Likely benign	Yes
Renal tumors	
Nephrectomy	Rarely and usually only after neoadjuvant chemotherapy
Partial nephrectomy	Rarely and usually only after neoadjuvant chemotherapy or small lesion detected on screening
Ovarian tumors	
Likely malignant	Yes, oophorectomy
Likely benign	Yes, ovary sparing
Rhabdomyosarcoma	
Site dependent	Yes, for bladder dome primary, some retroperitoneal tumors
Retroperitoneal lymph node dissection	Yes
Lung metastases	
Diagnostic intent	Yes
Therapeutic intent	Uncertain

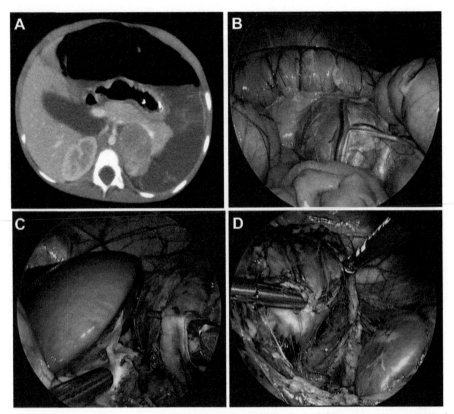

Fig. 1. Laparoscopic resection of a left adrenal neuroblastoma. (*A*) Preoperative computed tomography scan. (*B*) View of the tumor through the colon mesentery. (*C*) Isolation of the adrenal vein. (*D*) Elevation of the tumor from the left upper quadrant. (*Courtesy of* Harold N. Lovvorn, III, M.D).

factors (ie, L2 tumors), the role of MIS is uncertain because these tumors usually encase vital vascular structures. Because R0 resections are not required (or achievable) for L2 lesions, these tumors can be removed piecemeal and leave some residual disease behind. Therefore, some surgeons may undertake resections of L2 tumors, according to their experience and expertise, but most surgeons perform open resections of L2 tumors (**Fig. 2**).

Neuroblastic tumors can occur in the posterior mediastinum. These neoplasms are particularly well-suited for a thoracoscopic approach that avoids posterolateral thoracotomy, which, even with a muscle-sparing maneuver, may increase the risk of scoliosis development in pediatric patients. Tumors at the apex of the chest are particularly well-visualized with a thoracoscopic approach (**Fig. 3**). Thus, an increasing number of neuroblastic tumors are being removed with MIS.[9,10] Recently, Gurria and colleagues, along with the American Pediatric Surgery Cancer Committee published a comprehensive review of the role of MIS in the surgical management of neuroblastoma in children.[11]

Using MIS for neuroblastic tumors is in marked distinction to that for adrenocortical carcinomas (ACC) because adjuvant therapy is not very effective for ACC tumors and complete resection without spill or positive margins is critical for favorable oncologic

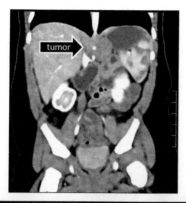
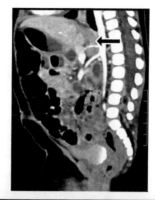

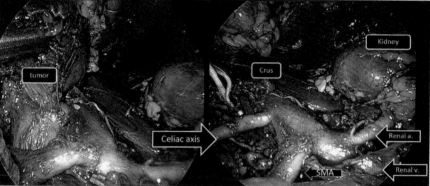

Fig. 2. Neuroblastoma with an image-defined risk factor (L2, encasement of the celiac axis) shown on coronal (*top, left*) and sagittal (*top, right*) views of the preoperative computed tomography scan. Laparoscopic mobilization of the tumor (*bottom, left*) and resection bed (*bottom, right*). (*Courtesy of* Harold N. Lovvorn, III, M.D.)

outcomes. Moreover, lymphadenectomy should be performed. Many studies now recommend that suspected ACC tumors should not be removed with a minimally invasive approach.[12,13] These are very friable tumors that can frequently rupture upon manipulation. Therefore, MIS should be discouraged when patients have an adrenal tumor and evidence of metastatic disease in the lung because such tumors are most likely ACCs. Other preoperative factors suggesting malignant tumors and thereby discouraging an MIS approach include large tumor size (>10 cm), local invasion, and lymph node involvement. However, minimally invasive approaches can generally be safely used for small, well-circumscribed, and most likely benign adrenal tumors. This approach can either be transperitoneal or retroperitoneal. MIS can also be used for the resection of pheochromocytomas after appropriate preoperative preparation and with careful intraoperative vascular control.

Renal Tumors

The most common renal tumor histology in children is a Wilms tumor, but other histologies include renal cell carcinomas, clear cell sarcomas of the kidney, rhabdoid tumors of the kidney, and mesoblastic nephromas. Uniformly, for all of these histologies the goal of surgery is complete resection, generally in the upfront setting, with negative margins and without tumor spill, and sampling of lymph nodes, even if

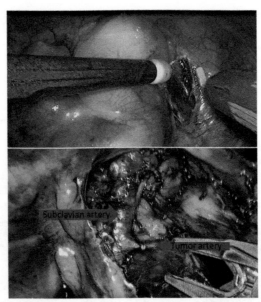

Fig. 3. Apical neuroblastoma before and after removal. (*Courtesy of* Hafeez Abdelhafeez, M.D.)

not apparently involved. This is especially important for Wilms tumor. Although not recommended by the Children's Oncology Group (COG) or the International Society for Pediatric Oncology, some surgeons elect to perform laparoscopic nephrectomies, particularly if the tumors are small and centrally located (and perhaps even surrounded by healthy kidney tissue).[14–16] A systematic review of MIS for pediatric renal tumors was published recently by Malek and the American Pediatric Surgical Association Cancer Committee.[17] Importantly, the recommended approach for treating Wilms tumors by the COG differs from that of the International Society for Pediatric Oncology. Specifically, the COG recommends upfront nephrectomy, whereas the International Society for Pediatric Oncology recommends nephrectomy after neoadjuvant chemotherapy. This difference affects the number of cases that may be amenable with a laparoscopic approach, with the International Society for Pediatric Oncology treatment strategy resulting in smaller, firmer tumors at the time of resection, which may be more suitable for an MIS approach.

Despite the enthusiasm for minimally invasive nephron-sparing surgery in adult patients with renal cell carcinoma, laparoscopic nephron-sparing surgery is rarely performed in children because of the risk of upstaging the tumors, thereby necessitating additional cytotoxic chemotherapy and radiation therapy.[18] Anatomically favorable (eg, polar or exophytic) pretreated tumors or small tumors found on surveillance imaging of syndromic patients may be the rare circumstance in which MIS may be attempted. However, Schmidt and colleagues[19] have suggested that, when a minimally invasive or open partial nephrectomy is considered, open partial nephrectomy should be favored to facilitate the preservation of long-term renal function.

Ovarian Tumors

The most common use for MIS in definitive solid tumor resection in children is for ovarian tumors, largely because of the favorable anatomic location of the ovary. The goals of surgery are different, however, depending on whether the tumor is malignant or benign. For malignant ovarian tumors, recommendations include performing a salpingo-oophorectomy on the ipsilateral side. For large tumors, a Pfannenstiel incision may be required to remove the tumor intact. In addition, inspection of the contralateral ovary, ipsilateral iliac lymph nodes, and omentum should be performed with biopsy of suspicious lesions in any of the sites and collection of ascites. This practice is distinct from the surgical management of benign ovarian tumors, in which ovarian-sparing tumor excision is now the standard of care (**Fig. 4**). Many investigators have found predictive criteria to assess the likelihood of whether a tumor is benign or malignant. The factors suggesting the likelihood of malignancy include tumor size greater than 10 cm, solid lesions (in contrast with cystic lesions), and elevated serum markers (alpha-fetoprotein and/or beta human chorionic gonadotropin).[20,21] For large cystic masses deemed benign, controlled drainage of the cyst can be performed to facilitate removal of the cyst wall through a very small incision. Other laparoscopic ovarian procedures include oophoropexy for girls or young women who will receive lower abdominal or pelvic radiation and ovarian tissue harvest for fertility preservation.

Lung Nodules

The most common use for MIS in pediatric patients with cancer is for the removal of lung nodules, most often to confirm the presence of metastatic disease or non-neoplastic etiologies, but occasionally as a therapeutic intervention. Because tactile sensation is lost during thoracoscopy, lesion localization may be required. The techniques for this include hook-wire, methylene blue, and ultrasound examination, among

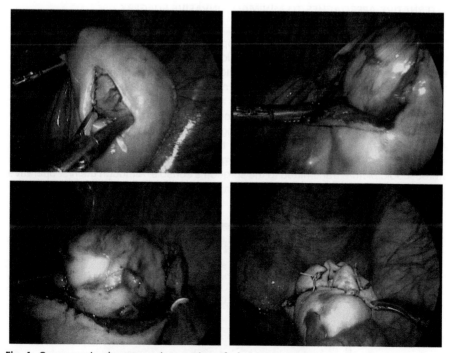

Fig. 4. Ovary-sparing laparoscopic resection of a benign ovarian tumor. The final view shows the edges of the normal ovary sewn over the raw surface at the site of tumor enucleation. (*Courtesy of* Harold N. Lovvorn, III, M.D.)

others. Occasionally, the removal of lung metastases may play a therapeutic role, particularly for tumor types that are relatively resistant to adjuvant therapies, such as osteosarcomas. However, whether thoracoscopy or thoracotomy should be used to manage pulmonary metastatic osteosarcoma is controversial because surgical clearance of all disease is required for potential cure. However, whether potentially delayed tumor clearance with multiple thoracoscopic procedures results in a survival disadvantage is unclear. To address this, COG surgeons plan to open a prospective, randomized trial of thoracoscopy versus thoracotomy for the resection of osteosarcoma metastases. Resection of solitary nodules with a thoracoscopic approach seems to be acceptable because additional metastases are unlikely to be present in this setting of minimal metastatic disease.[22]

Rhabdomyosarcomas

Rhabdomyosarcomas of the abdomen (eg, retroperitoneum or bladder) may be removed with a minimally invasive approach while maintaining the same surgical oncologic principles as for open resections. These procedures are usually performed after pretreatment with neoadjuvant chemotherapy and sometimes with radiation therapy. An additional indication is retroperitoneal lymph node dissection in boys older than 10 years with paratesticular rhabdomyosarcoma (**Fig. 5**). An MIS approach most likely spares the patient the postoperative discomfort associated with laparotomy and may prevent erectile dysfunction by providing a better visualization of pelvic nerves. New modifications to this approach, including limited lymph node sampling and sentinel lymph node biopsy, are currently being tested.[23]

ALTERNATIVE APPROACHES TO MINIMALLY INVASIVE SURGERY
Robotic-Assisted Surgery

Robotic surgeries are similar to laparoscopic and thoracoscopic surgeries because they both use small incisions through which specialized instruments are passed to enter a specific body cavity while monitoring the operation with a high-definition camera. In contrast with laparoscopic and thoracoscopic surgeries, robotic surgeries use instruments with a greater range of motion and precision. Laparoscopic and thoracoscopic instruments have only 4° of freedom, whereas robotic instruments typically have 7° of freedom, allowing a greater range of precise movements. Surgical robots also sense surgeon hand movements and translate and filter them electronically into smaller movements to manipulate the surgical instruments. The camera provides a stereoscopic picture transmitted to the surgeon's console. Although the first operative surgical robots in the United States were approved in 2000, they are not extensively

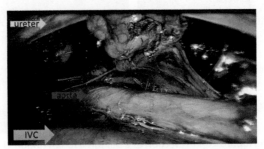

Fig. 5. Extraperitoneal exposure for retroperitoneal lymph node dissection in an older patient with paratesticular rhabdomyosarcoma. (*Courtesy of* Hafeez Abdelhafeez, M.D.)

used in pediatric surgical oncology because of the limited number of indications, cost, and instruments that are not well-suited for smaller patients.

Natural Orifice Transluminal Endoscopic Surgery

A relatively new approach to access the peritoneal cavity for performing surgery within the abdomen is via natural orifice transluminal endoscopic surgery, which accesses the abdominal cavity through a natural orifice under endoscopic visualization. Specifically, natural orifices are used to access intra-abdominal organs by passing an endoscope into the peritoneal space via a transgastric, transvaginal, transvesical, or transcolonic approach. Natural orifice transluminal endoscopic surgery is used in rare circumstances in adult surgical oncology for limited indications, including colorectal cancer, staging of gastrointestinal tumors, and splenectomy. However, to date, using natural orifice transluminal endoscopic surgery to manage solid tumors in children has not been reported.

ADJUVANTS TO MINIMALLY INVASIVE SURGERY
Three-Dimensional Visualization

Better visualization and preoperative planning using 3-dimensional (3D) imaging can improve surgical outcomes. Surgeons must mentally transform 2-dimensional images into 3D images, yet now this can be done by the imaging system, facilitating the surgeon's understanding of the tumor anatomy. Most radiology departments can provide 3D images during surgery, rotating the screen to improve anatomic understanding of the surgical field. With very limited resources, this process can be expanded to yield life-size 3D images and augmented reality images. The resection of renal tumors in which partial nephrectomy is warranted is a particularly useful application of 3D imaging. The incomplete resection rate is approximately 30%, and the resection rate of unilateral tumors with partial nephrectomy is less than 5%.[24–27]

With commercially available software and a 3D printer, life-sized models of the tumor, renal tissue, collecting system, and vessels in relation to each other can be rapidly produced (**Fig. 6**). Moreover, these models cost approximately $5 per model to print after a 3D printer is purchased.

The 3D Slicer software can create such 3D-printed surgical field models. This software package is free to use and reads MRI and computed tomography data. Either manual or semiautomatic segmentation techniques can be used to build the 3D models. The software allows for the export of standard 3D model formats, which are recognized by the 3D printer software. The dual extrusion Ultimaker S5 3D printer allows printing with multiple materials. The most common material (polylactic acid) is a

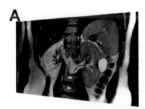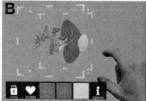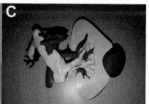

Fig. 6. (*Left*) The 3D model of a left sided renal tumor shown in 3DSlicer. (*Middle*) The same tumor visualized in augmented reality through a HoloLens. (*Right*) Again, the same patient's renal tumor as a life-size 3D printed model. (*From* Matthijs Fitski et al. MRI-Based 3-Dimensional Visualization Workflow for the Preoperative Planning of Nephron-Sparing Surgery in Wilms' Tumor Surgery: A Pilot Study; 2020: 2020; 3.)

standard plastic that facilitates printing without extensive knowledge. Other materials such as thermoplastic polyurethane (a flexible polymer) and polyvinyl alcohol (a soluble material) are more difficult to print, but are better for advanced 3D printing.

If 3D printing is not possible for a specific surgical field, 3D images can be used in a mixed reality device and viewed from all angles. This process permits the relation between the vessels and tumor to be assessed. Software can depict 3D anatomic images, and different anatomic and pathologic images can be switched on and off, or the transparency can be adjusted to yield various views of the surgical field. Additionally, MRI and computed tomography data can be shown in all 3 directions to correlate traditional imaging data with augmented reality images. This approach allows surgeons, patients, and families to more clearly understand the surgical process and goals.[28,29] The advantages of 3D printing are that it is reasonably inexpensive, has an acceptably short lead time for preoperative planning, is beneficial for advising patients and families when explaining procedures, and is real size, so that surgeons know the dimensions that can be expected. A disadvantage of the virtual modeling software is that the images can only be viewed by 1 person at a time, although multiple goggles can be synchronized. Another disadvantage of the virtual viewing technology is that some advanced knowledge of the hardware and software is needed; however, the hardware and software may become more accessible over time. In the near future, augmented reality may be used during operations by projecting augmented reality images of the kidney and overlaying them on the moving kidney of patients, making it possible to view the inside of the moving kidney during surgery.

Visual Field Augmentation

Another challenge that pediatric surgeons often face is that nearly all tumors are treated with preoperative chemotherapy, which makes it more difficult to discern malignant tumor tissue from scar tissue and benign tissue. To avoid unnecessary resection of healthy tissues and damage to vessels and organs, fluorescence-guided surgery improves the differentiation of tumors from the surrounding healthy tissue. Fluorescence-guided surgeries can be used in endoscopic and open surgery settings and may be used to determine the margins of resected tumors.[30,31]

The working mechanism of fluorescence is as follows. Characteristically, under the action of light, depending on wavelengths, the level of energy of the molecules increases; as soon as the level returns to its basal state, light is emitted. The difference between excitation and emission wavelengths is exploited thanks to cameras equipped with interferential filters to obtain the images. Fluorescent light emission is largely attenuated by hemoglobin and water as it traverses biological tissues. Hemoglobin strongly attenuates all wavelengths of light shorter than 700 nm, corresponding with the entire visible spectrum except deep red. Water is transparent in visible and near-infrared light, but attenuates wavelengths longer than 900 nm. Therefore, a window of wavelengths between the limits of deep red and near infrared (700–900 nm) wavelengths permits maximal tissue transparency. Because of this, indocyanine green (ICG) fluorescence can be detected as near-infrared light in tissues as deep as 10 mm from the surface.

Fluorescence can be used during sentinel lymph node resections in a similar method as conventional use of blue dyes. When using ICG for transecting lymph vessels, the whole operating field does not turn blue, as is the case with blue dyes, or green when the laser is switched off. Moreover, ICG does not permanently stain the skin, which can occur with blue dyes.[32]

However, using ICG during surgery does not preclude preoperative imaging with technetium, but may help in detecting lymph nodes that are superficially located.

ICG-guided near-infrared imaging has several advantages over that of other intraoperative detection methods. The maximum absorption (765 nm) and peak fluorescence emission (830 nm) wavelengths of ICG are in the near-infrared spectrum, permitting a depth of penetration of up to 10 mm and decreased background fluorescence. This factor enables the detection of tumor tissues even when obscured by blood or thin layers of tissue. In addition, ICG is relatively inexpensive and does not expose patients to ionizing radiation, in contrast with computed tomography scans or radiotracers. ICG is easy to use and does not interrupt the surgical workflow. The safety profile of ICG has been established in the pediatric population for other indications.

ICG can be administered intravenously to locate tumors and metastases in the lung, liver, and peritoneum. Because of the increased vascular permeability of ICG, it persists longer in tumor tissues than in healthy tissues. ICG injections are typically performed 24 hours before surgery to allow washout in healthy tissues and optimal tumor-to-background signal ratios. ICG use for hepatoblastoma tumor detection and resection is established, although the mechanism slightly differs from that of nonhepatic tissues. In hepatic surgeries, ICG is used to evaluate hepatic function and inform hepatectomy strategies for oncologic resections and transplants. After intravenous or direct intrabiliary injection of ICG, imaging allows for the visualization of the bile ducts and primary and metastatic liver tumors during surgery (**Fig. 7**).[33,34]

When ICG is administered intravenously before or during surgeries in variable time intervals, the liver surface is illuminated intraoperatively. Indeed, intravenous ICG administration of 0.25 to 0.50 mg/kg from 12 hours to 14 days before surgery helps to identify tumors by intraoperative fluorescence. After ICG injection, both healthy hepatocytes and tumor cells rapidly take up ICG. ICG is then excreted in the bile and dissipates from the healthy liver parenchyma within a few hours. In contrast, ICG persists in tumor cells and pathologic areas of the liver, particularly in the hypoactive hepatocytes located around nonhepatocellular tumors. Near-infrared cameras allow detection of hepatocellular (ie, tumor fluorescence) and nonhepatocellular tumors (ie, peritumoral fluorescence) because of retained ICG fluorescence. Similar to ICG, 5-aminolevulinic acid fluorescence can be used to discern glioma tumors from healthy brain tissue during neurosurgery.[35,36]

Intravenous ICG can also be used to visualize tissues at risk of hypoperfusion, such as difficult bowel anastomoses, free flap reconstructions, and extremity sarcoma surgeries in which 1 or more arteries are sacrificed.

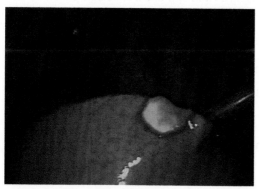

Fig. 7. Near-infrared image showing accumulation of ICG of a lung metastasis in a child being treated for hepatoblastoma. (*Courtesy of* Hafeez Abdelhafeez, M.D.)

Fluorophore-labelled antibodies can also be used to assist surgical oncology techniques as immune therapy becomes more prevalent and more tumor-specific antibodies become available. Fluorophore-labelled antibodies can be used to visualize tumor cells after intravenous injection of the tumor-specific antibody used for treatment. Preclinical trials of the use of nanobodies for this purpose are also ongoing.

Before the use of fluorescence in surgical oncology becomes widely disseminated in practice, several aspects regarding tumor type and specific applications must be addressed. First, optimal injection times to achieve the best tumor-to-background ratio must be established for various tumor types. Second, the implication of residual fluorescence in tissues after resection must be determined for distinct tumor types. Third, different protocols must be established for various fluorophores and their surgical applications. The optimal dosing of each fluorophore and application, depending on patient weight, must also be determined. Nevertheless, intravenous ICG doses up to 4 mg/kg seem to be safe for children. Last, the cost, service, and availability of support for surgical imaging equipment are important considerations. The decision of whether to buy a single or dual wavelength laser and the possibility of endoscopic use are particularly important factors to consider.

Targeted fluorophores are promising and may improve the specificity and precision of fluorescence-guided surgeries. Although ICG is generally nonspecific beyond its perfusion and clearance kinetics, some fluorophores can be activated only in tumor-specific environments. For example, 5-aminolevulinic acid is administered orally and metabolized within glioma cells to yield a fluorescent molecule that remains nonfluorescent in surrounding tissues.[36]

Studies of fluorophore-conjugated monoclonal antibodies targeting tumor-specific antigens are also ongoing.[37] Indeed, a first-in-human, proof-of-concept study recently demonstrated the usefulness of a fluorophore conjugated to an epidermal growth factor receptor antibody for localizing glioblastoma tumors during resection. First-in-human intraoperative near-infrared fluorescence imaging of glioblastoma using cetuximab-IRDye800.[38] The opportunities to expand the field of theranostics (ie, using therapeutic agents for diagnostic purposes) are nearly limitless.

SUMMARY

MIS has advanced the field of surgical oncology. Many widely accepted uses for MIS in pediatric surgical oncology that are largely tumor type specific now exist. In some cases, however, the appropriateness of MIS is uncertain and should be discouraged. In all cases, when using an MIS approach, oncologic principles should be maintained, and the procedures should be performed by surgeons trained and experienced in these techniques. Newer technologies and surgical adjuncts are certain to further increase the role MIS plays in pediatric surgical oncology practice.

ACKNOWLEDGMENTS

Thanks to Nisha Badders for editing of the article.

DISCLOSURE

Authors have nothing to disclose.

REFERENCES

1. Phelps HM, Lovvorn HN 3rd. Minimally invasive surgery in pediatric surgical oncology. Children (Basel) 2018;5(12):158.

2. Christison-Lagay ER, Thomas D. Minimally invasive approaches to pediatric solid tumors. Surg Oncol Clin N Am 2019;28(1):129–46.

3. Holcomb GW 3rd, Tomita SS, Haase GM, et al. Minimally invasive surgery in children with cancer. Cancer 1995;76(1):121–8.

4. Saenz NC, Conlon KC, Aronson DC, et al. The application of minimal access procedures in infants, children, and young adults with pediatric malignancies. J Laparoendosc Adv Surg Tech A 1997;7(5):289–94.

5. Ehrlich PF, Newman KD, Haase GM, et al. Lessons learned from a failed multi-institutional randomized controlled study. J Pediatr Surg 2002;37(3):431–6.

6. Cecchetto G, Riccipetitoni G, Inserra A, et al. Minimally-invasive surgery in paediatric oncology: proposal of recommendations. Pediatr Med Chir 2010;32(5):197–201.

7. Spurbeck WW, Davidoff AM, Lobe TE, et al. Minimally invasive surgery in pediatric cancer patients. Ann Surg Oncol 2004;11(3):340–3.

8. Abdelhafeez A, Ortega-Laureano L, Murphy AJ, et al. Minimally invasive surgery in pediatric surgical oncology: practice evolution at a contemporary single-center institution and a guideline proposal for a randomized controlled study. J Laparoendosc Adv Surg Tech A 2019;29(8):1046–51.

9. Boutros J, Bond M, Beaudry P, et al. Case selection in minimally invasive surgical treatment of neuroblastoma. Pediatr Surg Int 2008;24(10):1177–80.

10. Iwanaka T, Arai M, Ito M, et al. Challenges of laparoscopic resection of abdominal neuroblastoma with lymphadenectomy. A preliminary report. Surg Endosc 2001;15(5):489–92.

11. Gurria JP, Malek MM, Heaton TE, et al. Minimally invasive surgery for abdominal and thoracic neuroblastic tumors: a systematic review by the APSA Cancer Committee. J Pediatr Surg 2020;55(11):2260–72.

12. Delozier OM, Stiles ZE, Deschner BW, et al. Implications of conversion during attempted minimally invasive adrenalectomy for adrenocortical carcinoma. Ann Surg Oncol 2020. https://doi.org/10.1245/s10434-020-08824-9.

13. Hu X, Yang WX, Shao YX, et al. Minimally invasive versus open adrenalectomy in patients with adrenocortical carcinoma: a meta-analysis. Ann Surg Oncol 2020. https://doi.org/10.1245/s10434-020-08454-1.

14. Warmann SW, Godzinski J, van Tinteren H, et al. Minimally invasive nephrectomy for Wilms tumors in children - data from SIOP 2001. J Pediatr Surg 2014;49(11):1544–8.

15. Bouty A, Blanc T, Leclair MD, et al. Minimally invasive surgery for unilateral Wilms tumors: multicenter retrospective analysis of 50 transperitoneal laparoscopic total nephrectomies. Pediatr Blood Cancer 2020;67(5):e28212.

16. Eriksen KO, Johal NS, Mushtaq I. Minimally invasive surgery in management of renal tumours in children. Transl Pediatr 2016;5(4):305–14.

17. Malek MM, Behr CA, Aldrink JH, et al. Minimally invasive surgery for pediatric renal tumors: a systematic review by the APSA cancer committee. J Pediatr Surg 2020;55(11):2251–9.

18. Chui CH, Lee AC. Peritoneal metastases after laparoscopic nephron-sparing surgery for localized Wilms tumor. J Pediatr Surg 2011;46(3):e19–21.

19. Schmidt A, Warmann SW, Urla C, et al. Patient selection and technical aspects for laparoscopic nephrectomy in Wilms tumor. Surg Oncol 2019;29:14–9.

20. Ye G, Xu T, Liu J, et al. The role of preoperative imaging and tumor markers in predicting malignant ovarian masses in children. Pediatr Surg Int 2020;36(3):333–9.

21. Madenci AL, Vandewalle RJ, Dieffenbach BV, et al. Multicenter pre-operative assessment of pediatric ovarian malignancy. J Pediatr Surg 2019;54(9):1921–5.

22. Fernandez-Pineda I, Daw NC, McCarville B, et al. Patients with osteosarcoma with a single pulmonary nodule on computed tomography: a single-institution experience. J Pediatr Surg 2012;47(6):1250–4.

23. Mansfield SA, Murphy AJ, Talbot L, et al. Alternative approaches to retroperitoneal lymph node dissection for paratesticular rhabdomyosarcoma. J Pediatr Surg 2020. https://doi.org/10.1016/j.jpedsurg.2020.03.022.

24. Wilde JC, Aronson DC, Sznajder B, et al. Nephron sparing surgery (NSS) for unilateral Wilms tumor (UWT): the SIOP 2001 experience. Pediatr Blood Cancer 2014;61(12):2175–9.

25. Lupulescu C, Sun Z. A systematic review of the clinical value and applications of three-dimensional printing in renal surgery. J Clin Med 2019;8(7):990.

26. Davidoff AM, Interiano RB, Wynn L, et al. Overall survival and renal function of patients with synchronous bilateral Wilms tumor undergoing surgery at a single institution. Ann Surg 2015;262(4):570–6.

27. Richards MK, Goldin AB, Ehrlich PF, et al. Partial nephrectomy for nephroblastoma: a national cancer data base review. Am surg 2018;84(3):338–43.

28. Wellens LM, Meulstee J, van de Ven CP, et al. Comparison of 3-dimensional and augmented reality kidney models with conventional imaging data in the preoperative assessment of children with Wilms tumors. JAMA Netw open 2019;2(4): e192633.

29. Sánchez-Sánchez Á, Girón-Vallejo Ó, Ruiz-Pruneda R, et al. Three-dimensional printed model and virtual reconstruction: an extra tool for pediatric solid tumors surgery. European J Pediatr Surg Rep 2018;6(1):e70–6.

30. Nagaya T, Nakamura YA, Choyke PL, et al. Fluorescence-guided surgery. Front Oncol 2017;7:314.

31. Vahrmeijer AL, Hutteman M, van der Vorst JR, et al. Image-guided cancer surgery using near-infrared fluorescence. Nat Rev Clin Oncol 2013;10(9):507–18.

32. Govaert GA, Oostenbroek RJ, Plaisier PW. Prolonged skin staining after intradermal use of patent blue in sentinel lymph node biopsy for breast cancer. Eur J Surg Oncol 2005;31(4):373–5.

33. Yamada Y, Ohno M, Fujino A, et al. Fluorescence-guided surgery for hepatoblastoma with indocyanine green. Cancers 2019;11(8):1215.

34. Kitagawa N, Shinkai M, Mochizuki K, et al. Navigation using indocyanine green fluorescence imaging for hepatoblastoma pulmonary metastases surgery. Pediatr Surg Int 2015;31(4):407–11.

35. Cho SS, Salinas R, Lee JYK. Indocyanine-green for fluorescence-guided surgery of brain tumors: evidence, techniques, and practical experience. Front Surg 2019;6:11.

36. Schwake M, Schipmann S, Müther M, et al. 5-ALA fluorescence-guided surgery in pediatric brain tumors-a systematic review. Acta Neurochir (Wien) 2019;161(6): 1099–108.

37. Pèlegrin A, Gutowski M, Cailler F. Antibodies, tools of choice for fluorescence-guided surgery. Med Sci (Paris) 2019;35(12):1066–71.

38. Miller SE, Tummers WS, Teraphongphom N, et al. First-in-human intraoperative near-infrared fluorescence imaging of glioblastoma using cetuximab-IRDye800. J Neurooncol 2018;139(1):135–43.

Moving?

Make sure your subscription moves with you!

To notify us of your new address, find your **Clinics Account Number** (located on your mailing label above your name), and contact customer service at:

Email: journalscustomerservice-usa@elsevier.com

800-654-2452 (subscribers in the U.S. & Canada)
314-447-8871 (subscribers outside of the U.S. & Canada)

Fax number: 314-447-8029

Elsevier Health Sciences Division
Subscription Customer Service
3251 Riverport Lane
Maryland Heights, MO 63043

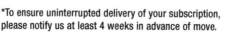

*To ensure uninterrupted delivery of your subscription, please notify us at least 4 weeks in advance of move.

Printed and bound by CPI Group (UK) Ltd, Croydon, CR0 4YY

03/10/2024

01040408-0004